Psychiatry as Cognitive Neuroscience
Philosophical perspectives

D1337917

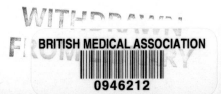

International Perspectives in Philosophy and Psychiatry

Series editors: KWM (Bill) Fulford, Katherine Morris, John Z Sadler, and Giovanni Stanghellini

Volumes in the series:

Forthcoming volumes in the series:

Psychiatry as Cognitive Neuroscience
Philosophical perspectives

Edited by

Matthew R. Broome

Lisa Bortolotti

OXFORD
UNIVERSITY PRESS

OXFORD
UNIVERSITY PRESS

Great Clarendon Street, Oxford OX2 6DP
Oxford University Press is a department of the University of Oxford.
It furthers the University's objective of excellence in research, scholarship,
and education by publishing worldwide in

Oxford New York

Auckland   Cape Town Dar es Salaam   Hong Kong   Karachi
Kuala Lumpur Madrid Melbourne Mexico City   Nairobi
New Delhi Shanghai Taipei Toronto
With offices in
Argentina Austria Brazil Chile Czech Republic France Greece
Guatemala Hungary Italy Japan South Korea Poland Portugal
Singapore Switzerland Thailand Turkey Ukraine Vietnam

ISBN 978-0-19-923803-3

Printed in the United Kingdom by
Lightning Source UK Ltd., Milton Keynes

For Louisa, Edward, and Matilda
For Adalberto and Ennia
In memory of Susan Hurley, 1954–2007

Contents

Section 4 **Psychiatry and the neurosciences**

Section 5 **Phenomenology and scientific explanation**

Section 6 **Delusions and cognition**

Section 7 **Moral psychology and psychopathology**

Conclusion

Acknowledgements

The editors of this volume are very grateful to all those who have given their time to them during the preparation of this book. In particular, they would like to thank Carol Maxwell and Martin Baum of Oxford University Press and Bill Fulford, co-editor of the 'International Perspectives in Philosophy and Psychiatry' series. They would also like to thank Martin Davies for his constant encouragement and for very helpful comments on an earlier draft of the introduction, and all the contributors to this volume for making the whole experience of editing it so interesting and so pleasant.

The editors owe a debt to Susan Hurley: in her dedication to neuroscience and philosophy, she inspired them and they hope this book would have been of interest to her. Susan gave Matthew his first opportunity to present a paper at a philosophy conference and later she spoke at the Philosophy, Psychology, and Psychiatry Conference organized by Lisa at the University of Birmingham in 2006 and sponsored by the Royal Institute of Philosophy. On both occasions, Susan's charm, intelligence, collegiality and ability to synthesize data from a variety of empirical disciplines set her out as a leading philosopher and as a bright light in drawing philosophy into engaging with science at a high level.

Matthew would like to thank all those philosophers who gave time over the years for the questions of a naïve junior psychiatric researcher: in particular, he would like to thank Anita Avramides, John Campbell, Havi Carel, Rachel Cooper, Simon Critchley, Steve Crowell, Peter Hacker, Dan Lloyd, Matthew Ratcliffe, and Tim Thornton. Matthew would also like to express his gratitude to the Maudsley Philosophy Group, and in particular Robert Harland, Gareth Owen, Richard Kanaan, and Argyris Stringaris. He would also like to thank the clinicians and academics who trained him, and with whom he worked, at the Institute of Psychiatry, the Maudsley and Bethlem Royal Hospitals, and the National Hospital for Neurology and Neurosurgery: Mick Brammer, Tony David, Paul Fearon, Dan Freeman, Cindy Fu, Philippa Garety, David Hemsley, Rob Howard, Philip McGuire, Robin Murray, Emmanuelle Peters, Larry Rifkin, Maria Ron, Eric Taylor, and Steve Williams. Many of their ideas and their attitudes of optimism and scepticism in clinical practice and science are what inspired his interest in philosophy and in the methods appropriate to a scientific psychopathology. He would also like to thank all those in the OASIS clinical and research team and the Section of Neuroimaging at the Institute of Psychiatry, particularly Paul Allen, Stefan Borgwardt, Fern Day, Paolo Fusar-Poli, Deanna Hall, Ollie Howes, Louise Johns, Marco Picchioni, Paul Tabraham, Isabel Valli, Lucia Valmaggia, Sandra Whitehead, and James Woolley. Most of all he would like to thank Lisa. He met her at an Institute of Psychiatry journal club he chaired several years ago. Since then, Lisa has been the perfect collaborator, co-editor, and a dear friend.

Lisa would like to thank Martin Davies and John Campbell for having inspired her to work in the philosophy of psychology and psychiatry with their lectures in Oxford during her B.Phil years in 1998–2000, and for having introduced her to the psychiatric literature. In the final stages of editing this volume, she visited the Macquarie Centre for Cognitive Science at Macquarie University in Sydney, as a 2008 Endeavour Research Fellow. Her time at Macquarie has been extremely valuable. Her gratitude goes to Max Coltheart, Robyn Langdon, Amanda Barnier, John Sutton, Peter Menzies, Rochelle Cox, Michael Connors, Neralie Wise, and all the participants in the Delusion and Hypnosis Reading Group, where some of the chapters in this collection were discussed. Lisa would also like to acknowledge the support of her colleagues in the Philosophy Department at the University of Birmingham, especially Helen Beebee and Yujin Nagasawa, and the members of the Psychiatrists' Philosophy Club in Birmingham, especially Femi Oyebode and Lenia Constantine. For philosophical discussion and moral support, she is grateful to Matteo Mameli, Jordi Fernández, Philip Gerrans, and Edoardo Zamuner.

Most of all, she would like to thank Matthew. His qualities as a collaborator and as a friend make him the ideal person to work with. He is extremely knowledgeable and generous with his time, organized, patient, and enthusiastic. It was fortunate for Lisa to meet him, and hopefully they will work together for many years to come.

Notes on Editors

Matthew Broome is Associate Clinical Professor of Psychiatry at the University of Warwick (UK), Honorary Senior Lecturer at the Institute of Psychiatry, Kings College London (UK) and Consultant Psychiatrist to the Coventry Early Intervention Team, Coventry and Warwickshire Partnership Trust. He is chair of the Philosophy Special Interest Group at the Royal College of Psychiatrists and founder member and trustee of the Maudsley Philosophy Group. His research has focused on the prodromal phase of psychosis, functional neuroimaging, and delusion formation. He is currently co-editing *The Maudsley Reader in Phenomenological Psychiatry*.

Lisa Bortolotti is Senior Lecturer in Philosophy at the University of Birmingham (UK). Her main interests are in the relationship between rationality, intentionality, and self-knowledge in philosophy and cognitive science, and in the ethical issues surrounding scientific research and reproduction. She is the author of *An Introduction to the Philosophy of Science* (Polity Press, 2008) and the editor of *Philosophy and Happiness* (Palgrave Macmillan, 2009). She has written many articles in the philosophy of psychiatry for journals such as *Mind & Language* and *Philosophical Psychology*, and she is currently writing a monograph on delusions for Oxford University Press.

Notes on Contributors

Anne M. Aimola Davies is University Research Fellow in Neuropsychology in the Department of Experimental Psychology, NIHR Biomedical Research Centre and Faculty of Philosophy at the University of Oxford (UK) and Senior Lecturer in the Department of Psychology, The Australian National University (Australia). She has interests in the directional and non-directional aspects of attention, inattentional blindness and unilateral neglect, the neural and cognitive basis of anosognosia, and neurorehabilitation.

John Campbell is Willis S. and Marion Slusser Professor of Philosophy at the University of California, Berkeley (US). He was Wilde Professor of Mental Philosophy at the University of Oxford. He is the author of *Reference and Consciousness* (2002) and *Past, Space and Self* (1994). He is currently working on causation in psychology.

Rachel Cooper is Senior Lecturer in Philosophy at Lancaster University (UK). She conducts research in the philosophy of science and medicine. Her publications include *Classifying Madness* (2005) and *Psychiatry and Philosophy of Science* (2007).

Martin Davies is Wilde Professor of Mental Philosophy at the University of Oxford (UK) and a Fellow of Corpus Christi College. His research interests lie in philosophy of psychology and cognitive science, philosophy of mind and language, and epistemology. He has published many articles in these areas and, with Lawrence Weiskrantz, edited *Frontiers of Consciousness: Chichele Lectures* (2008).

Keith Frankish is Senior Lecturer in Philosophy at The Open University (UK). He is the author of *Mind and Supermind* (2004) and *Consciousness* (2005), as well as numerous articles and book chapters. His research spans debates about the nature of belief, the structure of the mind, consciousness, and dual-process theories of reasoning. He is co-editor with Jonathan Evans of *In Two Minds: Dual Processes and Beyond* (2009).

KWM (Bill) Fulford is Fellow of St Cross College, Member of the Philosophy Faculty and Honorary Consultant Psychiatrist at the University of Oxford, and Professor of Philosophy and Mental Health, University of Warwick (UK). He is co-editor of the journal *Philosophy, Psychiatry, and Psychology*, and of the OUP book series, *International Perspectives in Philosophy and Psychiatry*.

Shaun Gallagher is Professor of Philosophy and Cognitive Sciences, Senior Researcher at the Institute of Simulation and Training at the University of Central Florida (US) and Research Professor of Philosophy and Cognitive Science at the University of Hertfordshire (UK). His recent books include *How the Body Shapes the Mind* (2005), and *Brainstorming* (2008).

Philip Gerrans is a Reader is the Philosophy Department at the University of Adelaide. His main research interest is the interdisciplinary study of abnormal psychology. He has written on developmental disorders (autism and Williams syndrome), cognitive neuropsychiatry, and, more recently, on moral psychopathologies (such as psychopathology) and the emotions. In each case he is interested in the role cognitive models play in bridging neurobiological and psychological explanations.

George Graham is Professor of Philosophy at Georgia State University in Atlanta (US), having previously taught at the University of Alabama at Birmingham and at Wake Forest University (US). He has published widely in the philosophy of mind and on philosophical issues connected with psychopathology. He is the author of a forthcoming book entitled *The Disordered Mind*.

Jeanette Kennett is Principal Research Fellow at the Centre for Applied Philosophy and Public Ethics, The Australian National University, and Charles Sturt University (Australia). She is the author of *Agency and Responsibility* (2001) and publishes in meta-ethics, moral psychology, and applied ethics. Her work has appeared in *Analysis, Ethics, The Journal of Philosophy, Philosophical Psychology,* and *Philosophical Quarterly*.

Iain Law is Senior Lecturer in Philosophy at the University of Birmingham (UK). He previously held posts at the Universities of Bristol and St Andrews (UK). He has published mainly in ethics: moral psychology, moral theory, and meta-ethics. He has also recently been working on the philosophy of health and disease in collaboration with his colleague at Birmingham, Heather Widdows.

Dan Lloyd is the Thomas C. Brownell Professor of Philosophy and a Professor in the Program in Neuroscience at Trinity College (Connecticut, US). He is the winner of the first 'New Perspectives in Functional MRI Research Award' given by the *Journal of Cognitive Neuroscience*, and the author of numerous articles and books, including *Simple Minds* (1989) and *Radiant Cool: A Novel Theory of Consciousness* (2004).

Steve Matthews is Senior Research Fellow at the Centre for Applied Philosophy and Public Ethics, and teaches in the philosophy program at the School of Humanities and Social Sciences, both at Charles Sturt University (Australia). He writes on issues of personal identity and agency, and in applied ethics. His work has appeared in *Philosophical Studies, Philosophical Psychology, Philosophy, Psychiatry, and Psychology,* and *The Monist*.

Dominic Murphy is Senior Lecturer in the Unit for History and Philosophy of Science, University of Sydney (Australia). He works mostly in the philosophy of the cognitive and biological sciences. He is the author of *Psychiatry in the Scientific Image* (2006). He is currently writing a book on theories of the self and self-knowledge in philosophy and cognitive science.

Hanna Pickard is Fellow of All Souls College, Oxford (UK), and a therapist at the Complex Needs Service, a NHS Therapeutic Community for people with Personality Disorder in Oxford. She has published articles on the emotions, other minds, body awareness, and action. Her current research aims to integrate clinical data with the philosophy of mind and psychiatry.

Matthew Ratcliffe is Reader in Philosophy at Durham University (UK). Most of his recent work addresses issues in phenomenology, philosophy of psychology, and philosophy of psychiatry. He is author of *Rethinking Commonsense Psychology: A Critique of Folk Psychology, Theory of Mind and Simulation* (2007) and *Feelings of Being: Phenomenology, Psychiatry and the Sense of Reality* (2008).

Richard Samuels is Professor of Philosophy at Ohio State University (US). His primary areas of research are the philosophy of mind and philosophy of psychology. He has published extensively on various topics in the foundations of cognitive science, including the modularity of mind, the notion of innateness, and the philosophical implications of empirical research on reasoning. He is currently finishing a book on cognitive architecture.

Norman Sartorius is the President of the International Association for the Improvement of Mental Health Programmes and he holds professorial appointments at the Universities of London, Prague, Zagreb, and at several other universities in the US and China. He was the principal investigator of major international studies on schizophrenia, depression, and health service delivery. He is the author of *Fighting for Mental Health* (2002).

Dan J. Stein is Professor and Chair of the Department of Psychiatry and Mental Health at the University of Cape Town (South Africa). His work ranges from basic neuroscience through to epidemiology, and he is particularly enthusiastic about the possibility of integrating theoretical concepts and empirical data across different levels. He is the author of *Philosophy of Psychopharmacology: Smart Pills, Happy Pills, and Pep Pills* (2008).

G. Lynn Stephens is Professor of Philosophy at the University of Alabama at Birmingham (US). He has published widely on philosophical issues connected with psychopathology. He also works in the philosophy of mind, history of American philosophy, and philosophy of religion. With George Graham, he co-authored *When Self-Consciousness Breaks* (2000).

Tim Thornton is Director of Philosophy and Professor of Philosophy and Mental Health at the University of Central Lancashire (UK). As well as contemporary philosophy of thought and language, his research concerns conceptual issues at the heart of mental health care. He is author of *Essential Philosophy of Psychiatry* (2007), and co-author of the *Oxford Textbook of Philosophy and Psychiatry* (2006).

Psychiatry as cognitive neuroscience: An overview

Matthew R. Broome and Lisa Bortolotti

Aims of the volume

The unifying philosophical theme of this volume is how psychopathology is studied scientifically within psychiatry and psychology through the paradigms of cognitive neuroscience and cognitive neuropsychiatry. Topics addressed in the volume include: the nature of psychiatry as a science; the compatibility of the accounts of mental illness derived from neuroscience, information-processing, and folk psychology; the nature of mental illness; the impact of contemporary methods in neuroscientific investigation, such as functional neuroimaging, neuropsychology, and neurochemistry, on psychiatry; the relationship between phenomenological accounts of mental illness and those provided by naturalistic explanations; the status of delusions and the (dis)continuity between delusions and ordinary beliefs; and the interplay between clinical and empirical findings in psychopathology and accounts of virtue and responsibility in moral psychology and ethics.

Several of the questions addressed by the contributors span the topics listed above. Given their importance to the debate on whether psychiatry has scientific status, it is worth making these questions explicit. What are the respective roles of neuroscience and scientific psychology in informing psychopathology? Are folk-psychological categories, such as 'belief' and 'responsibility', misleading or necessary to the scientific understanding of mental illness? Are normative concepts legitimately used in both neuroscientific and psychiatric explanations? Do naturalistic and folk-psychological accounts of psychopathology neglect the basic features of human existence?

It is an open question how much philosophers can learn from the study of psychopathologies. For instance, some use anecdotal evidence of delusional reports as a source of imaginative examples to illustrate the extent to which some beliefs resist revision. Similarly, data on psychopathy or addiction can be taken to exemplify the extent to which behaviour can deviate from socially acceptable norms and how it can fail to be guided by autonomous thought and to qualify as morally virtuous. These are 'thin' uses of the empirical literature to be contrasted with the methodological stance according to which evidence collected in the context of psychopathology needs to be taken into account whenever, say, a theory of normal belief generation and evaluation, or a theory of moral responsibility and moral virtue are formulated. These latter projects strengthen the collaboration between philosophers and cognitive or neuroscientists, by providing new models for phenomena that are not accounted for by the available theoretical frameworks, and drawing on the authors' complementary areas of competence (e.g. Coltheart and Davies, 2000).

To what extent can philosophical theories be conceived as independent of data in the empirical sciences? Can philosophy tell us merely how to think clearly and how to make the concepts we use more precise? Or can it also contribute in unveiling truths about the world which need to be compatible with and supplemented by the picture of the world we get from the sciences? In this volume, we have splendid examples of 'thick' uses of the empirical literature in philosophy in the work of Gallagher, Frankish, and Aimola Davies and Davies on the (dis)continuity between delusions and beliefs; and in the work of Law, Kennett and Matthews, and Pickard on the morally relevant aspects of psychopathology.

A family of debates, more modest in scope but of extreme importance for the status of psychiatry and psychology as sciences, is centered on the way in which traditional notions in the philosophy of the natural sciences (i.e. causation, natural kinds, classification) can be applied to the domain of psychopathology (see Cooper, 2008). Many of the contributors to this volume have actively participated in these debates. Murphy discusses two different approaches to mental illness: diseases can be identified on the basis of their symptoms or of their underlying causes. By reference to the empirical literature on delusions, Campbell suggests that there can be causal connections between propositional attitudes that are not rational. Cooper asks whether traditional demarcation criteria for natural or social sciences meaningfully apply to psychiatry. Samuels defends the thesis that delusions constitute a natural kind by addressing common objections.

Another common concern is the necessity to reconcile different research traditions in the study of psychopathology. In contemporary psychiatry, one of the main paradigms is that of cognitive neuroscience. Halligan and David define cognitive neuropsychiatry as 'a systematic and theoretically driven approach to explain clinical psychopathologies in terms of deficits to normal cognitive mechanisms'. They continue: 'A concern with the neural substrates of impaired cognitive mechanisms links cognitive neuropsychiatry to the basic neurosciences' (Halligan and David, 2001, p. 209). The authors go on to describe the methodology of such a paradigm, according to which psychiatric disorders need to be understood within the framework of cognitive psychology and by referring to the pathology of brain structures.

This approach not only suggests immediate links to functional neuroimaging through its use of the term 'neural substrate' and brain structure, but also contains several assumptions regarding psychology, psychopathology, and neuroscience that may benefit from being considered in greater detail. Explicitly, such an approach seeks to understand psychopathology through the models and tools provided by cognitive neuropsychology, and in turn relate such an understanding back to the anatomy of the brain. Further, it characterizes the symptoms of mental illnesses as being consequent to deficits and biases of normal psychological function, and thus due to qualitatively similar mechanisms. Examples of contributions from the volume addressing these issues include those by Lloyd, Stein, and Stephens and Graham. Lloyd examines the use of functional magnetic resonance imaging (fMRI) in the study of temporality and schizophrenia and suggests that analyses based around connectivity rather than local activations support phenomenological accounts of the experience of time. Stein argues that diagnosis and treatment in psychiatry can be enhanced by cognitive-affective neurogenetics, but that a given psychopathology can only be understood by referring to a whole range of considerations, and cannot simply be reduced to a particular genetic polymorphism. Stephens and Graham argue that a purely neuroscientific description is unable to offer the normative information required to make a judgement regarding the presence of addiction, and possibly other disorders. As such, the findings of cognitive neuroscience cannot be imported into psychiatry uncritically.

Next, we précis the papers in the order in which they appear in the volume. Although we have arranged chapters thematically, many of them in fact contribute to more than one theme. All chapters are stand-alone contributions and can be read in any order.

Guide to contents

Psychiatry as science

In this section we are interested in the claim that psychiatry is a science, and focus on the questions whether psychiatry can satisfy the demarcation criteria for science and whether the entities theorized about in psychiatry, such as delusions, can be described as natural kinds.

Does it make sense to examine the status of psychiatry as a science? Rachel Cooper argues that the general demarcation question is outdated and uninformative and that we should concentrate instead on what makes research in psychiatry special and controversial (e.g. the co-habitation of different styles of explanation and the plurality of methods of empirical investigation) in order to better understand and assess its epistemic status. One of the very interesting features of Cooper's argument is that it can generalize from the case of psychiatry to all types of research that can be viewed as either scientific or pseudoscientific, because it is grounded in the view that 'science' is a family resemblance term and not a concept that can be captured by a list of necessary and sufficient conditions. The case of psychiatry proves to be the perfect illustration of how the traditional debates on demarcation are unable to account for the evolving conception of scientific research that cuts across disciplines.

Bill Fulford and Norman Sartorius offer an intriguing account of the direct influence of the philosophy, and philosophers, of science on psychiatry and its classificatory systems. They concentrate on logical empiricism, the work of Carl Hempel and the distinction between descriptive statements and statements of theory. However, the traditional account of Hempel as advocating a descriptive, symptom-based classification is undermined by documents from the World Health Organization (WHO) meetings which suggest that this move was inspired by Aubrey Lewis, an influential psychiatrist from the Maudsley Hospital. Lewis offered a distinction between 'public' and 'private' classification and suggested that, for the WHO, which wanted a system that can be employed internationally in epidemiological research, such a 'public' classification may be more successful if it avoids categories dependent on theoretical concepts. Hempel, rather than criticizing psychiatry for moving too swiftly from a descriptive to an aetiological classification, argued for the appropriateness of using theoretical terms, such as those employed in psychoanalysis, in classificatory systems. Fulford and Sartorius utilize these historical data to offer some suggestions for the future of psychiatric classification drawing on Hempel's criticism of operationalism and Lewis' conception of a family of different classificatory systems.

Richard Samuels discusses the thesis that delusions constitute a natural kind. He clarifies what the constraints for being a natural kind are, and presents some *prima facie* reasons for supposing that delusions satisfy these constraints. Next, he reviews some of the most common arguments against the natural-kind conception of delusions. The continuity objection purports to show that delusions are not a natural kind because they are continuous with other phenomena. A family of mind-dependent objections seeks to show that delusions cannot be a natural kind because the notion of a delusion is either an artefact of our folk psychology, or culturally relative, or normative. Samuels argues that such objections fail to undermine the natural-kind conception of delusions, and concludes by recommending the adoption of the natural-kind conception of delusions as a working hypothesis.

The nature of mental illness

Papers in this section address the nature of mental illnesses, and in particular investigate whether a general account of disorder or illness is appropriate in the case of psychopathologies.

Hanna Pickard considers Szasz's view according to which 'mental illness' is a misnomer. Although conditions such as schizophrenia are characterized by a deviation from social, ethical, and legal norms, calling them 'illnesses' suggests that they involve a deviation from normal physiological structure or biological function. Pickard makes a very useful distinction between the superficial properties by which a condition is identified, which can be seen as deviations from social, ethical, or legal norms, and the physical or biological underlying properties of the condition. As current research stands, schizophrenia has no clearly identified underlying physical or biological properties, but there are clusters of symptoms within schizophrenia which can be subject to scientific explanation, and this is a promising start. Pickard asks what this implies for the status of personality disorders, which are often depicted as moral failings. She concludes that, although science can help explain their occurrence, their manifestations concern the sphere of morality and social relations, and successful therapy might require patients to experiment with new forms of participation in a socially shared space, such as an NHS therapeutic community for people with personality disorders.

Dominic Murphy also deals with the suitability of the medical model, in its different versions, for the classification and explanation of psychiatric conditions. The medical model can come in weak and strong versions. For instance, Guze thinks that in order to fit the medical model it is sufficient that psychiatric conditions have characteristic symptoms which are used to group patients together, whereas Andreasen believes that it is necessary that specific pathophysiologies are identified. Murphy argues for the strong reading of the medical model via a theory of the normal function of ideal cognitive systems which provides the framework for identifying and explaining pathologies.

Reconciling paradigms

Tim Thornton, John Campbell, and Philip Gerrans are reconciling paradigms. Thornton's paper addresses the interface between personal-level explanation and sub-personal level explanation; Campbell examines the relationship between rationally connected attitudes and neuroscientific explanation; Gerrans brings together empirical findings of dopamine release and attributions of salience, and the accounts of delusional subjects as deficient in mental time travel.

The interface problem is the need to reconcile within psychiatry, explanation at the personal level, which often appeals to normative properties, and explanation at lower levels, which can be formulated in the language of the natural sciences. Thornton argues that neither broad dualist approaches nor physicalist ones will do. Dualism surrenders to the interface problem by postulating two radically heterogeneous levels of discourse and being, whereas physicalism in all its incarnations is unable to offer a satisfactory deflationary account. Thornton concludes that the interface problem cannot be successfully and globally solved by armchair philosophy. But, once the assumptions that seem to make a global solution necessary have been rejected, the interface problem can be more fruitfully approached locally, by identifying in each case, ways in which two potentially autonomous languages and levels of explanation relate to, and interface with, one another.

Campbell is also interested in the relation between different levels of explanation, and challenges the view according to which explanation at the neuroscientific level needs to replace explanation at the psychological level when no rational relations can be found between the propositional attitudes of people reporting delusions. This view is based on the Davidsonian assumption that there needs to be a rationality constraint on the way propositional attitudes relate to each other: if causal relations can be identified between propositional attitudes, then these are deemed to be rational relations. Non-rational causal relations could occur outside the realm of the mental. Campbell thinks this is a problem because the case of delusions shows that there are causal connections between propositional attitudes that are not rational connections. Instead of upholding the rationality constraint in the face of the evidence, we should opt for an account of causation that makes sense of this observation, and Campbell argues that we should view propositional attitudes as control variables in the mental life of subjects with delusions. This allows us to talk about causal relations that operate at the psychological level and turn to neuroscience for an account of the mechanisms that underpin them.

For Gerrans, context-independent dopamine release and dysregulation, and the attribution of salience, do not just support inferential accounts of delusions, but are also instrumental in the construction of unreliable autobiographical narratives. Gerrans challenges the view of delusional subjects as scientists who have access to biased evidence in support of their hypotheses ('the inferential conception') and proposes an alternative analysis. Delusional subjects think and act on the basis of inaccurate information about themselves, because the account of their past experiences (as reconstructed through memory), and hence their autobiographical narrative, is compromised. That is why they benefit from cognitive behavioural therapy when they are offered the opportunity to 're-weave their stories'.

Psychiatry and the neurosciences

Dan Lloyd and Dan Stein both attempt to reconcile neuroscience with clinical psychiatry. They recognize the positive contributions of neuroscience to psychiatry and both suggest that sophisticated scientific methodologies may do greater justice to clinical findings. Lynn Stephens and George Graham highlight the limitations of an account of disorder framed in purely cognitive neuroscientific terms.

Lloyd proposes a hypothesis about the nature of schizophrenia which is compatible both with neuroimaging data and the behavioural manifestations of the condition in patients who seem to suffer from failures of self-understanding. Lloyd argues that the neuropsychological changes in schizophrenia are not functionally localized, but involve the dysregulation of a recurrent network, which in normal functioning is likely to be responsible for an awareness of time. Lloyd presents data suggesting that subjects with schizophrenia demonstrate dysregulation whose effects include a faulty representation of temporal context, which is responsible for the subject failing to maintain a sense of time and losing the capacity to anticipate the behaviour of other people and objects. Temporality, for Husserl and Lloyd, is an essential feature of perception and is ubiquitous, and a disorder of the representation of time may explain the puzzling experiences in schizophrenia.

Stein addresses the effects of a new paradigm in psychology, namely cognitive-affective neuroscience as combined with neurogenetics, on explanations of psychiatric disorders, psychiatric diagnosis, and intervention. The advantage of this new paradigm is that it does not attempt to oversimplify mind/body relations and that, although it seeks the real psychobiological mechanisms responsible for psychopathology, it does not try to reduce subjects to their underlying physical or biological properties, but takes into serious consideration personal-level properties too, such as the character of one's experience. Stein employs the paradigm afforded by cognitive-affective neurogenetics to adjudicate debates in psychiatry including the nature of mental illnesses, what an explanation in psychiatry should look like, and whether we should treat psychiatric disorders. This scientific approach may yield important gains for ontology, epistemology, and ethics in the philosophy of psychiatry.

Stephens and Graham are interested in the contribution of neuroscience to psychiatry and focus on the case of addiction. Definitions of addiction are characterized by the notion of compulsion, but can neuroscience distinguish behaviour that is compulsive from behaviour that is not, in a way that sheds light on pathologies such as drug addiction? The authors are sceptical about the possibility of a neuroscientific account of addiction and the pathological nature of addictive behaviour, because neuroscience is a purely descriptive science that cannot further elucidate normative notions. And normative notions are needed to explain how casual drug taking differs from drug addiction, in the sense that an instance of behaviour needs to be classified as being 'rational', 'prudent', or 'desirable'. For addiction, descriptions of neural states, that are normatively neutral, are insufficient to warrant the attribution of an addiction disorder and as such, Stephens and Graham suggest that the offerings of cognitive neuroscience to psychopathology be viewed with 'caution and analysis'.

Phenomenology and scientific explanation

Matthew Ratcliffe first characterizes phenomenological understanding by distinguishing it from psychological and personal understanding. He then offers a phenomenological analysis of depression in order to illustrate the need for phenomenological understanding in psychiatry. This leads on to a discussion of the relationship between phenomenology and neuroscience. Phenomenology consists of a set of methods for exploring aspects of experience that are obliviously presupposed by most philosophical, scientific, and everyday thinking. For example, phenomenologists study a sense of reality and of belonging to a world that scientific conceptions of mind and world seldom recognize. Ratcliffe argues that phenomenology can inform scientific explanation of psychiatric disorders by discriminating between different types of experience that need to be taken into account when looking for neural correlates. At the same time, scientific studies can bring about conceptual distinctions that impact on phenomenology. However, although phenomenology and science can interact in ways that are mutually illuminating, there is no hope for a naturalization of phenomenology, as naturalistic accounts of mind and world presuppose rather than incorporate the sense of reality that phenomenologists seek to describe.

Shaun Gallagher provides an alternative account of delusions from the standard bottom-up and top-down approaches by taking seriously the relations between brain, body, and environment. According to bottom-up accounts, delusions are due to cognitive errors, and manifest themselves as 'experiential irrationality'. According to top-down accounts, delusions are due to 'inferential mistakes made on the basis of higher-order introspective or perceptual self-observations'. Neither bottom-up nor top-down accounts can explain why the delusion has the thematic content that it does. Gallagher's preferred multiple-realities model, instead, sees delusional reality as one of many (virtual reality, fictional reality, etc.) that can be more or less at odds with everyday reality and explains the delusional subject experiencing feelings of unfamiliarity. Further, he takes seriously the phenomenological experiences offered by deluded patients who describe the different worlds they live in with different meanings and affordances for action. According to Gallagher, this model can also solve the problem of the specificity of the delusional content, which would be taken from 'the experiential presence of social or environmental factors encountered in everyday reality'. This personal-level explanation of delusions has implications for neuroscience and clinical practice and suggests that we view delusions as a more global phenomenon (thinking about body, affect, social world, and environment) than is conventional in the doxastic accounts focused on belief, reasoning, and experience.

Delusions and cognition

Questions about the nature of delusions, and especially about what it is that makes them puzzling or irrational, are central to an understanding of how people affected by psychopathologies are conceived by others. Can they be considered as intentional systems who represent more or less accurately the reality surrounding them? Or are they simply defective physical systems to be fixed? Many of these questions cannot be settled without deciding whether delusions are beliefs, or belief-like enough, to justify the claim that there is continuity between normal and abnormal cognition.

Keith Frankish attempts to answer the question whether delusions are beliefs. He observes that the traditional doxastic account of delusions runs into difficulties, because it cannot explain why delusions sometimes behave differently from typical beliefs. For instance, delusions can be cognitively or behaviourally inert. Frankish argues that there are two types of mental states that we ordinarily call 'beliefs': (1) non-conscious, passive, and graded dispositional states; and (2) conscious, controlled, and binary functional states. According to Frankish, delusions have most of the characteristics of the second type of mental states (level 2 beliefs or acceptances), in that they are 'policies' that are in the subject's control and that the subject has a non-conscious desire to adopt. Some of delusions are doxastic acceptances, and some non-doxastic ones, where the difference is that the latter will not be available to empirical scrutiny. Frankish ends the chapter by exploring the consequences of his approach for the study of delusions, and of beliefs in general.

Anne Aimola Davies and Martin Davies make significant progress in the articulation of the two-factor model of delusions developed by Max Coltheart and colleagues (Coltheart, 2007). They propose that the cognitive functions required for belief evaluation involve working memory and inhibitory executive processes and that, in individuals with delusions, these functions are impaired as a result of right frontal lobe dysfunction or damage. They support their argument by drawing on a range of studies utilizing reasoning, neuropsychology, and functional neuroimaging. The account is compelling. Aimola Davies and Davies offer us an account of parametric variation within the two-factor explanatory framework. A first factor – varying from delusion to delusion – accounts for the initial formation of a delusion. A second factor explains why the false belief is not subsequently rejected. The second factor involves failures to inhibit preponent responses and to assess alternative hypotheses and these failures result from impairments of working memory and executive function. Working memory, and its role in predicting clinical course and 'caseness' in populations is of increasing importance in contemporary psychosis research and hence this contribution links in explicitly to many themes currently under investigation.

Moral psychology and psychopathology

The virtuous person and the morally responsible person have certain characteristics, and on the basis of these we relate to them and form expectations concerning their behaviour. We expect the virtuous person to be motivated to do good, and the morally responsible person to reflect about her beliefs and desires and act in a way that corresponds to her values. But in psychopathology, these views about what counts as virtuous, or morally responsible, are challenged and we remain confused about how to integrate the mentally ill into the moral community. The papers in this section address two main questions: (1) can people affected by conditions such as dissociative disorders and depression be morally virtuous, or morally responsible for their actions? (2) How do we go about establishing whether they are virtuous or morally responsible? The methodological concern is close to the authors' hearts in this section as in any of the previous ones. Once we have a good philosophical theory about which capacities make one virtuous or morally responsible, we examine whether people with psychopathologies retain those capacities. And this investigation will have to be conducted empirically and scientifically. At the same time, the ethical analysis can contribute positively to the common and scientific conception of the mentally ill, and to aspects of the required treatment.

Jeanette Kennett and Steve Matthews apply their view of moral responsibility to psychiatric disorders, and argue that one cannot be morally responsible unless one has a capacity for self-control. In turn, this capacity depends on mental time travel – the ability humans typically have to remember their past experiences as theirs and to project themselves into the future. In people who suffer from dissociative disorders, frontal lobe damage, and amnesia, mental time travel is impaired, which means that normative reasons for acting in a certain way, in accordance with a desirable self-image, cannot be accessed, and the coordination and self-regulation required to carry out long-term projects is also negatively affected. The authors draw interesting conclusions about the moral responsibility and also the liability for criminal acts of people with dissociative disorders (when they are in their alter states) and psychopaths.

Iain Law notices how in the ethical literature, the example of depression has been used to argue for a specific view of virtue. For the Kantian, the virtuous person is the one who acts out of duty, thereby bringing one's desires in accord with one's beliefs. For the Humean, the virtuous person has a desire to do good, and acts on it, but beliefs and desires can go their separate ways. For the Aristotelian, appropriate desires accompany correct beliefs. The depressive has been characterized in the ethical literature as someone with unchanged beliefs and values, but different motivation: this reading of depression would favour the Humean. But Law argues that this is not the reading that fits the evidence: even the system of beliefs and values changes in the depressive (e.g. the belief that one lacks self-worth emerges). As a consequence of scarce confidence in themselves, people with depression do not do what they feel is the right thing to do, and have no motivation to do the right thing, apart from feeling that it is the right thing to do. This means that people with depression lack virtue, and they might not be entirely mistaken when they perceive their state as a character flaw rather than an illness. This does not mean that they are to be blamed, or to be made to feel even worse about themselves than they already feel. Law suggests that during cognitive therapy, mental health and virtue can be re-gained simultaneously.

References

Coltheart, M. (2007). Cognitive neuropsychiatry and delusional belief. *Quarterly Journal of Experimental Psychology*, **60**, 1041–1062.

Coltheart, M. and Davies, M. (2000). *Pathologies of Belief*. Oxford, Blackwell.

Cooper, R. (2008). *Psychiatry and Philosophy of Science*. Chesham, Bucks, Acumen.

Halligan, P. W. and David, A. S. (2001). Cognitive neuropsychiatry: towards a scientific psychopathology. *Nature Reviews Neuroscience*, **2**, 209–215.

Section 1

Psychiatry as a science

Chapter 1

Is psychiatric research scientific?

Rachel Cooper

Abstract

It is generally assumed that asking whether psychiatric research can be scientific is a reasonable question to ask and that the answer matters. In this chapter I contest both these claims.

I start by arguing that the search for a 'demarcation criterion' that would distinguish science from non-science has failed. I then defend the claim that 'science' is best considered a family resemblance term. This suggests that whether psychiatric research is scientific may be a fuzzy matter, and that psychiatric science might be like the more paradigmatic sciences in some respects but unlike them in others. As psychiatric research tackles diverse problems in diverse ways, assessing whether it is empirically and conceptually sound will be a piecemeal and difficult task.

1.1 Introduction

Lots of people want to know whether psychiatric research is scientific (e.g. Faust and Ziskin, 1988; Reznek, 1991; Cawley, 1993; Chur-Hansen and Parker, 2005). Opinions vary and tempers flare but participants in the debates have taken two points for granted: first, all of them assume that asking whether psychiatric research can be scientific is a reasonable question to ask. Second, all consider that whether or not psychiatric research is scientific matters. In this chapter I contest both these claims.

I start by reviewing the work of those philosophers of science who sought a 'demarcation criterion' that would distinguish science from non-science. Philosophers of science now generally agree that the search for a demarcation criterion has failed. However, in other disciplines the search for a means of distinguishing science from pseudoscience continues. I review the current debate in psychology and psychiatry. Then, returning to philosophical work, I discuss and support accounts according to which 'science' is best considered a family resemblance term. This suggests that whether psychiatric research is scientific may be a fuzzy matter, and that psychiatric science might be like the more paradigmatic sciences in some respects but unlike them in others. Instead of asking whether psychiatric research is scientific, we would do better to ask more specific questions, such as: what are the forms of explanation used in psychiatry? Are they like those used in other sciences? Are mental disorders natural kinds? Can psychiatric theory be reduced to more fundamental theories?

Furthermore, as 'psychiatric research' is diverse, these questions may themselves be too broad – different areas of psychiatric research plausibly use different forms of explanation, some types of mental disorder may be natural kinds while others are not, and so on. In general, the best questions to ask should be very particular. Instead of asking whether psychiatric research is scientific, we should ask questions like: given what we know about schizophrenia, does it seem to be a natural kind? Might cognitive theories of autism be reduced to theories that posit neurological problems?

Finally, I shall briefly consider why it is that the question of whether psychiatry is a science is so popular. If the question is malformed, what accounts for its enduring appeal?

The remainder of the chapter falls into the following sections:

♦ Work on demarcation within philosophy.

♦ The debate in psychology and psychiatry.

♦ Returning to philosophy: 'science' as a family resemblance term.

♦ Asking better questions.

♦ Demanding higher epistemic standards across the board.

♦ Why have people wanted to know whether psychiatry is a science?

1.2 **Work on demarcation within philosophy**

When considering philosophical work on the demarcation problem, we should start with the work of Karl Popper (1963). Karl Popper was one of the greatest philosophers of the twentieth century and wrote extensively on demarcation. Popper was greatly impressed by the physics of his time and sceptical of other popular contemporary theories, in particular, Freudian psychoanalysis. Popper sought a criterion that would demarcate the theories of physics from those of psychoanalysis and more generally distinguish science from pseudoscience. In his theory of falsification, Popper thought he had found what he was looking for. According to Popper, scientific theories are those that can be falsified – that is, if they are false, it is possible for this to be revealed by empirical evidence. Pseudoscientific theories, on the other hand, are not falsifiable – whatever happens, the theory will be able to come up with some explanation.

Using his criterion of falsifiability, Popper classified the theories of relativity as science and those of psychoanalysis as pseudoscience. Let us consider the relativity theory first: relativity theory can be used to make highly specific predictions, for example, it predicts that the light from the stars is bent by the mass of the sun. During a solar eclipse, it is possible to measure this bending and as it happens, the observed effect fits with that predicted. For Popper, the noticeable thing about relativity theory is that it commits itself to making specific empirical claims. In doing this, it runs the risk of being shown wrong by events. The theory is falsifiable and therefore counts as science according to Popper. On the other hand, Popper claims that psychoanalysts have an answer for every eventuality – if an analysand accepts an interpretation, then it is proved right, but if they deny it the analyst can simply excuse this by saying that they are in denial. As Popper thinks that psychoanalysis cannot be proved wrong, he considers it to be unfalsifiable and therefore pseudoscience.

Popper's demarcation criterion is still widely discussed in medical and lay debates about the scientific status of psychiatry and psychoanalysis (e.g. Grant and Harari, 2005), but has now largely been abandoned by philosophers. Philosophers have rejected Popper's demarcation criterion because it runs into various well-known problems, perhaps the greatest of which is the Quine–Duhem problem (a similar if not identical problem is also sometimes known as 'the experimenters' regress') (Duhem, 1954; Quine, 1961; Collins and Pinch, 1993). The problem is that theories only make concrete predictions in concert with various auxiliary hypotheses. Popper says that scientists should come up with theories and then see if experiments falsify them. However, when an unexpected observation is made, although this might be because the theory is false, it might also be because something has gone wrong elsewhere – maybe some part of the experimental apparatus has broken, or maybe the statistics have been analysed incorrectly. Even when all imaginable sources of error have been checked out, the theory may still actually be true in spite of the results not being as expected. This is because in some cases factors that are as yet unknown might be interfering with the results.

A consequence of the Quine–Duhem problem is that a theory can never be conclusively falsified. When an experiment gives an unexpected result, the problem may always lie somewhere other than in the theory. Popper knew about the Quine–Duhem problem and modified his account to deal with it. He says that good scientists should agree before an experiment which auxiliary hypotheses they will check if they face an unexpected result (so, they agree to check that the wires have not fallen off and to repeat any statistical analyses, but they do not resort to positing that unknown factors are interfering with their results) (Popper, 1959 §20). However, Popper's modified account is much less attractive than the simple criterion of falsification. With the modifications, distinguishing between science and pseudoscience is no longer a simple matter. It no longer depends simply on the question of whether a theory makes empirical predictions that might turn out to be false, but also on whether the practitioners have the correct 'scientific' outlook – whether they only check auxiliary hypotheses to an extent that is 'reasonable'.

Of course, philosophers of science other than Popper have also proposed demarcation criteria. Perhaps most influentially, Thomas Kuhn suggested that a field becomes a science when it finds its first 'paradigm' (1970). A Kuhnian paradigm is a commonly agreed framework for doing research in some area. Scientists who share a paradigm will agree on the questions that should be addressed, on the methods that should be used, and on what counts as good research in a particular area. Once a field has found its first paradigm, scientists in that area can begin to practise 'normal science' – that is, puzzle solving within the taken-for-granted framework of the paradigm. So, physicists working within the paradigm of Newtonian mechanics, for example, can spend time worrying about how to apply the laws of mechanics to collisions involving multiple bodies or the flow of liquids, but they never question the fundamental correctness of the Newtonian framework. The puzzle solving that is characteristic of normal science practised within a paradigm is of central importance for Kuhn because it is what enables a science to make progress.

However, Kuhn's demarcation criterion is also inadequate. As Paul Feyerabend points out, puzzle solving within some commonly accepted framework is not solely characteristic of science (1970). For example, organized crime shares this feature – once a criminal mastermind has come up with something that works, other criminals content themselves with developing variations on the theme. Similarly, theologians, and philosophers working within particular schools, work on intellectual puzzles set out within a particular intellectual tradition.

1.3 The debate in psychology and psychiatry

Philosophers have now fairly much given up on demarcating science from pseudoscience, but the demarcation problem remains a live issue in other areas of the academy. In psychology in particular, a large body of work addresses the issue of what is it that makes work scientific or pseudoscientific. In recent years, a number of writers within psychology have become concerned that psychology is being brought into disrepute by practitioners who engage in pseudoscience. Some worry about the range of dubious therapies that are now offered to the public (Lilienfeld *et al.*, 2003). Others think that the debates over multiple personality disorder, the detection of child abuse, and the possibility of recovered memories are suspect and have led the field into crisis (Tavris, 2004).

These concerns have led to an attempt within psychology to identify science and pseudoscience and to cleanse psychology of its more dubious theories and practitioners: a number of books on this theme have been published, most notably Lilienfeld, Lynn, and Lohr's (2003) *Science and Pseudoscience in Clinical Psychology*; a new journal, *The Scientific Review of Mental Health Practice* (SRMHP), has been set up with the explicit aim of distinguishing the scientific wheat from the pseudoscientific chaff in clinical psychology, psychiatry, and allied disciplines; and there have been calls for psychology undergraduates to be taught courses that will help them distinguish science from pseudoscience (Lilienfeld *et al.*, 2001).

In contrast to the earlier philosophical attempts at demarcation, in the psychological literature most writers have not sought to define science or pseudoscience in terms of necessary and sufficient conditions. Rather, writers have tended to provide lists of criteria that make a field more or less scientific. These lists are highly reminiscent of the lists of symptoms that are used to identify psychopathology. In the same sort of way that a patient with a number of depressive symptoms is considered more likely to suffer from depression, a field that shows a number of specified signs is considered more likely to be a pseudoscience.

Different writers provide various different lists of the symptoms of pseudoscience and science. Tavris (2003) notes that in contrast with pseudoscience, sciences tend to be characterized by a willingness to question received wisdom and rely on gathering empirical evidence to determine whether a prediction or belief is valid. In addition, she notes that scientific claims tend to be falsifiable in Popper's sense.

Lilienfeld *et al.* (2001, p. 182) provide a longer list of criteria. They think that the difference between science and pseudoscience is a difference of degree rather than kind, but think that pseudoscientific claims often have a number of markers:

> Among these characteristics are (a) unfalsifiability (Popper, 1959), (b) absence of self-correction (Herbert *et al.*, in press), (c) overuse of ad hoc immunizing tactics designed to protect theories from refutation (Lakatos, 1978), (d) absence of 'connectivity' (Stanovich, 1998, p. 116) with other domains of knowledge (i.e., failure to build on extant scientific constructs; Bunge, 1967), (e) the placing of the burden of proof on critics rather than on the proponents of claims (Shermer, 1997), (f) the use of obscurantist language (i.e., language that seems to have as its primary function to confuse rather than clarify; Hockenbury & Hockenbury, 1999; van Rillaer, 1991), and (g) overreliance on anecdotes and testimonials at the expense of systematic evidence (Herbert *et al.*, 2000)[1].
>
> (Lilienfeld *et al.*, 2001, p. 182)

The point of such lists is to enable pseudoscience to be identified and done away with, and indeed a number of papers have used such lists to condemn specific practices as pseudoscientific. For example, Herbert *et al.* (2000) examine the technique of 'eye movement desensitization and reprocessing' (EMDR), a supposed treatment for anxiety disorders. They spot the symptoms of pseudoscience and thus dismiss the technique. Similarly, papers in Lilienfeld, Lynn, and Lohr's (eds.) (2003) *Science and Pseudoscience in Clinical Psychology* use lists of criteria that make a field pseudoscientific, in their attempt to root out dubious therapies.

Distinguishing scholarly research from rubbish is important. However, I shall argue that it is a mistake to try and diagnose pseudoscience in a way analogous to the manner in which a clinician diagnoses psychopathology. Looking at Lilienfeld *et al.*'s criteria, I have several worries. First, it is unclear how the criteria are to be weighted: is obscure language as big a sin as unfalsifiability? How is a reliance on anecdotes to be weighted against an absence of 'connectivity'?

My more serious worry is that considered individually, each of the criteria is insufficient to indicate that a discipline has problems. Depending on the context, unfalsifiability, or obscure language, or meeting any of the other criteria may not be indicative of pseudoscience. I will show this by considering each criterion in turn.

Unfalsifiability – As mentioned earlier, the Quine–Duhem problem means that conclusive falsification is always very difficult (if not impossible). In addition, as pointed

---

[1] In a later book, *Science and Pseudoscience in Clinical Psychology* (2003), Lilienfeld *et al.* present the same list of criteria but also add:

h. evasion of peer review (2003, p. 6)

i. emphasis on confirmation rather than refutation (p. 7)

j. absence of boundary conditions – they claim that 'most well-supported scientific theories possess boundary conditions, that is, well-articulated limits under which predicted phenomena do and do not apply' (p. 9)

k. the mantra of holism 'proponents of pseudoscientific claims . . . typically maintain that scientific claims can be evaluated only within the context of broader claims and therefore cannot be judged in isolation' (p. 9).

out by Larry Laudan, certain statements that are surely scientific are not candidates for falsification. In particular, many existential statements are unfalsifiable. For example, 'There was a missing link between apes and humans', 'There are black holes' (Laudan, 1996 p. 218).

Absence of self-correction – Sometimes, a field will not self-correct because it is right – thus, geometrical optics has not progressed for centuries.

Overuse of *ad hoc* revisions – This criterion is of little use for spotting pseudoscience. Revisions will only be considered to be 'overused' and '*ad hoc*' if they are independently considered problematic.

Absence of 'connectivity' – Many scientifically accepted phenomena cannot be connected into a satisfactory world theory because there is as yet no understanding of how they occur. For example, there is as yet no commonly accepted way of making sense of EPR correlations in quantum mechanics.

Placing the burden of proof on critics – Oddly, this criterion conflicts with the first one, that is, unfalsifiability. The falsificationist thinks that a scientist should be free to propose any hypothesis so long as it has empirically testable consequences, and that the task of science is then to seek to demonstrate the falsity of the theory. In lay terms, Popper's theory of falsificationism places the burden of proof on critics!

Use of obscurantist language – Again, this criterion is of little use – whether language is considered 'obscurantist' or of 'necessary theoretical complexity' depends on whether one considers the theory plausible or not.

Overreliance on anecdotes and testimonials – Again, only someone who considers a theory problematic will think that it displays an 'overreliance' on single case studies. Depending on the question, the use of single case studies may be appropriate. Although a single case study is seldom sufficient to show that an effect will always, or even normally, occur, it often will be adequate for showing that something is possible. Take, for example, the much reported single case study of D.F. – the woman who can guide her hand through a vertical or horizontal slot without having conscious awareness of the slot's orientation (Goodale and Milner, 1996). This single case is sufficient to make it conceivable that vision for action and for recognition can come apart.

I conclude that each of the seven criteria fails when considered individually. At this, Lilienfeld and colleagues may not be too distressed. Their criteria are not intended to offer a foolproof way of spotting pseudoscience when considered individually, but are instead taken to be diagnostic of a problem when they co-occur in a particular field. Similarly, sadness when considered alone may not be indicative of depression but if it lasts for a considerable time and co-occurs with psychomotor retardation and sleep-related problems, then it suggests that there is a problem.

However, claiming that pseudoscience is only to be suspected when a certain number, say four, of the seven criteria are met will not do. I will argue that in some cases a claim may not meet any criteria and yet still plausibly be 'pseudoscientific'. Conversely, in other cases a claim may meet multiple criteria and yet still be scientifically respectable. Here, I will discuss each possibility in turn.

1.3.1 Lilienfeld *et al.*'s criteria give rise to false negatives

In some cases, we may want to consider a claim pseudoscience even though it fails to meet any of the seven criteria. Consider the field of ufology – the study of UFOs. Some practitioners in the field are keen to meet standards of scientific acceptability. They publish in peer-reviewed journals, avoid obscure language, and pride themselves in seeking to test their claims empirically and applying standard statistical tests of significance (Cross, 2004). Let us suppose that an ufologist is investigating the trauma that can be suffered by 'alien abductees'. The researcher suspects that different types of aliens have different types of transport and are differentially likely to harm abductees. Such a researcher may come up with the following hypothesis:

> People who have been abducted by UFOs with flashing lights are more likely to suffer post-abduction trauma than those who are abducted by UFOs with constant lights.

The ufologist's hypothesis is not obscure. It is falsifiable. The ufologist may seek to assess the claim empirically, for example, by studying a sample of abductees and examining whether there is a statistically significant correlation between reports of flashing lights and trauma. Keen to adhere to the standards of scientific acceptability, the ufologist may send the resulting paper off to an appropriate peer-review journal – say, *The Journal of UFO Studies*.

The ufologist fails to meet Lilienfeld *et al.*'s criteria for pseudoscience. And, yet, I suggest, the odds are that they are a crank. The fundamental problem is not methodological, however. The basic problem is that a fundamental assumption on which their research is based – that aliens frequently come to earth – is highly unlikely to be true. As the methods employed by ufologists are similar to those used by reputable scientists and yet ufology is a paradigmatic example of pseudoscience, I conclude that displaying Lilienfeld *et al.*'s hallmarks of science is not sufficient to render a field scientific.

1.3.2 Lilienfeld *et al.*'s criteria give rise to false positives

Conversely, some claims that we would normally consider scientifically respectable meet several of Lilienfeld *et al.*'s criteria for pseudoscience. Consider the following claim:

> There are brocken spectres.

Brocken spectres are rare phenomena. They sometimes occur when a mountaineer gets above the clouds and his shadow is cast on the clouds below creating the appearance of a spectre. The claim 'There are brocken spectres' is unfalsifiable (if I go looking for a brocken spectre and do not see any, this does not mean that they do not occur). The language is somewhat obscure. The evidence for the existence of brocken spectres is anecdotal and testimonial. There is an 'absence of self-correction'. At least until it was discovered what caused brocken spectres, there was an 'absence of connectivity' with other scientific claims. And yet, brocken spectres do occur and the claim is scientifically respectable despite the fact that it displays many of

Lilienfeld *et al.*'s signs of pseudoscience. Applying Lilienfeld *et al.*'s criteria gives rise to false positives.

We have already seen that Lilienfeld *et al.*'s criteria cannot distinguish science from pseudoscience when applied singly. Now we have seen that they cannot distinguish science from pseudoscience when applied in concert either.

1.4 **Returning to philosophy: 'science' as a family resemblance term**

Recent philosophical work presents a picture of the distinction between science and pseudoscience that is somewhat similar to that presented in the psychological literature. In philosophy too, attempts to define 'science' and 'pseudoscience' in terms of necessary and sufficient conditions have been largely abandoned. Here, though, the similarity ends. Philosophers and psychologists tend to draw quite different consequences from the idea that 'science' cannot be precisely defined. Psychologists have sought to use lists of possible symptoms to diagnose pseudoscience. Philosophers have tended to conclude that seeking to demarcate science from pseudoscience is a mistake. Here I examine in greater detail recent literature from the philosophy and history of science and then ask why it is that the projects of psychologists and philosophers have diverged.

Recently, a number of philosophers of science have suggested that seeking a demarcation criterion is misguided. Rather than it being possible to define 'science' in terms of necessary and sufficient conditions, these philosophers suggest that science is best conceived of as a family resemblance term (Dupré, 1993; Pickstone, 2000) in the sense introduced by Ludwig Wittgenstein. In the *Philosophical Investigations*, Wittgenstein asks us to consider what games have in common. He suggests that there is no one feature that they all share. Many games are competitive, but some are not (ring-a-ring-a-roses). Some games are fun, but others are not (I spy is quite dull). Many have rules, but some do not (playing cops and robbers). Most involve other people, but some can be played alone (Patience). Wittgenstein concludes that:

> if you look at them you will not see something that is common to all, but similarities, relationships and a whole series of them at that . . . I can think of no better way to characterise these similarities than 'family resemblances'; for the various resemblances of a family: build, features, colour of eyes, gait, temperament, etc etc. overlap and criss-cross in the same way – And I shall say: games form a family.
>
> (Wittgenstein, 1953, §66)

Similarly, the various sciences can be seen as forming a family. There is no one feature that they all share, but rather a network of resemblances unites them. Many sciences make predictions, but others do not. Some posit unobservable entities, some do not. Some, but not all, involve experiments. The claim that there is no one feature that all sciences have in common is made all the more plausible when we consider the wide range of activities that are classified as 'science' The activities of theoretical physicists, evolutionary biologists, natural historians, game theorists, epidemiologists, neuropsychologists, and materials scientists all get classified as scientific. However, there is plausibly no one feature that all these areas share.

John Pickstone's (2000) *Ways of Knowing* develops the thesis that there are many different types of scientific activity. Different sciences in different times seek to understand the world in different ways. Some sciences have depended on natural history – the describing and classification of things. Others have focused on analysis – looking within phenomena and breaking them down to fundamental elements. Others have learnt through experiments – they have sought to control phenomena and to create novelties. Pickstone thinks that methods come to be used in different areas at different times, and that the importance of the different methods varies with subject and period. Looking to the future, he expects new methods to become available – he cites simulation as a method that may hold future promise.

Pickstone's picture of science stresses the diversity of the activities that we consider 'scientific'. Arguing along similar lines, Larry Laudan concludes that:

> The evident epistemic heterogeneity of the activities and beliefs customarily regarded as scientific should alert us to the probable futility of seeking an epistemic version of a demarcation criterion.
>
> (Laudan, 1996, p. 221)

What is more, such a view also brings out the fact that the same methods that are used within the sciences can also be used in fields that we would not normally classify as 'sciences'. Consider the skills used to analyse statistical data – the same skills of sampling and extrapolation are needed by the market researcher, or the ecologist, or in social science. Similarly, the skills of the natural historian – collecting and classifying – can be employed by those who order collections of beetles, as well as by those who order collections of wine.

One moral that I think we can draw from this picture of science is that asking whether a field is scientific will seldom be the right question to ask. As Pickstone shows us, the methods that are used in the sciences are often also employed elsewhere, and whether a field gets counted as 'science' or not often depends on contingent historical factors. Thus, instead of asking 'Is psychiatric research scientific?', we would do better to ask questions like 'What are the methods that have been used in addressing the research question?' and 'Are these methods generally reliable and appropriate in the case at hand?'.

Writing in the psychological literature, McNally has drawn much the same conclusion. As he puts it:

> Rather than asking, Is this pseudoscience or genuine science? we should ask, What arguments and evidence support this clinical claim? We should be concerned with belief-worthiness, epistemic warrant, evidential basis, empirical support (pick your favourite locution), rather than attempting to determine whether the theory or practice falls on the proper side of a demarcation criterion that separates science from pseudoscience.
>
> (McNally, 2003, p. 4)

1.5 Asking better questions

I conclude that 'science' is a family resemblance term and that asking whether psychiatric research is scientific is thus not a very useful question. Rather than asking whether psychiatry is a science we would do better to ask finer-grained questions: what methods does psychiatry use to explain and predict phenomena? Are these methods generally reliable? Are they appropriately applied in psychiatry? What is more, although these questions are better questions than asking 'Is psychiatric research scientific?' we would do still better to get more refined. Psychiatry is a diverse field – the sorts of questions that research psychiatrists ask and the methods that they employ vary wildly across different areas. Consider the sorts of research that are published in psychiatry journals:

- randomized controlled trials (RCTs) to test drugs and psychological treatment efficacy;
- papers that compare rates of disorder with other factors and examine, for example, whether place of residence, or drug abuse, increases the risk of disorder;
- papers that assess patient satisfaction with facilities;
- papers that look at the physiological, or neuropsychological, or cognitive correlates of disorder;
- brain imaging studies;
- cluster-analytic studies; and
- studies that assess whether diagnostic criteria can be reliably applied.

And, of course, this list is not exhaustive. It merely acts as a reminder of the range of research conducted by psychiatrists. The methods used by research psychiatrists are diverse. Some of the methods used are similar to those used in other disciplines. So, for example, the statistical methods employed in RCTs were originally developed for comparing seed varieties and fertilizers in agriculture. The methods used in cluster analysis were first used by biologists – especially bacteriologists. Other methods may be unique to psychiatry.

Depending on the methods employed, different questions may be asked about the research at issue. Some questions will be largely empirical or mathematical – for example, determining how large a sample needs to be before statistical methods yield robust results. Other questions about methods may be philosophical. For example, the methodology used in RCTs commits one to certain views about the foundations of probability theory, and whether these assumptions are acceptable is a question that is explored by philosophers (amongst others) (Ashcroft, 2004). As another example, elsewhere I have argued that certain interpretations of cluster-analytic studies commit one to certain views about the nature of properties (Cooper, 2005). The sociology and history of science also have work to do if we want to know which methods are likely to produce reliable results under which circumstances. For example, the history of psychiatry shows us that new treatments have often been introduced by overenthusiastic proponents, and that the reports of the initial users of a treatment cannot be relied on for assessing treatment efficacy.

Not only are the methods that psychiatrists employ diverse, so too are the conditions that they research: some psychiatric research examines genetically caused disorders like Down's syndrome. Other work looks at conditions that appear clearly pathological but where no biological cause is known, for example, schizophrenia. Some disorders appear to vary radically with social environment, for example, multiple personality disorder. Some psychiatric research examines conditions that are not clearly pathological at all, but that might be normal under certain conditions, for example, suicidal thoughts, or hearing voices.

Depending on the type of condition under consideration, very different conceptual issues are raised. In the case of suicidal thoughts, one might worry about the relevance of Donald Davidson's claims that rational thoughts are necessarily holistically connected (Davidson, 1970). Maybe this means that rational thoughts of suicide will resist reduction, for example. Here we will not get drawn into considering the acceptability and implications of Davidson's claims, but will just note that any such concerns could only affect rational thoughts, and would leave work on non-rational mental states, such as feelings of panic or nightmares, untouched. Other worries specifically concern disorders that appear subject to 'looping effects', in the sense introduced by Ian Hacking (1995a, b). The symptoms of certain disorders appear to be affected by our descriptions of them – so the symptoms of multiple personality disorder have plausibly altered as the media presentations of the condition have changed. Disorders that display such effects pose specific problems. Hacking argues that in such cases, epidemiological studies will make little sense, for example, as the disorder is necessarily a moving target that shifts as it is studied. Once again, such worries are specific. Certain conditions and certain conditions only can be expected to be affected by such concerns.

Thinking about the diversity of research methods that psychiatrists employ and the range of phenomena that they examine makes it plausible that there will not be very much that one can say about the standing of psychiatric research in general. If there are conceptual problems with the use of certain methods, or with certain types of investigation into certain conditions, there is no need to think that this implies there will be problems with other types of psychiatric research.

1.6 Demanding higher epistemic standards across the board

If we cease to consider the distinction between science and non-science as being of any importance, we can concentrate instead on more significant questions – such as how best we can find out truths. In all areas where people purport to be seeking truths, they should be expected to conduct their research in epistemically responsible ways. Most obviously, this will lead us to demand more from research in areas that have been traditionally regarded as non-scientific. For example, at present when a philosopher or historian presents figures and discusses trends, they can just give tables of raw figures (as I do in Cooper, 2005, p. 116, for example). However, we may well decide that statistical techniques that are good in fields traditionally regarded scientific are also good elsewhere, and demand that all of those who discuss 'trends' supply robust evidence that the trends under discussion are actually statistically significant. Similarly, the methods of systematic review might usefully be employed in disciplines outside the traditional sciences.

However, it's not only 'non-scientific' work from which we should expect more. In the non-sciences we accept that the epistemic status of many claims depends on the personal integrity of the expert in question. So, if we want a builder's opinion on a job we typically worry a lot about whether the builder we ask is honest. We are more likely to trust someone who we know and with whom we are likely to have continued contact, we may ask for multiple quotes and compare them, and we may seek advice from someone who has nothing to gain personally from the answer that we are given.

In science, on the other hand, I suggest that the thought that there is a 'scientific method' which turns raw data into reliable facts has led to a neglect of the question of personal trustworthiness. We have a picture whereby the 'scientific method' works well regardless of who the researchers are or what their interests might be. However the idea that 'the scientific method' can operate regardless of the personal integrity of researchers should be rejected. Work by historians and sociologists of science has shown that it is an essential part of scientific practice that scientists make judgements about the trustworthiness of different practitioners. Harry Collins, for example, has provided numerous cases where judgements as to whether an experiment has been performed correctly ultimately come down to judgements of the personal integrity of the researchers involved (Collins, 1985). Science cannot work unless the scientific community can decide which results to believe and therefore judgements of trustworthiness play an essential role in the enterprise. For those who are unconvinced by Collins' work, it is also possible to argue that the allegiances of researchers matter more directly: take the data that is produced by RCTs in psychiatry. An RCT is 'scientific', if anything is. However, numerous studies have shown that the results that are found by an RCT depend on who is paying the bill. Researchers who are paid by drug companies find results that favour drug companies (Baker *et al.*, 2003; Perlis *et al.*, 2005). Here, we do not need to consider the mechanisms via which this occurs; we just need to note that it happens. The fact that findings vary with the researchers' allegiance is sufficient to show that the interests of the researchers matter. As such, in the same way that we seek out independent advice in non-scientific fields, we should also expect scientific researchers to be financially disinterested. In non-scientific fields, we expect that those who review products, for example, the people who test kitchen implements for consumer magazines, should have no financial incentive to deliver one judgement above another. We should extend the same demands to those who test drugs.

1.7 Why have people wanted to know whether psychiatry is a science?

In this chapter, I have argued that the question 'Is psychiatric research scientific?' is the wrong question to ask. What then accounts for its enduring appeal? I suggest that the attraction of asking whether psychiatric research is scientific has two explanations.

First, many people genuinely want to know what to make of psychiatric research. They want to know whether psychiatrists should be treated as experts or charlatans. Asking whether such research is scientific has been seen as a way of addressing this question. Roughly, if psychiatric research is scientific, then, it has been assumed, researchers in psychiatry should have the same expert status as other scientists – their findings will be trustworthy. If psychiatry is only a pseudoscience on the other hand, then what research psychiatrists say can be ignored. However, once one considers the diversity of psychiatric research and the diversity of the conditions that psychiatrists examine, the idea that one might reach a conclusion as to whether the whole lot is science (and so presumably decent stuff) or pseudoscience (and so presumably not worth listening to) seems laughable. Working out whether psychiatric research is empirically and conceptually sound will of necessity be a piecemeal and difficult job.

The second reason why asking whether psychiatry is a science has had broad appeal is that it has played a key role in the rhetoric associated with boundary drawing (as noted by Still and Dryden, 2004). When two parties wish to dismiss each others' claims, for one side to denounce the other as 'pseudoscience' operates as a way of rubbishing particular positions. Thus, the whole of psychiatry or psychology is denounced as pseudoscience by parties opposed to these disciplines, such as scientology. Or, at a finer grain, particular theories within psychology are denounced as pseudoscience by theorists who wish to exclude certain researchers. Calling an area pseudoscience has acted as a battle-cry. In this chapter, however, I have argued that science cannot be defined and is not necessarily epistemically superior to non-science. As such, the temptation to praise a field as scientific or denounce it as pseudoscience is not helpful and should be resisted.

1.8 Conclusion

In this chapter, I have argued that 'science' is a family resemblance term. Science has no defining features and asking whether a field is scientific is a red herring. Instead, we should ask more specific questions. We need to ask whether the methods used to address specific questions are appropriate. The research methods used by psychiatrists are diverse; so too are the conditions that they investigate. As such, there is likely to be little that can be said about the epistemology of psychiatry in general. The best questions to ask will be very particular. Instead of asking whether psychiatry is a science, we should ask questions like 'Given what we know about schizophrenia does it seem to be a natural kind?' or 'Might cognitive theories of autism be reduced to theories that posit neurological problems?' If we want to know which psychiatric claims to believe and how to interpret them, there are no short-cuts that can be made. Psychiatric research tackles diverse problems in diverse ways and assessing whether it is empirically and conceptually sound will be a piecemeal and difficult task.

Acknowledgements

A version of this paper was presented at the Philosophy of Psychiatry Work in Progress workshop held at Lancaster University, January 2008 and I am grateful for the comments of all those present. I am also grateful to Lisa Bortolotti, Matthew Broome, and the members of the Lancaster University Philosophy Department for comments on an earlier draft.

References

Ashcroft, R. (2004). Current epistemological problems in evidence based medicine. *Journal of Medical Ethics*, **30**, 131–135.

Baker, C., Johnsrud, M., Crismon, M., Rosenheck, R. A., and Woods, S. W. (2003). Quantitative analysis of sponsorship bias in economic studies of antidepressants. *British Journal of Psychiatry*, **183**, 498–506.

Cawley, R. H. (1993). Psychiatry is more than a science. *British Journal of Psychiatry*, **162**, 154–160.

Chur-Hansen, A. and Parker, D. (2005). Is psychiatry an art or a science? The views of psychiatrists and trainees. *Australasian Psychiatry*, **13**, 415–418.

Collins, H. M. (1985). *Changing Order: Replication and Induction in Scientific Practice*, Beverley Hills and London, Sage.

Collins, H. and Pinch, T. (1993). *The Golem – What Everyone Should Know about Science*, Cambridge, Cambridge University Press.

Cooper, R. (2005). *Classifying Madness*, Dordrecht, Springer.

Cross, A. (2004). The flexibility of scientific rhetoric: a case study of UFO researchers. *Qualitative Sociology*, **27**, 3–34.

Davidson, D. (1970). Mental events. Reprinted in Davidson, D. (1980) *Essays on Actions and Events*, pp. 207–227. Oxford, Oxford University Press.

Duhem, P. (1954). *The Aim and Structure of Physical Theory*, Princeton, NJ, Princeton University.

Dupré, J. (1993). *The Disorder of Things*, Cambridge, MA, Harvard University Press.

Faust, D. and Ziskin, J. (1988). The expert witness in psychology and psychiatry. *Science*, **241**(4861), 31–35.

Feyerabend, P. (1970). Consolations for the specialist. In *Criticism and the Growth of Knowledge* (eds. I. Lakatos and A. Musgrove), pp. 197–230. Cambridge, Cambridge University Press.

Fox, R. (1996). Charlatanism, scientism, and psychology's social contract. *American Psychologist*, **51**, 777–784.

Goodale, M. and Milner, A. (1996). Separate visual pathways for perception and action. In *Human Cognitive Neuropsychology: A Textbook with Readings*, (eds. A. Ellis and A. Young), pp. 395–407. Hove Psychology Press.

Grant, D. and Harari, E. (2005). Psychoanalysis, science and the seductive theory of Karl Popper. *Australian and New Zealand Journal of Psychiatry*, **39**, 446–452.

Hacking, I. (1995a). *Rewriting the Soul*, Princeton, NJ, Princeton University Press.

Hacking, I. (1995b). The looping effects of human kinds. In *Causal Cognition* (eds. D. Sperber, D. Premack, and A. Premack), pp. 351–394. Oxford, Clarendon Press.

Herbert, J., Lilienfeld, S., Lohr J., *et al.* (2000). Science and pseudoscience in the development of eye movement desensitization and reprocessing: implications for clinical psychology. *Clinical Psychology Review*, **20**, 945–971.

Kuhn, T. (1970). *The Structure of Scientific Revolutions*, Chicago, IL, University of Chicago Press.

Laudan, L. (1996). *Beyond Positivism and Relativism*, Boulder, CO, Westview Press.

Lilienfeld, S., Lohr, J., and Morier, D. (2001). The teaching of courses in the science and pseudoscience of psychology: useful resources. *Teaching of Psychology*, **28**, 182–191.

Lilienfeld, S., Lynn, S., and Lohr, J. (2003). *Science and Pseudoscience in Clinical Psychology*, New York, The Guilford Press.

McNally, R. (2003). Is the pseudoscience concept useful for clinical psychology? *The Scientific Review of Mental Health Practice*, **2**. Available at http://www.srmhp.org/0202/pseudo-science.html (accessed October 2008).

Perlis, R., Perlis, C., Wu, Y., Hwang, C., Joseph, M., and Nierenberg, A. A. (2005). Industry sponsorship and financial conflict of interest in the reporting of clinical trials in psychiatry. *American Journal of Psychiatry*, **162**, 1957–1960.

Pickstone, J. (2000). *Ways of Knowing*, Manchester, Manchester University Press.

Popper, K. (1959). *Logic of Scientific Discovery*, London, Hutchinson.

Popper, K. (1963). *Conjectures and Refutations*, London, Routledge and Kegan Paul.

Quine, W. V. O. (1961). Two dogmas of empiricism. In *From a Logical Point of View*, pp. 20–46. New York, Harper and Row.

Reznek, L. (1991). *The Philosophical Defence of Psychiatry*, London, Routledge.

Still, A. and Dryden, W. (2004). The social psychology of pseudoscience: a brief history. *Journal for the Theory of Social Behaviour*, **34**, 265–290.

Tavris, C. (2/28/2003) Mind games: Psychological warfare between therapist and scientists. *Chronicle of Higher Education*, **49**. Available at http://www.psych.utoronto.ca/users/pgsa/Course%20Readings/Clinical%20Issues/Mind%20Games.pdf (accessed October 2008).

Wittgenstein, L. (1953). *Philosophical Investigations*, Oxford, Blackwell.

Chapter 2

The secret history of ICD and the hidden future of DSM

KWM (Bill) Fulford and Norman Sartorius

Abstract

This chapter describes a key, but largely forgotten, episode in the early development of the *International Classification of Diseases* (ICD) and the *Diagnostic and Statistical Manual* (DSM) as descriptive (symptom-based) classifications of mental disorders. The received history has been that ICD-8 and its associated glossary, as the first firmly symptom-based classification, was based on a report to the WHO in the early 1960s by the British psychiatrist, Erwin Stengel, which was in turn based on a Logical Empiricist analysis of psychiatric classification developed by the American philosopher of science, Carl Hempel. Direct examination of the papers from this period, however, shows that although Hempel and Stengel were indeed highly influential, we owe the key move from earlier theoretical (aetiological) to descriptive (symptom-based) classifications to the British psychiatrist, Sir Aubrey Lewis. The final part of the chapter outlines the significance of this 'secret history' for the future of psychiatric classification as the basis of neuroscientific developments in psychiatric science.

2.1 **Introduction**

The development of modern descriptive (or symptom-based) classifications of mental disorders and the move away from earlier theoretical (or aetiology-based) classifications, has been widely attributed to the British psychiatrist, Erwin Stengel, building on the work of the American philosopher of science, Carl Hempel, in the late 1950s.

   The story has been that Stengel recommended the move to descriptive classification in a report that he prepared for the World Health Organization (WHO) in 1959 (Stengel 1959); and that Stengel based his recommendation, with due acknowledgement, on a paper that had been given by Hempel to a research group convened, under the auspices of the American Psychopathological Association, in New York earlier that year (see, for example, Kendell, 1975, chapter 7; and Sadler *et al.*, 1994, Introduction). Yet, if we go back to the actual documents, to Stengel's report (1959) and to Hempel's paper as it was subsequently published (1961), no such recommendation is to be found. It is true that Stengel, following Hempel, noted the difference between descriptive and theoretical sciences; and that Stengel, again following Hempel, emphasized the potential of operationalism in psychiatric science; but Stengel, still following Hempel, made no recommendation as such for a move to a descriptive classification.

So what really happened? How did we get our present firmly descriptive, atheoretical, and predominantly symptom-based classifications of mental disorders? In this chapter, we reveal the secret history behind the early development of Chapter 8 (the mental disorders section) of the WHO's *International Classification of Diseases* (the ICD); and we outline the significance of this secret history for the future development of psychiatric classification in the context of current revision processes that will lead to new editions both of ICD and of the American Psychiatric Association's *Diagnostic and Statistical Manual* (DSM).

2.2 **The received history**

The received history, then, runs thus. Immediately on its foundation in 1945, the WHO published a 6th revision of the *International List of Causes of Death* (WHO, 1948). This had previously been published by the French Government as the *Manual of the International Statistical Classification of Diseases, Injuries and Causes of Death*. The WHO edition included for the first time, a classification of mental disorders. However, while a large majority of chapters in the new classification, those dealing with bodily disorders, were well received and readily adopted around the world, the psychiatric section proved to be problematic. Eleven years later, it was found to have been adopted only in Finland, Peru, Thailand, and the United Kingdom.

It was in light of these difficulties that the WHO commissioned Stengel to look into what had gone wrong and that the 1959 research group was convened in New York with Hempel as an invited speaker. Hempel was one of the founders (and last great advocate, see later) of the model of science developed by what has become known as the Vienna Circle of philosophers, in the 1930s and 1940s, called logical empiricism. Closely related to positivism, the guiding aim of logical empiricism was to establish a sharp separation between observational or descriptive statements and statements of theory. Stengel was the first respondent to Hempel's paper and Hempel's insights into scientific classification, drawing on the Logical Empiricist separation of descriptive statements and statements of theory, subsequently appeared, with full acknowledgement, in key sections of Stengel's report to the WHO (Stengel, 1959).

ICD-8, as we describe in more detail below, consequently appeared in 1967 (WHO, 1967) and, with the publication of a glossary (WHO, 1974), became the first predominantly symptom-based modern classification of mental disorders (the mental disorders section of ICD-7 was identical to ICD-6). The American Psychiatric Association adopted the ICD-8 nomenclature in its DSM-II (American Psychiatric Association, 1968), abandoning, against much domestic opposition (Kendell, 1975, p. 94), the predominantly psychodynamic–theoretical basis of the original DSM (American Psychiatric Association, 1952). ICD-9, which largely incorporated the ICD-8 glossary, followed in 1978 (WHO, 1978). The DSM-III (American Psychiatric Association, 1980), developed by a task force chaired by Robert Spitzer, introduced clear inclusion and exclusion criteria. Finally, DSM-IV explicitly (American Psychiatric Association, 1994, p.xv), and ICD-10 implicitly (WHO, 1992), under the leaderships respectively of Allen Frances (DSM) and Norman Sartorius (ICD), established overtly evidence-based approaches to refining and modifying the categories in these classifications.

2.3 The gaps in the received history

The received history thus suggests a clear line of descent from the Logical Empiricist separation of descriptive statements and statements of theory in science, through Hempel to Stengel, and from Stengel's report for the WHO to the corresponding shifts in ICD and DSM from theoretical (or aetiology-based) to descriptive (or symptom-based) classifications of mental disorders. But what did Stengel really say? And what did Hempel really say?

2.3.1 Stengel's report to the WHO

Stengel's report, published in 1959, runs to 20 pages. It has much of enduring interest including a detailed comparative review of the many classifications of mental disorders available at the time in different parts of the world (reproduced in a 40-page Appendix). The key passage drawing on Hempel's paper comes in a short section of Stengel's report titled 'Principles of Psychiatric Classification' and subtitled 'General Principles' (Stengel, 1959, pp. 611–612). Stengel opens this section by referring directly to Hempel's 1959 oral presentation of his paper and he gives a synopsis of Hempel's account of scientific classification. 'Description and theoretical systematisation . . .' Stengel says, with clear reference to the logical separation of descriptive statements and statements of theory in logical empiricism, '. . . are two basic functions of . . . classifications.' He continues, 'In medical science there has been a gradual development from a predominantly descriptive, i.e. symptomatological, to a theoretical, i.e. aetiological emphasis.'

At this point in Stengel's report, then, we expect the key recommendation for a shift in psychiatric classification from an aetiological to a descriptive basis. But no such recommendation comes. Instead, Stengel moves directly to an account of the 'difficulties of using objectively verifiable concepts in psychiatry' and of the potential of 'operational definitions' for dealing with such difficulties. Again, we might be expecting Stengel to suggest that operationalism could be applied particularly fruitfully in the development of a descriptive classification. This is, after all, how it has subsequently been applied not only in psychiatric classifications but in diagnostic schedules such as the Present State Examination (PSE) (Wing *et al.*, 1974). But in what follows, Stengel refers not to descriptive but to theoretical science: he writes about the importance of 'the formulation of general principles which would provide a basis for *explanation*, *prediction*, and, in general, scientific *understanding*' (emphases added); and he gives a direct quote from Hempel's paper about a 'good taxonomic system' being based on 'a more or less comprehensive system of *laws*' (emphasis added).

Stengel returns to operationalism a little later in the section, after noting a number of particular difficulties with psychiatric classification. Again, though, there is no recommendation for a shift to descriptive classification. On the contrary, Stengel suggests that, properly understood, 'many of the present nosological concepts (in psychiatry) are (already) operational definitions.' 'Schizophrenia', he continues (anticipating current usage), understood 'as an operational concept, would not be an illness, or a specific reaction type, but an agreed operational definition for certain types of abnormal behaviour.'

What is needed, then, to solve the problems of international classification of mental disorders, Stengel continues, is not a change in the basis of the classifications of the day, but a change in how those classifications are understood. Stengel puts it thus: 'The question, therefore, which a person or group of persons trying to reach agreement on a national or international classification ought to answer is not what schizophrenia or psychopathy is, but what *interpretation* should be placed on these concepts for the purposes of diagnosis and classification . . . ' (p. 612, column 2, emphasis added). Stengel acknowledges that many psychiatrists, wedded to the idea that 'our diagnostic concepts stand for biological realities' will find this 'frankly practical and utilitarian attitude' difficult to accept. But he argues that it is entirely consistent with the approach taken in practice by one of the founders of current psychiatric diagnostic concepts, Emil Kraepelin. 'It is most unlikely', he concludes, 'that Kraepelin himself would have disagreed with the recent statement . . . that his [Kraepelin's] groups of clinical pictures are no more than conventions'; and he quotes Kraepelin as saying that '. . . "some of the clinical pictures outlined (by him) are no more than attempts at presenting part of the material observed in communicable form".'

As a rough audit of this section of Stengel's report to the WHO, then, we can say that Stengel draws appropriately on the distinction between description and theory outlined by Hempel; and that he agrees with Hempel that operationalism may be helpful. But he makes no recommendation for a move from a theoretical to a descriptive classification. Rather, he suggests that operationalism may be helpful in developing the theory underpinning psychiatry; and that, properly understood, many of the then current psychiatric diagnostic concepts were in fact already operational in form. Stengel consolidates his position in the final section of his report, when he returns to the 'Requirements of an International Classification of Mental Disorders' (pp. 618–620), by emphasizing that 'No psychiatric classification can help being partly aetiological and partly symptomatological, because these are the criteria by which psychiatrists distinguish mental disorders from each other.'

So, did Stengel misunderstand Hempel? What indeed did Hempel himself actually say?

2.3.2 Hempel's paper to the 1959 research meeting

Like Stengel's report, Hempel's paper is scholarly and detailed and we cannot do full justice to it here. It contains many insights that are directly relevant to the problems facing psychiatric classification today – we return to one of these insights (about the limits of operationalism) in the final part of this chapter.

The distinction between descriptive statements and statements of theory to which Stengel refers, is introduced early on (Hempel, p. 317[1]). Drawing directly on logical

---

[1] Page numbers refer to Hempel's paper as reproduced in full in an appendix to Sadler *et al.*, 1994.

empiricism, Hempel notes that 'the vocabulary of science has two basic functions: first, to permit an adequate description of the things and events that are the objects of scientific investigation; second, to permit the establishment of general laws or theories by means of which particular events may be *explained* and *predicted* and thus *scientifically understood*' (emphases in original). Stengel's terminology in the corresponding section of his report (noted above), thus repeats Hempel's almost word for word.

Stengel's debt to Hempel is evident, too, in the passage that immediately follows on the progression of sciences from descriptive to theoretical stages. The passage runs thus: '. . . granting some over simplification, the development of a scientific discipline may often be said to proceed from an initial . . . stage, which seeks to describe the phenomena under study and to establish simple empirical generalisations concerning them, to subsequent and more theoretical stages, in which increasing emphasis is placed upon the attainment of comprehensive theoretical accounts of the empirical subject matter under investigation' (Hempel, p. 318). Hempel goes on to give examples of theoretical terms in physics (electric and magnetic fields) and chemistry (valencies): these are theoretical terms in the sense that they refer to entities that have explanatory force but '. . . are more or less removed from the level of directly observable things and events.' Similarly in medical science, then, we have moved from the description of symptoms to a search for underlying causes (aetiology), broadly understood as '. . . a search for explanatory laws and theories . . . ' (Hempel, p. 318).

As with Stengel's report, then, the received history leads us to expect something at this point from Hempel about psychiatric classifications having got into difficulties because, essentially, they have moved too quickly from a descriptive to a theoretical stage, that is in the absence of an adequate (or at any rate agreed) underlying theory. But it is not so. Again, as faithfully reflected by Stengel, Hempel goes on more or less immediately to give, with apparent endorsement, examples of theoretical terms derived from psychodynamic theory as they appear in the then current (1952) edition of the DSM. The DSM, he notes by way of example, '. . . characterizes the concept of conversion reaction as ". . . the impulse causing the anxiety is 'converted' into functional symptoms . . . (which) . . . serve to lessen conscious (felt) anxiety and ordinarily are symbolic of the underlying conflict."' Clearly, Hempel concludes, 'the terms used in this passage refer . . . to theoretically assumed psychodynamic factors' (Hempel, p. 318).

In the next section of Hempel's paper, he introduces the concept of operationalism. Initially, this looks more promising. Thus, Hempel opens this section by noting that 'Science aims at knowledge that is *objective* in the sense of being inter-subjectively certifiable . . . [and] . . . This requires that the terms used in formulating scientific statements have clearly specified meanings . . . ' (p. 318, emphasis in original). He continues, 'One of the main objections to various types of contemporary psychodynamic theories . . . is that their central concepts lack clear and uniform criteria of application . . . ' It is here, he suggests, that the use of operational definitions, as introduced originally by the physicist P.W. Bridgman (1927), may be helpful. An operational definition, he explains, specifies an operational test; and he gives an example from mineralogy: an operational definition of 'x is harder than y', he says, could be that '. . . the operation of drawing a sharp point of x under pressure across a smooth surface of y has as its outcome a scratch of y, whereas y does not thus scratch x.' (p. 319).

Initially, then, the scene looks set for a recommendation to abandon, if not psychiatric theory as a whole, at least psychodynamic theory as a basis for psychiatric classification. Again, though, this is not the line that Hempel actually takes. True, he contrasts certain psychiatric diagnostic terms, such as 'praecox feeling', adversely with 'most diagnostic procedures used in medicine . . . ': the former is not, while the latter generally are, '. . . based on operational criteria . . . ' (p. 319). But the praecox feeling is not, uniquely, a term of psychodynamic theory. Further, Hempel then goes on to argue that a somewhat relaxed form of operationalism, one which allows 'mere observation' (p. 320) to have the status of an operational test, may have wide application in the social and psychological sciences.

Hempel, therefore, appears to be at the very least neutral on the question of whether psychodynamic theory is an appropriate theory on which to base a scientific classification of mental disorders. The point of applying operationalism to psychiatric classifications would not be to shift the basis of those classifications from theory to description, but rather to improve the objectivity (and hence scientific quality) of the theoretical statements, whether psychodynamic or neuroscientific, in terms of which the classifications themselves were couched. Towards the end of his paper, when Hempel, like Stengel, turns to the future of psychiatric classifications, this is indeed what he says. He starts by noting that 'It is not for me [Hempel] to speculate on the direction that theoretical developments in this field may take and especially whether the major theories will be couched in biophysiological or biochemical terms or rather in psychodynamic terms lacking in overall physiological or physiochemical interpretation.' Nonetheless, he continues 'Theoretical systems of *either kind* can satisfy the basic requirements for scientific theories' (p. 327, emphasis added).

2.4 **The secret history**

Nowhere then, either in Stengel's report to the WHO or in Hempel's paper on which he draws, is there a clear recommendation for a move from a theoretical (aetiology-based) to a descriptive (symptom-based) classification of mental disorders. Like an unfinished jigsaw, the pieces are all there – the distinction between description and theory, the progression of science from a descriptive to an increasingly theoretical stage, and the role of operationalism to improve the scientific quality of the relevant terms (whether, in Hempel's view, descriptive or theoretical terms) – but the pieces have not been assembled into the expected picture.

Two questions then arise. Who was it that suggested the move from a theoretical to a descriptive (symptom-based) classification of mental disorders? And how did the symptom-based glossary to ICD-8, as the first firmly descriptive international classification of mental disorders, come to be written?

2.4.1 **Who suggested the move to a descriptive classification?**

The answer to the first question is to be found in the discussion that followed Hempel's paper in the 1959 research meeting in New York. The discussion appeared alongside Hempel's paper when it was originally published (Zubin, 1961). It has generally been omitted from subsequent publications (e.g. as reproduced in the appendix to Sadler *et al.*, 1994). Yet, as we will see, it provides a crucial missing link between Hempel's logical empiricism and ICD-8.

Stengel opens the discussion. He thanks Hempel for his clear account of the issues and notes how important it is '. . . for psychiatrists to take great pains with their conceptual tools' (p. 23[2]). Consistent with the line that he was to take later that year in his report to the WHO, Stengel notes among the points he takes from Hempel's paper: 1) Hempel's prediction that '. . . in the taxonomy of mental disorders the conceptual basis will be increasingly determined by theoretical considerations' (p. 25), albeit 2) with a greater degree of agreement on the meanings of key classificatory terms, arrived at 3) through making explicit their true nature as operational definitions. Further interventions follow, raising, as is the way with such meetings, a number of individually important but largely unconnected issues, many of which resonate with current debates: the role of statistical analysis; the political aspects of classification; the practical problems raised by changing our classificatory concepts; resistance to philosophers and others from outside psychiatry telling psychiatrists what to do; differences between the needs of researchers and of clinicians in the field; and hopes for a future '. . . understanding of psychiatric maladies (at) a molecular level' (Dr Burdock, p. 32). But at no point is there a suggestion of the need for a move from a theoretical to a descriptive basis for psychiatric classification.

Then, from left field as it were, comes the key intervention. Hempel has just entered the discussion to develop, in response to an earlier point, a distinction he had noted briefly in his paper, between what he had called artificial and natural classifications. This prompts the first (and only) intervention from one 'Dr Lewis' (p. 34). Rather than artificial and natural classifications, Lewis suggests, '. . . we might properly distinguish between public classifications and private classifications.' 'Public classifications', Lewis continues, presumably with the ICD in mind, 'are the kind that are most valuable for epidemiological work, since we need to make comparisons of findings in different countries, and unless there is uniformity of usage, that is impractical.' Private classifications, by contrast, may be used by particular groups (including particular research groups, presumably) who have, '. . . a uniform background . . . and have agreed among themselves as to the usage of the [relevant classificatory] terms.' Lewis concludes:

> Therefore I would suggest that for the purpose of public classification we should eschew categories based on theoretical concepts and restrict ourselves to the operational, descriptive type of classification, whereas, for the purposes of certain groups, the private classification, based on a theory which seems a workable, profitable one, may be very appropriate.
>
> (Lewis, p. 34)

So, finally we have it. A clear suggestion that for the WHO's purposes of international comparative epidemiological statistics, psychiatric classification should, to repeat Lewis' words, 'eschew categories based on theoretical concepts' and be restricted to the 'descriptive type of classification.' This is an extraordinary intervention. We should expect no less, perhaps: the 'Dr Lewis' in question went on to become Professor Sir Aubrey Lewis as Head of the 'Maudsley School'. Lewis' intervention, moreover, did not come out of the blue. The distinction between descriptive and theoretical classifications, although presented particularly clearly by Hempel, had been discussed by others at

---

[2] Page references in this section are all to Zubin, 1961.

the time: Stengel, for example, notes among the classifications that he included in his review, one by Lecomte *et al.* (1947) that 'represents [an] attempt at classifying along two axes, i.e. the clinical and the aetiological' (Stengel, 1959, p. 615). All the same, Lewis' intervention is remarkable. In three short paragraphs, 1) he pinpoints the key Logical Empiricist distinction outlined by Hempel between theoretical and descriptive terms; but 2) he reverses the way both Hempel and Stengel applied the distinction; and 3) he suggests, cutting right across the discussion as a whole, the key move to a descriptive basis for ICD.

There was no applause! On the contrary, Lewis' suggestion was largely ignored, the focus of the discussion immediately shifting to a long exploration of the role of ostensive definition. Lewis' intervention is referred to favourably by one or two speakers later on in the discussion, notably Dr Pichot (p. 36/37: Pichot subsequently became highly influential in the development of French psychiatry), and, briefly, in the Chair's summing up (Dr Reid, p. 49). But the discussion in the remainder of the session is largely taken up with the advantages/disadvantages of mixed classifications, that is, of classifications combining in different ways, elements of description, aetiology, prognosis, and response to therapy. Lewis' suggestion is not referred to at all in a subsequently written summary (Dr Clausen, p. 50).

2.4.2 How did the glossary to ICD-8 come to be written?

Lewis's views did not go unnoticed in the WHO, however, and he went on to play a key role in the development of ICD-8 and its associated glossary, as the first firmly symptom-based classification of mental disorders.

What happened was this. In 1965, WHO launched a programme in psychiatric epidemiology led by Dr Tsung-yi Lin, a Taiwanese psychiatrist, a key component of which (its Programme A) dealt with the improvement of psychiatric diagnosis and classification (Lin, 1967; Sartorius, 1976; Cooper, 1999). The programme started by creating a 'nuclear group' of leading specialists in psychiatry, statistics, and public health from different countries, one of the members of which was Sir Aubrey Lewis.[3] The nuclear group met once every year, each time in a different country. At each meeting, specialists from that country were invited to meet with the nuclear group and to work with them on the classification of a major group of mental disorders. Most of the discussions were introduced by the presentation of case histories or video tape interviews (Sartorius, 1989). The results of these discussions, most of which were published (see, for example, Shepherd *et al.*, 1968), were used in developing the Eighth Revision of the chapter on mental disorder in the ICD.

The need for a glossary of terms used in the classification and description of cases was noted in several of the discussions of the nuclear group. Sir Aubrey Lewis was invited to Geneva to help in the development and production of the glossary, the first draft of which he produced in 1967. This was sent for comment to the members of the nuclear group mentioned above and to a number of other experts. A working party then met in

---

[3] Other members of the nuclear group were Eileen Brooke and M. Shepherd (UK); R. Sadoun (France); A.V. Sheznevski and Z. Serebrjakova (USSR); E. Gruenberg, M. Kramer, and J. Ewalt (USA); M. Kato (Japan); H. Rotondo (Peru); H. Strotzka (Austria); and G. Odegard (Norway).

Geneva in 1969 to consider the glossary and the comments received from the experts. Their recommendations guided the revision of the draft which was then brought to a meeting in London, chaired by Sir Aubrey Lewis and involving several members of the nuclear group as well as some other advisors – notably Professor Essen-Moller, whom Sir Aubrey particularly wanted to invite. That draft was then sent to numerous people in different countries to establish whether the definitions were easy to apply and whether they covered most of the conditions met in practice. The comments received were incorporated in the next draft, this time examined by a lexicologist (Mr Nicole) and finalized by Professor J.E. Cooper. One more review was done in London in 1972 and then the glossary was presented at the 8th meeting of the nuclear group in Geneva. It met with general satisfaction. Several annexes were added to it and then the glossary was made ready for publication by Professor Cooper who added an introductory section and notes for users of the glossary as it was finally published in 1974. It was from this glossary, as described earlier, that current descriptive international classifications of mental disorder, the ICD and DSM, are ultimately derived.

2.5 **The hidden future**

When symptom-based classifications of mental disorder first appeared, they were warmly welcomed. Chapter 5 of ICD-9, unlike its predecessors, was readily adopted by nearly all member states of the WHO (the corresponding chapter of ICD-6, as we noted earlier, was adopted in only four countries). During the 1960s and 1970s, indeed, there was a positive explosion of research aimed at operationalizing the descriptive basis of key psychiatric diagnostic concepts: the Philadelphia Study (Beck et al., 1962), the US–UK Diagnostic Project (Cooper et al., 1972), the subsequent International Pilot Study of Schizophrenia (WHO, 1973), and the PSE (Wing et al., 1974), are just a few of the classic publications that emerged from this period. Improved reliability, furthermore, was embraced not only by psychiatrists but by the wider public as the key to scientific advance: a 1963 article in the New York Post described the early research at Columbia University of Robert Spitzer, who was to go on to chair the DSM-III Task Force, as developing 'a tool that may become the psychiatrist's thermometer and microscope and X-ray machine rolled in to one.' (Spitzer, 1983).

Yet, over the years doubts have increasingly set in. Clinicians began to find many of the categories hard to apply: well-defined inclusion and exclusion criteria, for example, introduced in the DSM-III, appropriate as they might be in a research context and for improving the comparability of statistical information, seemed often artificially restrictive when applied in day-to-day clinical care. Many patients, similarly, resented what they felt were artificial and imposed labels that failed to capture what was important to them as individuals in their particular circumstances. Recently, indeed, echoing the extreme anti-psychiatric views of the 1960s and 1970s, some have come to reject psychiatric diagnosis as a whole (Kutchins and Kirk, 1997). Worse still, with the rise of the new neurosciences in the 1990s, researchers themselves, for whom a scientific classification of mental disorders might be thought to be most apt, have expressed increasing dissatisfaction (Hyman, 2002; Andreasen, 2007). The American psychiatrists, David Kupfer, Michael First, and Darrel Regier, make the point bluntly in their introduction to the American Psychiatric Association's authoritative edited collection, *A Research Agenda for DSM-V*, which was published in 2002 in anticipation of the launch of the DSM revision process. 'In the more than 30 years', they write, 'since the introduction of the Feighner criteria by Robins and Guze, which eventually led to DSM-III, the goal of validating these syndromes and discovering common etiologies has remained elusive. Despite many proposed candidates, not one laboratory marker has been found to be specific in identifying any of the DSM-defined syndromes.' (Kupfer *et al.*, 2002, p. xviii).

In this final part of the chapter, then, we will be considering the significance of the secret history of ICD outlined above for current concerns about psychiatric classification. Our aim will not be to consider particular concerns in detail. Rather, we will be indicating the importance of the secret history for three general issues underpinning many of these particular concerns. The three general issues can be characterized as: 1) big ideas, big trouble; 2) guarding the gate of observation; and 3) a third limit of operationalism.

2.5.1 Big ideas, big trouble

Many of the concerns among different stakeholders in psychiatric classification about current editions of both ICD and DSM, arise not from the principle of symptom-based classification being wrong, but from such classifications being used for purposes for which they were not originally intended.

Recall, here, Lewis' very clear comments in this respect: it was, he said, specifically for the purpose of *public* classifications that descriptive (symptom-based) classifications were appropriate. What Lewis had in mind, then, and what WHO had in mind in publishing ICD-8, was a classification that could be used to improve the comparability of statistical information about rates of mental disorders between different parts of the world. Yet ICD, and then DSM, have increasingly been used for purposes well beyond this original well-defined focus. The ICD is used in many countries for administrative purposes, for example, including determining access to clinical care. DSM, similarly, has been used in legal proceedings (a use specifically proscribed by DSM itself (American Psychiatric Association, 1994, p. xvii)). Moreover, and in stark contrast with Lewis' suggestion that there was a need for 'private classifications' for particular groups, including therefore particular research groups, the DSM, a victim of its own success in this respect, has become the gold standard for research of all kinds and in most parts of the world (Kuper *et al.*, 2002, p. 15).

The ever-widening use of descriptive classifications beyond their originally intended purpose is an example of what the psychiatrist and historian, Paul Hoff, has called psychiatry's tendency to succumb to one or another 'single message mythology' (Hoff, 2005). We start out, that is to say, with a perfectly good idea and then run into trouble by trying to make it into the 'big idea', a cure-all. What is needed, then, to return to Lewis' original suggestion, is not to abandon symptom-based classifications but to limit their use to the purposes for which they are appropriate while at the same time recognizing that *other* classifications (Lewis' 'private classifications') will be needed for *other* purposes. Encouragingly, there have been developments in this direction already: WHO has been developing a family of classifications including, for example, a classification for use in primary care (WHO, 2003) which has been translated into many languages, and a classification of functioning (WHO, 2001). The ICD itself has a multi-axial presentation (WHO, 1997) that includes an axis for environmental circumstances likely to be clinically significant. The DSM, similarly, has a number of axes (structured differently from those of ICD) that include along with Axis I (its symptom-based categories), a 'global assessment of functioning' (Axis V).

A natural objection to this approach – of adopting different classifications for different purposes – is that it might seem somehow 'unscientific'. How, it may be said, can a scientific classification properly reflect our purposes rather than the objective world 'out there'? After all, there is only one 'Periodic Table' in chemistry. This objection, however, reflects a misunderstanding of the nature of science. 'A classification' as one of us has put it elsewhere, 'is a way of seeing the world at a point in time' (Sartorius, 1992, p. vii). Hence, while a single classification (a single way of seeing the world) may be appropriate for certain sciences at certain times (as with the chemical Periodic Table), in other sciences at other times, more than one classification (more than one way of seeing the world) may be needed. A headline example of such a science at the present time is physics, traditionally the hardest of the hard sciences, and a science, surely, at the cutting edge. Yet, physics has had, since the early twentieth century, two entirely different, and indeed mathematically incompatible, ways of seeing the world – relativity (as a theory of the very large) and quantum mechanics (as a theory of the very small). The need, then, for more than one way of seeing the world scientifically, and hence for more than one classification, arises not from the discipline in question being unscientific, but rather from it being, like physics, a science at the cutting edge (Fulford *et al.*, 2006, chapter 1). We return to the significance of the parallels in this respect between psychiatry and physics later in the chapter.

2.5.2. Guarding the gate of observation

In the preface to ICD-9, Lewis, now recognized (in 1978) as a world leader in the field of psychiatric classification, welcomes the move to symptom-based categories as putting psychiatric science on a firmly observational basis. He warns, though, against psychiatry resting on its observational laurels. 'It would seem', he says, '. . . that accurate observation is still the gate that needs the closest guard.' (WHO, 1978, p. 5).

The importance of Lewis' warning is evident in current debates in, of all places, the American Psychiatric Association's *A Research Agenda for DSM-V*. The *Research Agenda*, as we noted earlier, provides an authoritative review of the range of empirical research topics that have an important bearing on the DSM revision process. Yet, in their introduction, the editors of the *Research Agenda*, Kupfer, First, and Regier, in calling for greater attention to validity, come close to abandoning the basis of observation in reliability. 'The major advantage', they argue (p. xviii), 'of adopting a descriptive classification was its improved reliability over prior classifications based on unproved aetiological assumptions.' So far, so good. But, they continue, 'From the outset, however, it was recognized that the primary strength of a descriptive approach was its ability to improve communication among clinicians and researchers, *not its established validity*' (p. xviii, emphasis added). We should be clear here. Kupfer, First, and Regier emphasize later on 'the value of having a well-described, well-operationalized . . . '

diagnostic system (p. xix). But it would be perilously easy, as Lewis' warning reminds us, to take from their contrast between reliability and validity, the implication that earlier gains in reliability had been achieved at the expense of validity.

It would be perilously easy, too, to take the same implication from Hempel's paper. As we noted earlier, Hempel had a good deal to say about operationalism as a way of improving the scientific usefulness of psychiatric concepts. Reliability, by contrast, is passed over relatively quickly. Hempel, moreover, as we saw, recommends operationalism equally for theoretical statements (hence validity) as for descriptive statements. Closer inspection of Hempel's paper, however, shows that as the *Oxford Textbook of Philosophy and Psychiatry* puts it, when it comes to the observational basis of science, '. . . operationalism gets the credit but reliability does the work' (Fulford *et al.*, 2006, p. 337). That it is reliability that does the work becomes clear when we look in detail at the more relaxed model of operationalism that Hempel says is needed if the approach is to be successfully transferred from physics to psychiatry. Thus, the required relaxation of operationalism, as we noted earlier, is that 'mere observation' has to be allowed to count as an operational test. Hempel (1961, p. 10, Zubin edition) gives the example of 'endomorphy'. The criteria for endomorphy, Hempel says, although observational rather than operational criteria (in the sense defined originally by Bridgman), are capable of being used with 'high *inter-subjective* uniformity' (emphasis added). But Hempel's 'high inter-subjective uniformity' is, no more and no less, reliability (specifically, inter-observer reliability). So, it is not operationalism as such that is doing the work of putting psychiatry on a firm observational footing, according to Hempel's own account. Rather, operationalism, and a relaxed operationalism at that, is being used to improve the *reliability* of psychiatric assessment.

Clearly, this is not a 'knock down' argument for the importance of reliability in guarding Lewis' gate of observation. Certainly, we should be careful here, for reliability, according to Hempel's Logical Empiricist model, is a stepping stone to validity: and, importantly in this respect, remember that Hempel advocated operationalism as a way of improving the scientific quality not only of descriptive but also of theoretical terms in psychiatry, that is, of just those terms that would be required for the improved validity to which Kupfer, First, and Regier (rightly) aspire. Logical empiricism, however, is not the last word as a model of science. Indeed, logical empiricism ultimately failed in its core aim of providing a sharp separation between descriptive statements and statements of theory, and this in turn has opened up a new and perhaps more sophisticated model of science that is highly relevant to the challenges facing psychiatric science (Fulford *et al.*, 2006, chapter 13, Part IV). This more sophisticated model includes work in the philosophy of science, drawing like Hempel's work particularly on physics, into the nature of validity (Fine, 1999). It also includes insights relevant to the translation of the results of scientific research into practice: work on clinical judgement, for example (Thornton, 2007, pp. 203–229); and on the particular and often surprising ways in which mental disorders are experienced by those concerned (Stanghellini, 2004).

So, while reliability is important, or at any rate not to be lightly thrown aside, there is more to guarding the gate of observation than reliability alone. Which is not to say that logical empiricism has nothing useful to offer. On the contrary, logical empiricism,

THE HIDDEN FUTURE | 41

particularly as applied by Hempel to psychiatric classification, remains a rich resource of lessons for psychiatric science. It is to one of these, to Hempel's account of the limitations of operationalism, that we turn next.

2.5.3 A third limit of operationalism

In his paper presented at the 1959 research meeting, Hempel, while advocating the use of operationalism in psychiatry, also pointed out three important limitations of the approach. Two of these are well recognized: the first is the limitation of 'mere observation' noted above; the second is the limitation of 'partial criteria application', that is, that any given operational definition can cover only a limited part of the range of any particular variable (we need different kinds of thermometers for different ranges of temperature, for example).

Hempel's third limitation of operationalism is less well known but perhaps even more fundamental to the application of operationalism in psychiatry. This limitation is what may be called the limitation of 'antecedently understood terms'. Hempel makes the point with his usual clarity. Immediately after his illustration (noted above) of the application of operationalism to endomorphy, and the need for 'high inter-subjective uniformity' (i.e. reliability) in the terms used for its specification, he continues: 'It would be unreasonable to demand, however, that all of the terms used in a given scientific discipline be given an operational specification of meaning, for then the process of specifying the meanings of the defining terms, and so forth, would lead to an infinite regress.' Hempel goes on to note that the need for antecedently understood terms is a feature of all definitions, not just of operational definitions. He gives no actual examples here but his earlier illustration of 'harder than' makes the point. His definition (as above) includes the terms 'sharp', 'point', 'pressure', 'smooth', and 'scratch', the meanings of which must already be understood (i.e. antecedently understood) if the operational test of 'harder than' is itself to be understood, and, hence, used with the (scientifically requisite) high inter-subjective uniformity (reliability) in practice.

Hempel is pressed on this third limitation of operationalism in the discussion and it is here that some of the cracks in logical empiricism, and the corresponding need for a more sophisticated understanding of the nature of science, begin to appear. Thus, Dr Gruenberg (p. 34) asks Hempel to explain how the non-operationally defined terms on which operational definitions depend are themselves defined, and what role such non-operational terms have in a scientific classification. Hempel replies by talking about ostension (i.e. learning the meaning of 'green', for example, by '. . . indicating various green objects', p. 35). He acknowledges that ostension might seem to involve a shift away from the objectivity to which science aspires. 'Fortunately for the objectives of science', however, he concludes, 'there is a vast array of terms which in these non-definitional ways we learn to use with high individual consistency and interpersonal uniformity; these terms may then be chosen as antecedently understood and may serve as a basis for specifying the meaning of scientific terms by actual definitions.' (p. 35, emphasis added.)

Here are the cracks, then. First, Hempel's answer begs the question. It is true, as he suggests, that for many operational definitions, the required antecedently understood terms show a high degree of uniformity of usage in practice. Thus, in his example of 'harder than', the required antecedently understood terms – 'sharp', 'point', 'pressure', 'smooth', and 'scratch', as above – generally show a sufficiently high degree of uniformity of usage not to cause difficulties in applying the operational test in practice. But this is precisely the point that lies behind Dr Gruenberg's question. Dr Gruenberg accepts Hempel's reassurances. But he should not have done. For Hempel's answer amounts to agreeing with Dr Gruenberg that, in practice, operational definitions only produce a high degree of uniformity of usage (reliability) because they employ non-operationally defined terms which, despite being non-operationally defined, themselves already show a high degree of uniformity of usage (reliability). WHO, indeed, aware of the potential criticism that operational definitions use terms that are not defined, has produced a series of glossaries – of psychiatric symptoms, of terms used in cross-cultural psychiatry, and of terms used in substance abuse – that have been translated into a number of languages (WHO, 1994), as well as many instruments for the assessment of such mental health variables as the clinical state, the level of disability and of personality disorder (Sartorius and Janca, 1996). All of which, as our repeated bracketed references to the equivalence between Hempel's 'high inter-subjective uniformity of usage' and 'reliability' are intended to indicate, underlines the point made in the last section, that, insofar as Hempel's account of the observational basis of science goes, while operationalism gets the credit, it is indeed reliability that is doing the work.

This may seem a somewhat theoretical 'crack' from the perspective of psychiatry. Hanging on to reliability, it may be agreed, is important if we are to guard Lewis' 'gate of observation': but that point has already been made. There is, though, a second and more fundamental crack in logical empiricism that is opened up by Hempel's response, a crack that leads directly to psychiatry's need for the more sophisticated model of science to which the failure of logical empiricism has led.

The second crack is this: it is simply not the case, as Hempel suggests, that the antecedently understood terms required by operational definitions are always in practice used with a high uniformity of usage. Again, physics, from which as we have several times noted operationalism is derived, and to which Hempel repeatedly turns for examples, is a case in point. In many areas of physics, the antecedently understood terms are indeed unproblematic. In mineralogy, no doubt, the operational definition of 'harder than' suggested by Hempel would be acceptable, because, or to the extent that, the required antecedently understood terms 'sharp', 'point', 'pressure', 'smooth', and 'scratch', are unproblematic. But if we move to the cutting edge of physics, to relativity and quantum mechanics, it is the antecedent terms themselves that are at the heart of the relevant research questions. Einstein employed what amount to (virtual) operational definitions of time and space (clocks and measuring rods, respectively) in developing the Special Theory of Relativity, not for purposes of improving the uniformity of usage (reliability) of these concepts, but in order to derive wholly new ways of understanding their meanings. Far from being antecedently understood, then, it was new understandings of the meanings of the terms 'time' and 'space' that led to the Special Theory of Relativity. Again, the failure of (mathematical) fit between relativity and quantum mechanics (noted above), arises, in part but importantly, from the very different (and incompatible) ways in which the concept of time is understood in the two theories. Indeed, quantum mechanics itself has generated a whole series of different (and highly contested) ways of understanding normally taken-for-granted antecedent terms such as 'object', 'event', and 'location' (d'Espagnat, 1976).

Such is the nature, then, of a science at the cutting edge: the research questions in such a science are questions as much about concepts as about data. And so it is with psychiatry. As one of us has described in detail elsewhere (Fulford and Sadler, forthcoming), the important advances achieved in the reliability of psychiatric diagnostic terms in the 1960s and 1970s, depended on an entirely *appropriate* use of operational definitions in Hempel's (relaxed) sense: and the apparent disillusionment with reliability (as reflected in the American Psychiatric Association's Research Agenda, above), reflects a corresponding failure to recognize that the same approach, the approach of using operationally defined terms, is equally *in*appropriate for tackling the problems (which are problems essentially of validity) raised by the antecedent terms (again, in Hempel's sense) on which our operational definitions depend. For example, the various particular kinds of delusion defined operationally in the PSE, show a high degree of Hempel's 'uniformity of usage', that is, of reliability (Wing *et al.*, 1974, chapter 5). But the antecedent terms on which these operational definitions depend have resisted operational definition: the definition of 'delusion' itself remains stubbornly elusive (Garety and Freeman, 1999). Similarly, further up Hempel's 'infinite regress' of definition as it were, are the equally elusive concepts of 'insight' (a concept that Lewis himself had trouble with, Lewis, 1934; see also, Amador and David, 2004) and 'psychosis' (Fulford, 1989, chapter 10). And the top concept of all, 'mental disorder' itself, as the authors of the DSM found (American Psychiatric Association, 1994, pp. xxi and xxii), has proved highly resistant to agreed, let alone operationally agreed, definition (Rounsaville *et al.*, 2002, pp. 2–7).

The difficulties of defining mental disorder, which bear a number of very different interpretations (Fulford, 2003), have been the basis through much of the twentieth century of deeply stigmatizing attitudes towards psychiatric science: 'They can't even say what mental disorder is!', we can hear someone say, contrasting the DSM's attempt to define mental disorder (American Psychiatric Association, 1994, pp. xxi and xxii) with the absence of any such attempt to define, say, 'cardiological disorder' in cardiological classifications. These attitudes, in turn, have been deeply prejudicial to psychiatry's effectiveness as a clinical discipline (Sartorius, 2004). Yet, the many parallels between psychiatry and physics noted above show that such attitudes are scientifically naïve. Cardiology is in this respect no more 'scientific' than psychiatry. It is rather that where cardiology is (scientifically) similar to mineralogy (as in Hempel's example of 'harder than') in the research questions with which it is concerned, psychiatry is (scientifically) closer to physics, and hence, like physics, in need of sharp conceptual tools alongside and as a full partner to rigorous empirical methods in its research paradigms.

Again, there are encouraging signs of developments along these lines: the American Psychiatric Association's Research Agenda, for example, although very much an agenda for empirical research, includes an extensive discussion of the conceptual problems facing psychiatric classification (Kupfer *et al.*, 2002, Introduction); there are rich methodological resources for conceptual research in the rapidly expanding philosophy of psychiatry (Fulford *et al.*, 2003, chapter 1); and there have been influential voices, particularly within the neurosciences, arguing the need for conceptual as well as empirical research in psychiatry (Andreasen, 2001; Kendler *et al.*, 2008). Such developments could play a key role in helping us to move past the still all too widespread stigmatizing attitudes of the twentieth century and to recognize psychiatry's proper place as a science, like physics, at the cutting edge.

2.6 **Conclusions**

In this chapter, we have described the secret history behind the early development of ICD. Contrary to the received history, there was no direct line of descent from Hempel's logical empiricism through Stengel's report to the WHO and from there to our current descriptive classifications. The Logical Empiricist distinction between descriptive statements and statements of theory was indeed influential. But it took the critical intervention of Aubrey Lewis, subsequently supported by the WHO, to achieve the clear shift from earlier theoretical (aetiological) to the descriptive (symptom-based) classifications that we have today.

This secret history, we have further argued, has important lessons for the future of psychiatric classification as one of the foundations of psychiatric science: it shows the need for a family of classifications adapted for different purposes rather than one dominant all-purpose classification; it reinforces the importance for psychiatry as an observational science, of building on rather than rejecting the gains in reliability achieved in recent decades by focusing on the symptoms of mental disorder; and it leads to an understanding of the nature of psychiatry as a science like physics at the cutting edge, and hence, like physics, in need of sharp conceptual thinking alongside, and as a partner to, rigorous empirical methods. This last point as we have indicated is given particular urgency by recent dramatic developments in the neurosciences.

In the Preface to the American Psychiatric Association's (2002) *Research Agenda for DSM-V*, to which we have referred several times, the editors, David Kupfer, Michael First, and Darrel Regier, call for a 'new paradigm' the nature of which, they say, is '. . . still undiscovered'. It is as a contribution to revealing the hidden future of that still undiscovered paradigm that the lessons to be taken from the secret history of ICD may prove to be important.

Acknowledgements

Some of the historical materials on which this chapter is based were published originally in chapter 13, Part I, of *The Oxford Textbook of Philosophy and Psychiatry*. We are grateful to Fulford's co-authors of that volume, Tim Thornton and George Graham, for permission to use them here. Our thanks go also to Giovanni Stanghellini for pointing out the quote from the *New York Post* about Robert Spitzer's early research.

References

Amador, X. F. and David, A. S. (eds.) (2004). *Insight and Psychosis*. Oxford, Oxford University Press.

American Psychiatric Association (1952). *Diagnostic and Statistical Manual of Mental Disorders* (first edition, DSM-I). Washington, DC, American Psychiatric Association.

American Psychiatric Association (1968). *Diagnostic and Statistical Manual of Mental Disorders* (second edition, DSM-II). Washington, DC, American Psychiatric Association.

American Psychiatric Association (1980). *Diagnostic and Statistical Manual of Mental Disorders* (third edition, DSM-III). Washington, DC, American Psychiatric Association.

American Psychiatric Association (1994). *Diagnostic and Statistical Manual of Mental Disorders* (fourth edition, DSM-IV). Washington, DC, American Psychiatric Association.

Andreasen, N. C. (2001). *Brave New Brain: Conquering Mental Illness in the Era of the Genome*. Oxford, Oxford University Press.

Andreasen, N. C. (2007). DSM and the death of phenomenology in America: an example of unintended consequences. *Schizophrenia Bulletin*, **33**(1), 108–112.

Beck, A. T., Ward, C., Mendelson, M., Mock, J., and Erbaugh, J. (1962). Reliability of psychiatric diagnoses: 2. A study of consistency of clinical judgements and ratings. *American Journal of Psychiatry*, **119**, 351–357.

Bridgman, P. W. (1927). *The Logic of Modern Physics*. New York, Macmillan Press.

Cooper, J. E. (1999). Towards a common language for mental health workers. In *Promoting Mental Health Internationally* (eds. G. de Girolamo, L. Eisenburg, D. P. Goldberg, and J. E. Cooper). London, Gaskell.

Cooper, J. E., Kendell, R. E., Gurland, B. J., Sharpe, L., Copeland, J. R. M., and Simon, R. (1972). *Psychiatric Diagnosis in New York and London*. Maudsley Monograph Series No.20. London, Oxford University Press.

d'Espagnat, B. (1976). *Conceptual Foundations of Quantum Mechanics* (second edition). London, W. A. Benjamin Inc.

Fine, A. (1999). The natural ontological attitude. In *The Philosophy of Science* (eds. R. Boyd, P. Gasker, and J. D. Trout), pp. 261–277. Cambridge, MA, MIT Press.

Fulford, K. W. M. (1989, reprinted 1995 and 1999) *Moral Theory and Medical Practice*. Cambridge, Cambridge University Press.

Fulford, K. W. M. (2003). Mental Illness: definition, use and meaning. In *Encyclopedia of Bioethics* (ed. S. G. Post), 3rd edition, pp. 1789–1800. New York, Macmillan.

Fulford, K. W. M. and Sadler, J. Z. (forthcoming) Mapping the logical geography of delusion and spiritual experience: a linguistic-analytic research agenda covering problems, methods and outputs. In *Religious and Spiritual Issues in Psychiatric Diagnosis and Classification* (eds. J. Peteet and F. Lu). Arlington, American Psychiatric Publishing Inc.

Fulford, K. W. M., Morris, K. J., Sadler, J. Z., and Stanghellini, G. (2003). Past improbable, future possible: the renaissance in philosophy and psychiatry. In *Nature and Narrative: An Introduction to the New Philosophy of Psychiatry* (eds. K. W. M. Fulford, K. J. Morris, J. Z. Sadler, and G. Stanghellini), pp. 1–41. Oxford, Oxford University Press.

Fulford, K. W. M., Thornton, T., and Graham, G. (eds.) (2006). *The Oxford Textbook of Philosophy and Psychiatry*. Oxford, Oxford University Press.

Garety, P. A. and Freeman, D. (1999). Cognitive approaches to delusions: a critical review of theories and evidence. *British Journal of Clinical Psychology*, **38**, 113–154.

Hempel, C. G. (1961). Introduction to problems of taxonomy. In *Field Studies in the Mental Disorders* (ed. J. Zubin), pp. 3–22. Grune and Stratton, New York. Reproduced in Sadler, J. Z., Wiggins, O. P., and Schwartz, M. A. (1994). *Philosophical Perspectives on Psychiatric Diagnostic Classification*, pp. 315–331. Baltimore, MD, Johns Hopkins University Press.

Hoff, P. (2005). Die psychopathologische perspektive. In *Ethische Aspekte der Forschung in Psychiatrie und Psychotherapie* (eds. M. Bormuth and U. Wiesing), pp. 71–79. Cologne, Deutscher Aerzte-Verlag.

Hyman, S. E. (2002). Neuroscience, genetics, and the future of psychiatric diagnosis. *Psychopathology*, **35**(2–3), 139–44.

Kendell, R. E. (1975). *The Role of Diagnosis in Psychiatry*. Oxford, Blackwell Scientific Publications.

Kendler, K., Appelbaum, P., Bell, C., *et al.* (2008). Issues for DSM-V: DSM-V should include a conceptual issues work group. *American Journal of Psychiatry*, **165**(2), 1–2.

Kupfer, D. J., First, M. B., and Regier, D. A. (2002). Introduction. In *A Research Agenda for DSM-V* (eds. D. J. Kupfer, M. B. First, and D. A. Regier), p. xv–xxiii. Washington, D.C. American Psychiatric Association.

Lecomte, M., Donney, A., Delage, E., and Marty, F. (1947). *Techniques Hospitalières*, **2**, 5.

Lewis, A. J. (1934). The psychopathology of insight. *British Journal of Medical Psychology*, **14**, 332–348.

Lin, T-Y. (1967). The epidemiological studies of mental disorder. *World Health Organization Chronicle*, **21**, 503–516.

Rounsaville, B. J., Alarcón, R. D., Andrews, G., Jackson, J. S., Kendell, R. E., and Kendler, K. (2002). Basic nomenclature issues for DSM-V. Chapter 1 in *A Research Agenda for DSM-V* (eds. D. J. Kupfer, M. B. First, and D. A. Regier), pp. 1–30. Washington, American Psychiatric Association.

Sadler, J. Z., Wiggins, O. P., and Schwartz, M. A. (eds.) (1994). *Philosophical Perspectives on Psychiatric Diagnostic Classification*. Baltimore, MD, Johns Hopkins University Press.

Sartorius, N. (1976). Classification of mental disorders: an international perspective. *Psychiatric Annals*, **6**, 22–35.

Sartorius, N. (1989). Recent research activities in the WHO's mental health programme. *Psychological Medicine*, **19**, 233–244.

Sartorius, N. (1992). In World Health Organization (1992) *The ICD-10 Classification of Mental and Behavioural Disorders: Clinical Descriptions and Diagnostic Guidelines* p. vii. Geneva, World Health Organization.

Sartorius, N. (2004). Psychiatry and society. *Die Psychiatrie*, **1**, 36–41.

Sartorius, N. and Janca, A. (1996). Psychiatric assessment instruments developed by the WHO. *Social Psychiatry and Psychiatric Epidemiology*, **31**, 55–69.

Shepherd, M., Brooke, E., Cooper J. E., and Lin, T. -Y. (1968). An experimental approach to psychiatric diagnosis. *Acta Psychiatrica Scandinavica*, **42** Supplement 201.

Spitzer, R. L. (1983). Psychiatric diagnosis: are clinicians still necessary? *Comprehensive Psychiatry*, **24**(5), 399–411.

Stanghellini, G. (2004). *Deanimated Bodies and Disembodied Spirits. Essays on the Psychopathology of Common Sense*. Oxford, Oxford University Press.

Stengel, E. (1959). Classification of mental disorders. *Bulletin of the World Health Organization*, **21**, 601–663.

Thornton, T. (2007). *Essential Philosophy of Psychiatry*. Oxford, Oxford University Press.

Wing, J. K., Cooper, J. E., and Sartorius, N. (1974). *Measurement and Classification of Psychiatric Symptoms*. Cambridge, Cambridge University Press.

World Health Organization (1949). *Manual of the International Statistical Classification of Diseases, Injuries, and Causes of Death (ICD-6)*. Geneva, World Health Organization.

World Health Organization (1967). *Manual of the International Statistical Classification of Diseases, Injuries, and Causes of Death (ICD-8)*. World Health Organization, Geneva.

World Health Organization (1973) *The International Pilot Study of Schizophrenia*. Vol. 1. Geneva, World Health Organization.

World Health Organization (1974). *Glossary of Mental Disorders and Guide to their Classification, for Use in Conjunction with the International Classification of Diseases, 8th Revision*. Geneva, World Health Organization.

World Health Organization (1978). *Mental Disorders: Glossary and Guide to Their Classification in Accordance with the Ninth Revision of the International Classification of Diseases*. Geneva, World Health Organization.

World Health Organization (1992). *The ICD-10 Classification of Mental and Behavioural Disorders: Clinical Descriptions and Diagnostic Guidelines*. Geneva, World Health Organization.

World Health Organization (1994). *Lexicon of Psychiatric and Mental Health Terms*. Geneva, World Health Organization.

World Health Organization (1997). *Multiaxial Classification of the ICD-10 for Use in Adult Psychiatry*. Geneva, World Health Organization.

World Health Organization (2001). *International Classification of Functioning, Disability and Health*. Geneva, World Health Organization.

World Health Organization (2003). *International Classification of Primary Care, second edition*, (ICPC-2). Geneva, World Health Organization.

Chapter 3

Delusion as a natural kind

Richard Samuels

Abstract

This chapter clarifies and defends what I call the NK thesis: the thesis
that delusions constitute a *natural kind*. In doing so, I spell out the
relevant notion of a natural kind and show why the most prominent
objections to the NK thesis are unsatisfactory. In addition, I present
some *prima facie* reasons for adopting the NK thesis as a working
hypothesis, and argue that careful reflection on the standard
objections to the thesis provides some insight into the sort of
natural kind that delusions constitute. Roughly put: if the NK thesis
is true, then we have reason to suppose that delusions constitute a
generic, multiply realized, cognitive kind.

3.1 Introduction

Though delusions are widely regarded as a central psychiatric phenomenon, their
nature and ontological status has, since the inception of modern psychopathology,
been the subject of concerted debate (Jaspers, 1914). One important aspect of this
debate concerns whether or not delusions constitute a *natural kind*. Crudely put: are
delusions a scientifically respectable kind in nature in the way that, say, molecules or
quarks appear to be? Or, are they more like days of the week or domestic pets, in being,
in one respect or another, inappropriate for the purposes of scientific enquiry? It is
this issue that I propose to discuss here. In particular, I defend what I will call the *NK
thesis* – the thesis that delusions constitute a natural kind.

Two clarifications are in order. First, I will not be concerned merely with the issue
of whether or not some *sub-types* of delusions are natural kinds. For instance, the issue
is not merely whether Capgras delusion, or persecutory delusions, or any of the myriad
sub-kinds of delusion are natural kinds. Rather, I am interested in the more general
issue of whether delusions *as such* – the entire category – constitute a natural kind.

Second, though the best argument for the existence of a natural kind is to provide
a detailed, well-articulated, and highly confirmed account of the kind in question,
no such account will be provided here. I would be delighted if such a proposal were

available; but contemporary scientific psychopathology affords no such account. Still worse, in recent years, the conception of delusions as a natural kind has been roundly rejected by many theorists, and for many different reasons. The following discussion, then, is largely a defensive one that seeks to clear the ground for the more ambitious project of saying what natural kind delusions are. With this in mind, I argue that the main extant objections to the NK thesis are unsatisfactory. But in addition to this, I develop two more positive lines of thought. First, I argue that there are some *prima facie* reasons for taking the NK thesis seriously. Second, I maintain that a careful consideration of the main arguments, for and against the NK thesis, suggest a range of conditions that delusions need to satisfy if they are to constitute a natural kind. In spelling out these conditions I seek to indicate what are likely to be the most fruitful avenues for future scientific enquiry.

Here is the game plan. In section 3.2, I consider the general issue of what a natural kind is and defend what is sometimes called a *homeostatic cluster* account of natural kinds (Boyd, 1991). The remainder of the chapter interleaves critical assessment of the main objections to the NK thesis with positive morals about how best to develop the thesis. In section 3.3, I consider a first criticism of the NK thesis – the *anti-essentialist objection*. Though widely endorsed, I argue that the objection is misdirected since it attributes to the NK thesis assumptions that it need not – and should not – endorse. Nevertheless, a consideration of this objection yields a range of positive morals, and provides some *prima facie* reason to take the NK thesis seriously. In section 3.4, I outline these morals and reasons. Then in section 3.5, I consider a second kind of objection to the NK thesis, which I call *continuity objections*. Such arguments purport to show that the NK thesis is false because delusions fail to constitute a kind of any sort, natural or otherwise. I argue that whilst these objections show something interesting – roughly, that delusions exhibit various kinds of symptomatic continuity with other phenomena – they fail to show delusions are not a natural kind because these kinds of symptomatic continuity are wholly consistent with the truth of the NK thesis. Next, in section 3.6, I consider a third family of objections, which purport to show that delusions are a *mind-dependent* kind and, hence, fail to constitute a natural kind. The apparent plausibility of such arguments, I maintain, result from collapsing some crucial and well-motivated distinctions. Given the appropriate distinctions, the arguments themselves collapse. In section 3.7, I consider a final class of objections – *heterogeneity arguments* – which purport to show that delusions are not a natural kind because they are in some sense too heterogeneous. In response, I point out that providing a satisfactory theory of a natural kind requires that we identify the relevant granularity of description. In view of this, I maintain that the heterogeneity arguments fail to establish that the NK thesis is false. Rather, they merely impose constraints on what the relevant grain of description must be. I conclude with a brief discussion of what I take to be the central empirical challenge for a natural kind conception of delusions – what I call the *unity problem*.

3.2 **What is a natural kind?**

In order to evaluate the NK thesis we need to clarify the notion of a natural kind; and this is not an easy task, since the notion has a long and checkered history in which it has been characterized many times over. Indeed for much of the twentieth century, the notion of a natural kind was considered little more than an artefact of an ancient and outmoded metaphysics.[1] But in recent years, the notion of a natural kind has regained philosophical respectability in large measure because it has proven useful to understanding some central aspects of contemporary scientific practice (Boyd, 1991; Griffiths, 1997).

3.2.1 Why natural kinds matter

Which scientific practices does the notion of a natural kind help clarify? Here are three central candidates.

1 *Inductive Generalization* The notion of a natural kind is intimately connected with the problem of induction (Quine, 1969; Boyd, 1990, 1991; Hacking 1991; Machery, 2005). In brief, inductive generalizations are formulated on the basis of observed instances of a category and yet purport to license inferences about unobserved instances as well. But for such purposes, not all categories are created equally. On observing 100 birds that have hearts, for example, it is reasonable to suppose that most – even all – unobserved birds also have hearts. In contrast, observing 100 things over 2 metres tall that are made of wood does not license the analogous inference – that (most) things over 2 metres tall are made of wood—since the co-variation between height and being made of wood is an *accidental* one. The notion of natural kind is relevant to this issue because it is supposed to effect a distinction between these two kinds of classes: those about which non-accidental, scientifically relevant, inductive generalizations can be formulated – atoms, molecules, and species, for example – and those about which few, if any such generalizations can be formulated – for example, things over 2 metres tall (Machery, 2005). Natural kinds permit this distinction because a central aspect of any natural kind is that its members share many non-accidentally related – though logically unconnected – scientifically important properties (or relations).

2 *Objects of Scientific Discovery* In part, because the formulation of non-accidental, inductive generalizations is central to scientific practice, many sciences aim to determine which classes of entities are natural kinds relative to their domain of enquiry. Biologists, for example, have identified cells, species, and strings of mRNA as kinds relevant to the formulation of inductive generalization, whilst rejecting élan vital and domestic animals as kinds of this sort. Notice that the acceptance of such kinds is typically determined *a posteriori*. That is, where a category is accepted as a kind over which scientific generalizations are made, it is very typically on the basis of empirical considerations; and when they are rejected for such purposes, the reasons are similarly empirical.

3 *Targets for Mechanistic Explanation* As noted earlier, natural kinds are supposed to underwrite a rich inventory of non-accidental, inductive generalizations because they are the kinds of categories whose members possess many non-accidentally

---

[1] Of which more in section 3.2.4.

related properties (or relations). But such properties are not *logically* related in the way that, for example, being red and being coloured are. Rather, they are contingently but non-accidentally associated. As Richard Boyd has put it, the instances of natural kinds have *contingently clustering families of properties* – properties that reliably, though need not invariably, co-vary (Boyd, 1991). Consider a paradigmatic example of a natural kind: water. Samples of water tend to possess a wide array of characteristics – transparency, potability, specifiable boiling and freezing points, and so on. Moreover, these characteristics are not logically (or conceptually) necessary properties of water samples in the way that, say, being unmarried is a necessary property of bachelors. Clearly, the existence of such property clusters call out for explanation. And, in fact, the provision of such explanations is a widespread scientific practice. Specifically, much science seeks to explain the existence of reliably co-varying property clusters by identifying and specifying the structures, processes, or mechanisms that – under appropriate circumstances – causally explain the contingent clusters associated with (natural) kinds. Again, the task of identifying and characterizing such structures, processes, and mechanisms is a largely an *a posteriori* matter. In the case of water, for example, the relevant explanatory factor (give or take a bit) turned out to be the chemical structure of water molecules, and was not discovered until substantial developments in chemistry had been made.[2]

3.2.2 Three further conditions on natural kindhood

So, the notion of a natural kind is important, in large measure, because it helps explain a range of central scientific practices. But given the role that natural kinds play in science, what characteristics must they possess? Let me start with three fairly obvious characteristics.

1 *Discreteness.* Given that natural kinds are *kinds*, they must be reasonably *discrete* classes of entities that can be demarcated from other phenomena. But it is important to note that insisting on discreteness is *not* the same thing as maintaining that kinds cannot be vague – that they must be wholly determinate categories without borderline cases. Children constitute a kind, as do red things, flat things, and hexagonal objects. But all these kinds are vague (Sorensen, 2006). So, for example, to our knowledge there is no precise age – specified, for example, in picoseconds – that marks a precise divide between childhood and other life stages. But this alone would be a poor reason for supposing that children are not a kind of any sort.

    Even so, one might think that natural kinds are different in this regard – that they must have strictly determinate boundaries. But this fits poorly with the facts about the kinds invoked in science. For many of the kinds that figure in scientific generalizations also exhibit vagueness. The point is well illustrated by biological kinds – tigers and apes, for example, but also eyes and hearts. These kinds are widely regarded as plausible candidates for natural kind status (Kripke, 1972; Putnam, 1975). Yet, they

---

[2] See Weisberg, 2005 for a more detailed discussion of the chemistry of water.

are also vague.[3] Indeed the assumption of absolutely strict boundaries is incompatible with the fact that biological entities evolve gradually over time (Dennett, 1995).

2 *Homogeneity.* A second characteristic of natural kinds is that they need to be fairly *homogeneous* kinds. Some classes of objects are just too heterogeneous to be natural kinds. Consider, for example, the class consisting of left knees, brown hairs, and chicken curries. Though it is a genuine class – one might even think it constitutes a kind – no one would suggest that it constitutes a *natural* kind. It is just too heterogeneous – too disjunctive – to figure in the sorts of scientific practices mentioned in section 3.2.1. For example, we would not expect to find many non-accidental, scientifically relevant, inductive generalizations that ranged over the members of this class. Nor would we expect to find some mechanism operating in all – or even most – of these cases that explained the co-variation of whatever properties members of the class happened to share. This contrasts sharply with the paradigmatic exemplars of natural kinds – water, for example – whose instances typically share many common characteristics. In short, and in contrast to many classes, natural kinds appear to possess real *unity*.

3 *Mind-independence.* At the very heart of the natural kind concept is the idea that some kinds are *real* kinds in nature, where 'real' does not merely mean that they exist, but that they are not *ideal* – i.e. their existence is in some appropriate sense mind-independent. So, for example, electrons are plausibly mind-independent in the relevant sense whilst Tuesdays are not. But *what* is this sense of mind-(in)dependence? Given that we are concerned with the status of a mental phenomenon – delusion – some comments are in order, if we are to avoid confusion later on. First, some comments on what the relevant notion of mind-(in)dependence is *not:*

- One might think that the distinction is simply the distinction between *psychological* kinds and *non-psychological* kinds. But this is clearly unsatisfactory. There are long-standing disagreements about the mind-dependence of theoretical entities – e.g. quarks, electrical fields, and chemical compounds – and whilst I am prepared to believe that some of the people engaged in such debates are confused, it is hard to accept that everyone is *so* confused that they are arguing over whether quarks (or chemical compounds etc.) are psychological kinds! This strains credulity. Similarly, the status of psychological kinds – beliefs, experiences, and, of course, delusions – is a long-standing issue in philosophy and psychology. But by the present standard, all such things are *trivially* mind-dependent and hence, non-natural kinds. So, if the present conception of mind-(in)dependence were the relevant one, all such debates would be trivial and *very* easily resolvable. Again, this strains credulity.

- Nor is the relevant distinction merely between those *entities whose existence metaphysically necessitates the existence of minds* and those that do not. Again, this would render all questions about the naturalness of psychological kinds trivial.

---

[3] Or to vary the diet of examples, consider some categories from materials science – e.g. glass and silica. These are plausibly natural kinds in the domain of materials science, and yet they are vague in a variety of respects.

For, clearly, the existence of beliefs (or desires, experiences, delusions, and so on) necessitates the existence of minds.

- Nor is the relevant sense of (in)dependence mere *causal (in)dependence*. The existence of toy poodles is causally dependent on mental activity. Had breeders not made whatever decisions and judgements were required to breed this family favourite, no such kind of dog would exist. The same is true, *mutatis mutandis*, of the radioactive chemical element, californium. But despite their causal dependence of mental activity, this in no way implies that such kinds are mind-dependent in the relevant sense.

So, what notion of mind-independence *is* relevant to the characterization of natural kinds? It is what Page (2006) calls *individuative independence*. Roughly put, a kind, K, is individuatively independent if it is circumscribed by boundaries that are totally independent of where we draw the lines. In other words, individuatively independent kinds are the sorts of kinds whose existence does not (metaphysically) depend on how we categorize things.[4] Perhaps stars or oxygen atoms are individuatively independent. At any rate, it is plausible that had we never engaged in the cognitive activity of categorizing some things as stars and others as oxygen atoms, those kinds of things could still have existed. In contrast, constellations appear to constitute an individuatively *dependent* kind. As Page puts it:

> We individuate the night sky into constellations. We, or more specifically our ancestors, determined which stars comprise which constellations. We can come up with new constellations whenever we like simply by pointing out a few stars and giving the cluster a name. Furthermore, the boundary between a constellation and its surroundings is very much a function of where we draw the lines (or more aptly, how we connect the dots). Though it is prima facie plausible that reality is individuated intrinsically into stars, reality is not individuated intrinsically into constellations, since it is people who divide the night sky into constellations.
>
> (Page, 2006, p. 328)

The present suggestion, then, is this: natural kinds are mind-independent in the sense that they are individuatively independent. The NK thesis is thus committed to the view that delusions are individuatively independent – that they are more like stars and oxygen atoms than they are like constellations.

3.2.3 Homeostatic property clusters

Given the discussion so far, we are in a position to see that natural kinds tend to possess at least the following characteristics:

- They are discrete, though not necessarily determinate categories.
- They are mind-independent – i.e. individuatively independent – kinds.

---

[4] Even this might be too strong a condition. For example, currency is surely a kind of economics; and yet, the existence of currency depends on the existence of minds that can think of some things as currency *as such*. For present purposes, however, I ignore this concern since a) the kinds of economics are contentious candidates for natural kind status for exactly this sort of reason; and b) the present condition, in fact, makes my case *harder* to sustain and not easier.

- They can figure in scientific, inductive generalizations.
- They are associated with contingent clusterings of properties.
- They are empirically discoverable.
- They are associated with empirically discoverable structures, processes, or mechanisms that explain the occurrence of contingent clusterings.
- They are homogeneous.[5]

With these characteristics in mind, there is, I maintain, a plausible general characterization of natural kinds that fits well with scientific practice. The view in question – the *homeostatic cluster* account – is perhaps the most popular proposal to have emerged from the philosophy of science in recent years. Roughly put, what it maintains is that a kind, K, is natural if:

H1 It is associated with a contingent property cluster – a range of characteristics or symptoms which tend to be co-instantiated by instances of the kind, but need not be genuine necessary conditions for membership.

H2 There is some set of empirically discoverable causal mechanisms, processes, structures, and constraints – a *causal essence*, if you will – that causally explains the co-variation of these various symptoms.

H3 To the extent that there is any real definition of what it is for something to be a member of the kind, it is not the symptoms, as such, but the causal essence that defines membership. More precisely, to the extent that natural kinds have definitions, it is the presence of a causal essence producing (some of) the symptoms that comprise the property cluster that defines kind membership.[6]

Consider an illness such as influenza. Influenza is, on the homeostatic cluster view, a plausible candidate for natural kind status. First, it is associated with a range of characteristic symptoms – coughing, elevated body temperature, and so on – even though these symptoms do not *define* what it is to have flu. Second, there is a causal mechanism – roughly, the presence of the flu virus – whose operation explains the occurrence of the symptoms. Finally, to the extent that influenza has a definition, it is the presence of the virus – or better, the presence of the virus producing some of the symptoms – but not the symptoms as such, that make it the case that one has flu.

Notice that the homeostatic cluster view does a good job of accommodating the features of natural kinds mentioned earlier. First, on the present view, instances of a natural kind will (more-or-less by definition) tend to exhibit a contingently co-varying cluster of properties. Second, because natural kinds exhibit such property

---

[5] What is the status of these characteristics of natural kinds? Clearly, they are important aspects of natural kinds and their role in scientific practice. But are all (or some) of them necessary conditions on natural kindhood; or, are they merely typical, though unnecessary, features of natural kinds? These are interesting questions, though not the ones I address here. All I am assuming for present purposes is the following principle: all else being equal, an account of natural kinds that explains these characteristic features of natural kinds should be preferred to one that does not explain them.

[6] See Boyd, 1990 and 1991, for more extensive characterizations of the homeostatic cluster view.

clusters, they will, as required, be able to figure in non-accidental, scientifically relevant, inductive generalizations. Third, on the present view, contingent property clusters are causally explained by empirically discoverable casual essences. Thus it is trivially the case that natural kinds are associated with mechanisms or processes that explain the occurrence of contingent clusterings. Fourth, since empirically discoverable causal mechanisms and processes are mind-independent, natural kinds will also be mind-independent and empirically discoverable. Fifth, on the present view, kinds will tend to be homogeneous in two different respects: a) the fact that the members of a natural kind tend to exhibit a contingent property cluster means that most members of the kind will be similar in this regard; b) because members of the kind tend to share a causal essence, there will also be significant homogeneity at the level of causal mechanism as well. Finally, on the present view, natural kinds will be discrete, though not necessarily wholly determinate. In particular, discreteness derives from the causal essence producing some aspect(s) of the contingent property cluster. What this means is that other phenomena – even phenomena that are very similar or indeed wholly overlapping in manifest properties – will not be entirely continuous with members of the kind since they will lack the appropriate underlying causal essence.

3.2.4 Essentialism and austerity about natural kinds

The homeostatic cluster view does a good job of accommodating the central characteristics that categories need to possess in order to play their requisite role in scientific practice. This, I maintain, provides good reason to endorse it as an account of natural kinds – at least if by 'natural kinds' one is concerned with the sorts of categories that figure prominently in science. Nevertheless, some philosophers have suggested that the homeostatic cluster view is too permissive, and should be rejected in favour of some more austere view of natural kinds. Of these more austere views, the most commonly endorsed is *essentialism* about natural kinds, which imposes a range of requirements wholly lacking in the homeostatic cluster view (Ellis, 2001).

Traditional essentialism about natural kinds can be traced back to Aristotle and Locke and is suggested by the work of twentieth-century philosophers such as Kripke and Putnam (Kripke, 1972; Putnam, 1975). It has four main tenets:

E1 All and only the members of a kind share a common essence.

E2 The essence is a property, or a set of properties, that all the members of a kind must have.

E3 The properties that comprise a kind's essence are intrinsic – i.e. non-relational – properties.

E4 A kind's essence causes the other properties associated with that kind.

For example, the essence of the natural kind gold is gold's atomic structure. That atomic structure is an intrinsic property possessed by all and only pieces of gold. That structure is a property that all gold must have as opposed to such accidental properties as being valuable to humans. Finally, the atomic structure of gold causes pieces of gold to have the properties associated with that kind, such as dissolving in certain acids and conducting electricity (Ereshefsky, forthcoming).

Traditional essentialism and the homeostatic cluster views have much in common. Both maintain that natural kinds possess *some* sort of essence; that essences causally explain the other properties associated with the kind; and that they are relevant to determining kind membership. Where they differ, however, is in their conception of essences. Traditional essentialism is committed to what have been called *sortal essences*, whereas the homeostatic cluster view is committed only to *causal essences* (Gelman and Hirschfeld, 1999). As I use the terms, all sortal essences are causal essences but not *vice versa*. For, in addition to figuring in causal explanations, a sortal essence consists of intrinsic properties, and as a matter of metaphysical necessity, is possessed by all and only the members of the kind. In contrast, causal essences imply no such commitments. Causal essences need not be intrinsic. They need not be possessed by all members of the kind. (There may, for example, be deviant, abnormal, or borderline kind members that fail to instantiate the relevant process, mechanism, or structure.) And where present, it need not be metaphysically necessary that a member of the kind instantiate the causal essence. (It may, for example, only be nomologically necessary.)

Which conception of essences is most relevant to providing an account of natural kinds? Traditional essentialism – and the sortal essences it assumes – applies well to some of the categories that figure in scientific explanations. For instance, gold and other elements in the periodic table appear to conform to traditional essentialism. But if we aim to characterize the kinds that figure more generally in scientific practice, then an insistence on sortal essences is overly restrictive. One problem is that many kinds are not characterizable in terms of intrinsic properties. Biological kinds appear to be of this sort, as do some of the kinds of psychology, materials science, and arguably, physics.

Even if we reject the assumption that sortal essences consist only of intrinsic properties, the requirement that each natural kind has a sortal essence is still overly restrictive. What such essentialism implies is that there are necessary and sufficient conditions for kind membership, and moreover, these conditions are also the causally relevant properties of kind members. But this is overly restrictive because there appear to be many kinds that figure in scientific generalization, which do not satisfy these conditions. Biological kinds are the most widely discussed example. The category of dogs, for example, appears not to be definable in terms of some set of necessary and sufficient conditions that explain the other properties associated with dogs. There seems, for example, to be no phenotypic trait possessed by all and only dogs; and nor does there seem to be a genetic 'essence' possessed by all and only dogs. Indeed, the process of natural selection appears to work against the production of such stable sortal essences. As a consequence, many philosophers and biologists have rejected the thesis that species have essences (Ereshefsky, forthcoming). Nevertheless, biological kinds are still appropriate for the purposes of formulating robust empirical generalizations, and to that extent are natural kinds of the sort that concern us.

In addition to being overly restrictive, the sortal essentialist conception of natural kinds is unmotivated. This is because a kind does not need to possess a sortal essence in order to play its characteristic scientific roles. Consider the functions mentioned in section 3.2.1. First, in order to effect the distinction between kinds about which non-accidental, scientifically relevant, inductive generalizations can be formulated, and those about which few, if any such generalizations can be formulated, natural kinds need not have sortal essences. All that is required is that, as the homeostatic cluster view maintains, kind members share many non-accidentally related – though logically unconnected – properties (or relations). Second, in order for kinds to be objects of empirical discovery, they need not have sortal essences. All that is required is that it is an empirical matter whether such kinds can figure in robust generalizations and/or that have empirically discoverable causal mechanisms that explain the contingent property clusters associated with (prototypical) kind members. Again, the homeostatic property cluster view accommodates this without the need for sortal essences. Finally, natural kinds need not possess sortal essences in order to underwrite to project of mechanistic explanation – i.e. the search for causal essences. Now it may be that some causal essences are also sortal essences, as in the case of chemical elements. But there is no reason to suppose that this must generalize to all putative natural kinds. So, for example, to the extent that the kind *neuron* is definable by a set of necessary and sufficient conditions, it is that all and only members of the kind are conducting cells within the nervous system. But this definition does not provide a characterization of the properties in virtue of which neurons possess their characteristic properties. In this case, then, it would seem that defining features and causal essence come apart.

So, essentialism about natural kinds is unattractive for a variety of reasons. Nevertheless, one might still be inclined to argue, on the basis of other considerations, that the homeostatic cluster view is unduly permissive. Most obviously, one might claim that the account is overly permissive because it permits paradigmatic examples of non-natural kinds – most obviously, social kinds or human kinds – to be natural kinds as well. But this objection strikes me as unconvincing. First, though the account, taken in isolation, is *consistent* with the claim that social kinds are natural kinds, the same is also true of every other remotely plausible account of natural kinds as well – including the more austere ones. So, for example, taken in isolation, traditional essentialism also fails to preclude the possibility of social-cum-natural kinds. So, if the worry is a serious one, it is one that applies to accounts of natural kinds quite generally and not only to the homeostatic cluster view.

Second, whilst the homeostatic cluster view is consistent with the possibility of social-cum-natural kinds, it is also wholly consistent with their *impossibility* as well. For it may be that there are facts about each social kind – or about social kinds as such – which make it impossible for them to be natural kinds. To put the point another way: the homeostatic cluster view does not imply the possibility of social-cum-natural kinds. Rather, it merely fails to rule out this possibility by point of definition. Finally, the fact that an account of natural kinds fails to preclude social-cum-natural kinds as a point of definition is not grounds to reject the account. On the contrary, this is as things should be. For, if natural kinds in general are, as I have argued – and virtually everyone accepts – determined *a posteriori*, then – absent some good argument to the contrary – it should also be an *a posteriori* matter whether or not *social* kinds are natural kinds.[7]

3.2.5 Semantics and natural kinds

We have seen that the notion of a natural kind is important to the understanding of scientific practice. But the class of natural kind *terms*, such as 'water', 'gold', and 'tiger' – terms which purport to refer to natural kinds – have also been the object of sustained attention in linguistics and the philosophy of language. This is a rich and complex area of enquiry that we do not have the time to discuss in detail here. Nevertheless, there are two widely accepted characteristics of natural kind terms that I need to flag since they will be relevant to the discussion later on.

First, a very widespread view about natural kind terms is that they are not synonymous with the description of (prototypical) characteristics that speakers associate with kinds (Kripke, 1972; Soames, forthcoming). For example, the term 'water' is associated by speakers with a description. It is the kind of stuff that boils and freezes at certain temperatures, that is clear, potable, and necessary to life, etc. (Soames, 2008). Even so, the term 'water' is not synonymous with such a description; and we can see this because speakers are prepared to apply the predicate 'is water' to quantities that lack characteristics specified by the associated description.

A second and related feature of natural kind terms is that they are amenable to substantial conceptual revision. In particular, we routinely accept substantial modifications in the extension of natural kind terms on the basis of empirical enquiry. To take a well-known example: the extension of 'fish' was until relatively recently taken to include whales and other marine mammals. But developments in biological systematics undermined this claim. Similarly, at one time Kant could confidently claim that gold is a yellow metal is an analytic, hence, *a priori*, truth. Yet, in the light of empirical enquiry, we now suppose that many instances of gold are not yellow – e.g. white gold – and that many samples that superficially resemble gold to a high degree are not gold at all. Precisely how best to explain such phenomena is a point of ongoing debate, which for present purposes we need not address. Nevertheless, as we will see,

---

[7] I suppose that one might revise the complaint: the problem is not so much that the homeostatic cluster view fails to preclude the possibility of social-cum-natural kinds but that the account – being relatively permissive – makes it too easy for social kinds to be natural kinds. But we need not take this seriously. First, the complaint is *ad hoc*. The homeostatic cluster view is defended on independent grounds – viz. its power to explain the role of natural kinds in scientific practice. If it makes it easier than one expects for social kinds to be natural ones, so much the worse for the prejudice that it should be harder. Second, it is far from obvious that it is 'too easy' – whatever exactly that means – for social kinds to satisfy the conditions imposed by the homeostatic cluster view. Indeed, it is far from clear that any of the prototypical examples of social kinds – e.g. sociological groups – satisfy the relevant conditions. So, for example, if the above arguments are correct, then homeostatic clusters are both individuatively independent and have a causal essence: two features that prototypical social kinds are widely believed not to possess.

the existence of such phenomena will be relevant to addressing some common objections to the NK thesis.

3.3 **The anti-essentialist objection**

With a clearer conception of natural kinds in hand, we are now in a position to consider objections to the NK thesis. The first objection I discuss purports to show that delusions are not a natural kind because they fail to share an essence. Here is the argument in skeletal form:

1 There is no essential criterion for being a delusion.

2 But natural kinds must have essences.

3 So, delusions are not a natural kind.

According to the argument, then, the NK thesis is false,

Response: Though commonplace in recent discussion (see, for example, Zachar, 2000; Ghaemi, 2004), the present argument is misguided. The main problem is with the second premise. The notion of essence in play here is clearly the notion of a *sortal* essence – one that is necessary and sufficient for kind membership. Here is what Ghaemi (2004) has to say on the matter:

> There simply is no essential feature of delusions. We need to be clear about this fact, accept it deep in our souls, live with it, and go on from there in our work. This is, in my adaptation of Daniel Dennett's (1995) phrase, 'Darwin's dangerous method.' Darwin's key innovation was in realizing that species are not essentialistic; there is no single aspect of the nature of species that necessarily and sufficiently characterizes them . . . I suggest that many notions in biology and medicine (including psychiatry) are not essentialistic. Peter Zachar (2001) has shown, forcefully in my judgment, that psychiatric diagnoses should not be conceived as natural kinds with essential features, but rather as pragmatic kinds. . . . If psychiatric diagnoses are not essentialistic, it is plausible that neither are delusions. Delusions are not characterized by any single essential feature; so much the worse for essentialism. Now let's move on.
>
> (Ghaemi, 2004, p. 50)

Ghaemi's claim that many kinds do not have sortal essences – characteristics that are necessary and sufficient for kind membership – is plausible. But contrary to what he suggests, this in no way undermines the claim that delusions constitute a natural kind. As we saw in section 3.2, an adequate account of natural kinds need not insist on sortal essences. Rather, one need only insist on the existence of causal essences. Species and geological formations are plausibly natural kinds. But there are no known sets of necessary and sufficient conditions for such things. *Mutatis mutandis* for delusion. Thus the mere fact that they fail to share a sortal essence is no reason to deny that they constitute a natural kind.

So, the argument fails; and not because of what it says about delusions but because it recruits a flawed conception of natural kinds. Still, the first premise of the argument deserves some comment. According to this premise, there is no essential criterion or set of criteria for being a delusion. But why accept this? To my knowledge, the most plausible reason is the dismal track record of past efforts to define 'delusion'. (For a useful review, see Garety and Hemsley, 1994.) By way of illustration, consider what is arguably the most influential approach to defining delusion – what we might call the *standard account of delusion*. Though there are many slightly different versions of the standard account, what they share is a commitment to the idea that delusions are a species of *belief*, which possess the following characteristics:

1 *Falsity:* A delusion is a *false* belief.

2 *Entrenchment:* Delusions are *firmly held* by the patient.

3 *Doxastic Isolation:* A patient's delusion is not accepted by other members of the person's culture or subculture.

4 *Resistance to Rational Persuasion:* Delusions cannot be dispelled by argument – including *good* argument – to the contrary.

5 *Resistance to Incompatible Information:* Delusions are maintained in the face of incompatible information that is available to the patient.

Definitions of 'delusion' that cite these sorts of characteristics are widespread in psychiatry and clinical psychology.[8] Nevertheless, as an attempt to specify necessary and sufficient conditions for being a delusion, the standard account is unsatisfactory. First, many – perhaps all – the above are not necessary conditions for being a delusion. So, for example:

- Though delusions are very typically false, they are not invariably so. For example, there are reported cases of hypochondriacal delusions with the content *I am mentally ill*. The belief is true, but for all that, it is still a delusion. (See Fulford, 1994 for further details.)

- Delusions are not always doxastically isolated. Sometimes – as in the case of folie à deux – the very same delusion can be held by multiple individuals.

Similar points can be made about the other criteria.

It is also far from clear that the conditions specified by the standard account are jointly *sufficient* for delusion. By way of illustration, consider the case of a rather stubborn professor who is deeply invested – personally and professionally – in a false, pet theory that they alone defend. Philosophy is, I suspect, replete with such figures! Suppose further that the pet theory was arrived at by faulty reasoning, and maintained in the face of strong argument and evidence to the contrary. Perhaps we have a Lewis-like figure who maintains that there exists an uncountable infinity of concrete universes (Lewis, 1986); or an Unger-ish professor who maintains that they, themselves, do not exist (Unger, 1979).[9] Even so, no psychiatrist would return a diagnosis of psychosis. Pet theories – even false, implausible, and singularly held theories – are

---

[8] The standard account is nicely illustrated by the definition of 'delusion' in DSM IV: A delusion is a 'false belief based on incorrect inference about external reality that is firmly sustained despite what almost everyone else believes and despite what constitutes incontrovertible and obvious proof or evidence to the contrary. The belief is not ordinarily one accepted by other members of the person's culture or subculture (e.g. it is not an article of religious faith)' (DSM IV, p. 821).

[9] Of course, I do not mean to suggest that the real Lewis or Unger resemble deluded subjects. I would not dream of impugning the quality of reasoning found in the work of these excellent philosophers!

part and parcel of contemporary academia. The standard conditions for delusion are met, but the attribution of delusion is withheld. It would seem, then, that the standard account provides neither necessary nor sufficient conditions for delusion.[10]

Let us return to the anti-essentialist objection. Earlier, we saw that the argument fails because it incorrectly assumes that the instances of a natural kind must share a sortal essence. We have now seen that the most widespread approach to defining delusion – the standard account – is unsatisfactory – it fails to specify necessary and sufficient conditions for delusion. But on reflection, this should be unsurprising, if the NK thesis is true. What the NK thesis is committed to is that an underlying mechanism explains the typical co-variation of a property cluster. Moreover, to the extent that anything is determinative of kind membership it is – as in the case of water – the instantiation of a causal essence. But the standard account clearly does not specify any such causal essence. Rather it characterizes delusion in terms of a cluster of superficial properties that delusions often possess but, as we have seen, need not invariably possess. On the assumption that delusion is a *bona fide* natural kind, then, it should be unsurprising that the standard account fails to provide an accurate account of the kind.[11]

3.4 **Some provisional, positive morals**

Does this mean that if the NK thesis is correct, then the standard account has no bearing whatsoever on a theory of delusion? I think not. Indeed our discussion of the standard account yields a number of positive morals.

Positive moral # 1: The standard account specifies (part of) the property cluster associated with delusions. As already noted, natural kinds have an associated syndrome: a cluster of properties that tend to co-vary with each other despite being neither logically related nor definitive of the kind. But if this is so, then delusions must have an associated syndrome if they are to constitute a natural kind. What might this syndrome be? An obvious and plausible suggestion is that the characteristics identified by the standard account at least partially specify the relevant syndrome.[12] That is: delusions tend to possess – though need not invariably possess – the properties

---

[10] The point is not, of course, that there are no differences between stubborn professors and delusional patients. Rather, the point is that the standard account fails to mark such a distinction. Of course, one might try to shore up the standard account by adding further conditions. But this has been tried without much success. So, for example, one might suggest that the deluded subject, in contrast to the Ungerish academic, *lives* their beliefs – that they are rationally and coherently interfaced with their actions. But the problem with adding this condition to the standard account is that it is not a necessary one. Whilst some deluded individuals live their beliefs, not all do. (For further discussion see Buchanan and Wellesley, 2004.)

[11] A related point: the standard account is perhaps best viewed as an attempt to provide a nominal definition – an account of what our word 'delusion' means – as opposed to a real definition. But due to space limitations, I propose to put this issue to one side.

[12] It is worth stressing that according to a natural kinds conception of delusions, there may of course be other – empirically discoverable – properties in the cluster. I discuss some candidates later in the chapter.

of falsity, entrenchment, doxastic isolation, resistance to rational persuasion, and resistance to available incompatible information. On this view, then, the error of the standard account is not that the features it specifies are irrelevant to an account of delusions but that the logical character of these features has been misconstrued. They are not conceptually or metaphysically necessary conditions for being a delusion, but aspects of the syndrome associated with delusions.

Positive moral # 2: We have prima facie reason to adopt the default assumption that delusion constitutes a natural kind. If delusions are a natural kind for which we currently possess no good theory, then we should expect that scientific and medical practices concerning delusion would follow the pattern characteristic of other examples of natural kinds. This expectation appears to be met in at least the following respects:

1 *Co-variation.* Natural kinds possess an associated cluster of properties that whilst logically independent and empirically dissociable, very often co-vary. As I argued earlier, this seems to be true of delusions. Although the criteria identified by the standard account are logically independent and empirically dissociable, they often co-vary with each other. Indeed, they tend to co-vary in precisely those cases that clinicians and psychopathologists construe as paradigmatic examples of delusion. It would seem, then, that delusion, like many other putative candidates for natural kind status – water, dogs, chlorine, and so on – possess an appropriate cluster of associated properties.

2 *Anti-descriptivist Semantics.* As mentioned earlier, a very widespread view about natural kind terms is that they are not synonymous with the description of (proto-typical) characteristics that speakers associate with the kind (Kripke, 1972; Soames, 2008). For example, the term 'water' is associated by speakers with a description. It is the kind of stuff that boils and freezes at certain temperatures, that is clear, potable, and necessary to life, etc (Soames, 2008). Even so, the term 'water' is not synonymous to such a description; and we can see this because speakers are prepared to apply the predicate 'is water' to quantities that lack characteristics specified by the associated description. What of 'delusion'? Given what I have said so far, it is plausible that 'delusion' is relevantly similar to 'water' in the above respects. For as we have seen, it is not synonymous with the description that clinicians associate with delusion – i.e. the description specified by the standard account. Moreover, as in the case of water, this is clear from the fact that, as indicated in section 3.3, clinicians are prepared to apply the term to phenomena that fail to satisfy the description. In short, the term 'delusion' possesses precisely the semantic character we should expect it to exhibit on the assumption that it is a natural kind term.

3 *Reliable Tracking.* In the history of science many of the most plausible candidates for natural kind status – water, gold, lead, dogs, monkeys, etc. – have paradigmatic instances that are reliably – though not, of course, invariably – identifiable, even in the absence of any good theory or definition for the kind. There is an obvious rea-son for this. Good theories and definitions are not the starting point for science but the *end product.* In which case, if, as we suppose, natural kinds, are the sorts of things whose causal essences are empirically discoverable by the scientific community,

they must be kinds whose instances can be reliably tracked by the community *prior* to possession of a good theory. Notice that this implies not merely that some members of the relevant community can on some occasions identify instances of the kind, but also that there is a high degree of inter-rater reliability regarding which things are instances of the kind. When such reliability is absent, the standard methods of science simply will not work. *Prima facie*, this point applies to delusion. As many theorists have lamented, no good theory or definition, of what delusions are, currently exists. But despite this, there seems to be high levels of inter-rater reliability within the relevant scientific communities – e.g. psychiatry and clinical psychology – when it comes to identifying instances of delusion (Bell *et al.*, 2006a). It is not merely that psychiatrists, when exercising their clinical judgement, tend to agree. Rather, it seems that quite different methods for assessing delusion – e.g. clinical interview and various standardized scales – reliably converge (Bell *et al.*, 2006a). In short, assessments of delusion appear to exhibit precisely the sort of reliability that we would expect on the assumption that they constitute a natural kind.

4 *Empirical Regularities:* Let me add one final consideration that is largely independent of the discussion so far. If the NK thesis is true, then we should expect appropriate methods of enquiry to yield a body of empirical regularities concerning delusions. Though it is too early to tell with any certainty, there are grounds for optimism on this score. For over the past two decades or so, a wide range of results has emerged regarding delusions. So, for example, there is now considerable evidence of various abnormalities in the reasoning, attention, metacognition, and attributional tendencies of delusional patients (Bell *et al.*, 2006b) Some of these phenomena will be discussed briefly in section 3.7; though for reviews of some relevant results see Garety and Hemsley (1994); Garety *et al.* (2001); Bell *et al.* (2006b); Freeman and Garety (2006); and Freeman (2007).

What follows from the above? Though such considerations clearly fail to provide strong grounds for accepting the NK thesis, I maintain that they do give us *prima facie* reason to take the claim seriously. After all, the scientific practices surrounding delusion appear to exhibit precisely those characteristics that we should expect them to exhibit if the NK thesis were true. To put the point another way: Though such grounds for accepting the NK thesis are eminently defeasible, they still provide reason to adopt it as a working hypothesis. In view of this, one question that requires our attention is this: are there any good reasons for rejecting the *prima facie* plausible assumption that delusions are a natural kind? Most of the remainder of the chapter is concerned with this issue.

3.5 Continuity objections

So far, our discussion has proceeded under the assumption that delusions are a kind of some sort, even if they do not constitute a natural kind. But in fact, one prominent kind of objection to the NK thesis purports to undermine even this weaker assumption. According to such objections, delusions do not constitute a kind of any sort, natural or otherwise.

3.5.1 **Vagueness and delusions**

Let us start by disposing of a red herring. One might be inclined to argue that delusions are not a genuine kind, natural or otherwise, on the grounds that the category of delusion has vague boundaries – roughly put, there are entities for which it is indeterminate whether or not they are delusions. But as we saw in section 3.1, mere vagueness does not suffice for rejecting the existence of a kind. Children really do constitute a kind even though it is a kind that lacks precise borders. Nor is vagueness a reason to deny that a kind is a genuine natural kind. On the contrary, many plausible candidates for natural kind status have borderline cases. Eyes, for example, plausibly constitute a natural kind; and yet it does not have determinate boundaries. Consider, for example, a structure that biologists call 'pit-eyes': simple eye-spots of approximately 100 cells, set into a pit to reduce the angles of light that enters the eye-spot. Are such structures *eyes*? It is, I take it, utterly unclear how to categorize such a case. And if you think they are clearly categorizable as eyes, then what of eye-spots not located in pits? So far as we know, there are no clear answers regarding how best to classify such examples.

3.5.2 **Continuity with normal experience**

So, mere vagueness or indeterminacy does not suffice to undermine the NK thesis. It is simply beside the point. But another more interesting line of argument is that delusions do not constitute a kind because they are literally *continuous* with other non-delusional phenomena (Strauss, 1969; van Os, 2003; Freeman and Garety, 2006). On this *continuity view*, the right way of thinking about delusions is as a range on a continuum for which there exists no discrete boundaries at all, vague or precise. On such a view, the complaint against the NK thesis is not merely that delusions comprise a kind with vague boundaries but that there are no well-motivated points at which to draw the distinction between delusions and other phenomena. And since kinds are supposed to be discrete this would suffice to undermine the NK thesis.

Though the present objection comes in a variety of forms, the most plausible and popular version seeks to defend a continuum account of delusions on the grounds that they are continuous with normal, non-pathological experience (van Os, 2003; Freeman and Garety, 2006).[13] But what is the evidence for such continuity supposed to be? Much of the putative evidence comes from epidemiological studies. So, for example, in one well-known study involving over 7000 people in the Netherlands, it was found that 3.3% of the population had a 'true' psychiatrist-rated delusion whilst 8.7% had a 'not clinically relevant' delusion (van Os *et al.*, 2000; Johns and van Os, 2001). Similarly, in a study on delusional ideation in primary care patients, it was found that delusional ideation was frequent in those with no psychiatric history.

---

[13] It has also been suggested, though never presented as an objection to the NK thesis, that delusions are hard to discriminate from other pathological phenomena – e.g. over-valued ideas (David, 1999). Nevertheless, there is good reason to suppose that the patterns of characteristics associated with delusion are readily distinguishable from those associated with over-valued ideas (Jones, 1999).

For example, 10% of participants with no psychiatric history reported that they had at some point felt as if there was a conspiracy against them (Verdoux *et al.*, 1998).

Such data are interesting, perhaps even surprising. But it in no way adjudicates between kind and continuity conceptions of delusion. In order to see this, we need to look more closely at the character of the inference from the data. What the epidemiological data strongly suggests is that delusional phenomena are prevalent not merely among those with a psychiatric history but also amongst the population at large. But how does this cut in favour of a continuum conception of delusions? The idea, in brief, is that it supports a continuum hypothesis because according to such a view 'psychotic symptoms should be present not only in subjects identified as "cases of psychosis", but also in a proportion of subjects from the general population that does not fulfill the clinical criteria of "case of psychosis"' (Verdoux and van Os, 2002). In contrast, a kinds conception of delusion makes no such prediction. So, the continuum hypothesis wins.

The present issues and evidence are important and intriguing. Nevertheless, as an argument against the NK thesis it is far from overwhelming. First, the present data are wholly *compatible* with a kinds conception of delusions, including the NK thesis itself. In order to see this, consider the following – mutually compatible – possibilities. First, it is quite possible that psychotic pathology is more widespread than initially supposed. That is, what the data may in part reflect is the (rather unsurprising) fact that the general population contains people with psychotic symptoms who have not (as yet) acquired a documented psychiatric history.[14]

Second, the claim that delusions constitute a natural kind in no implies that delusions are *only* present in pathological cases. Instead, it may be that someone can be both deluded and not mentally disordered. By widespread consensus, having a mental disorder or psychopathology presupposes that some *evaluative* condition is met. So, for example, according to one prominent view, mental illness or mental disorder requires that the state is in some way *harmful* (Wakefield, 1992). But notice, if delusions are a natural kind, then this creates the possibility of some – indeed many – delusions that are not harmful, either to the deluded subject, or to anyone else for that matter. That is, there may be people who meet the following conditions:

• they exhibit the characteristic pattern of properties associated with delusions;

• the presence of the property cluster is explained by the activity of some mechanism, which in the case of delusions, is responsible for the covariation of the property cluster; but

• there are no harmful effects either for the individual or for those around them.

Under these conditions, someone would have a genuine delusion and yet fail to be mentally disordered.

Finally, it is important to be clear on the sort of continuity that the available evidence supports. At most, what the data suggest is a *symptomatic* continuum: non-pathological

---

[14] As Matthew Broome has pointed out to me, the general population clearly contains such people. After all, on first becoming ill, a person will lack a psychiatric history even though he/she still has a clear-cut psychotic illness.

subjects – and those with mood disorders – exhibit delusion-like states; states that possess properties that are very similar to, or overlap with, those associated with the psychotic delusions (Verdoux and van Os, 2002). But the existence of such symptomatic continuity is wholly consistent with the NK thesis. Recall that according to the NK thesis, symptoms, as such, are not definitional of having a delusion. Rather it is the instantiation of the salient causal essence that determines category inclusion. But what this means is that there can be many phenomena that are superficially very similar to delusions and yet are not delusions because the manifestation of the symptoms fails to depend on the appropriate kind of underlying causal mechanism. The point is in no way specific to delusions. It applies quite generally to natural kinds. So, for example, influenza is symptomatically quite similar to many other illnesses. For example, there are many diseases that characteristically involve an elevated body temperature, congestion, sore throat, and so on. But that does not mean that a continuum theory of influenza should be adopted. Rather, such continuity in symptomology between flu-sufferers and others is to be explained by the fact many mechanisms can produce flu-like symptoms. Despite this, only those people who exhibit such symptoms as a consequence of the activity of a flu virus have flu.

So, it would seem that the current evidence for continuity is compatible with the NK thesis. Nonetheless, one might think that a continuum view is at an advantage because it predicts the epidemiological data, whereas a kinds view of delusion does not. But in fact, the continuum hypothesis does not do such a good job of predicting the extant data. What the data suggest is not merely that delusion-like symptoms are present in a proportion of subjects from the general population. It also suggests that 'true' psychiatrist-rated delusions are present in the general population. The continuum model predicts the former fact. But it does not predict the latter. At best, it is silent on the matter. Indeed, one might think that it fits most naturally with the converse prediction. For, on perhaps the most natural way of formulating the continuum hypothesis, it should in fact be *surprising* that non-pathological populations manifest 'true' delusions. Specifically, what the continuum approach is widely thought to imply is that 'delusions are not qualitatively different from normal beliefs, but simply represent a more extreme end of the population spectrum or distribution of anomalous mental phenomena' (Bell *et al.*, 2006b). But if this is so – if delusions are just the tail of the curve – then one would expect 'true' delusions to be those found amongst those people with the most anomalous mental lives – i.e. those who comprise the clinical population.

Still, does not the continuum approach have the advantage of predicting the fact that delusion-like phenomena are found in the population at large? Yes, but it is only a very slight advantage. The reason is that the NK thesis, when combined with additional plausible assumptions, also makes the same prediction. Earlier, I commented that many different putative natural kinds bear striking symptomatic similarities to other kinds. The symptoms of influenza are remarkably similar to those of many other illnesses. Likewise, the superficial properties of gold are very similar to those of various compounds. Jadeite and nephrite are superficially very similar. And so on. Now the mere fact that these things are natural kinds in no way *implies* that such syndrome overlaps exist. But the fact that so *many* natural kinds exhibit such overlaps is inductive grounds for supposing that delusions would exhibit symptomatic continuities and overlaps, if the NK thesis were true. Thus, the NK thesis plus this apparent fact about natural kinds render symptomatic continuity unsurprising, if not probable.

3.6 Mind-dependence objections

Let us turn to a different sort of objection to the NK thesis: one that purports to put pressure on the assumption that delusions constitute a mind-independent kind. Though the objection comes in a number of forms, in what follows I consider what I take to be the three most plausible versions.

3.6.1 Delusion as a folk psychological kind

According to one version of the objection, delusions are not a natural kind but an artifact of our folk psychology: our commonsense mode of thought about the mental. Murphy (2006) expresses the position as well as anyone:

> [W]hether or not something is a delusion is a matter of how it strikes us, and that depends on how well it comports with our understanding of what people are like, both in general terms and within our culture. It does not depend on some psychological mechanism or a formal property of beliefs. Even if we can identify belief formation mechanisms, it is unlikely that any mechanism has *completely* broken down even when subjects are delusional, since even in the maddest psychotics we find some preservation of normal reasoning alongside the delusional reasoning.
>
> (Murphy, 2006, p. 180)

Murphy is not claiming that delusions are not a natural kind merely because they are a part of our folk conception of the world. This would be an obviously poor argument since there is no incompatibility between the naturalness of a kind and it being a kind identified in our folk conception. Water is plausibly a natural kind, though 'water' and the concept it expresses are part of commonsense. Similarly, species terms and the concepts they express are thoroughly folkish, but that alone does not mean that dogs or cats do not constitute natural kinds. Rather, it might be – and plausibly is the case – that some of our folk concepts pick out natural kinds.

Why, then, would one think that the present consideration threatens the NK thesis? According to the present view, it is because *what it is to be* a delusion is determined by how it strikes us. That is, being a delusion is a *response-dependent* property. In the present case, the claim is that how something strikes beings like us – beings with our commonsense psychology – is metaphysically determinative of what it is to be a delusion. But if this is so, then delusions will not constitute a natural kind. Natural kinds are supposed to be discoverable, mind-independent kinds whose existence is not parasitic on our taxonomic practices. But, according to the present view, being a delusion is metaphysically determined by our folk psychological classificatory practices. In which case, delusions will be mind-dependent in a way that precludes them from constituting a natural kind.

Response: The present line of reasoning conflates the metaphysics of delusion with its epistemology. The relevant metaphysical issue concerns the nature of delusions: roughly, what is it to be a delusion. The relevant epistemic question concerns the evidential basis for our judgements about delusion: roughly, the sorts of evidence we invoke in judging that someone is deluded. What is right about the present objection is that our judgements about delusion are not based on some scientific account of either the mechanisms on which delusions depend or the formal properties of belief. Instead, the judgements of clinicians depend largely on the sorts of evidence that are available on the basis of commonsense psychological considerations alone – e.g. the reasonableness of the belief, its failure to conform to cultural norms, the extent to which it is resistant to countervailing evidence, and so on. But it clearly does not follow from this epistemic point alone that the *nature* of delusion is exhausted by how things strike us. On the contrary, it is wholly compatible with a conception of delusions as a natural kind. Compare this with the fact that our standard methods of determining whether something is water are made on the basis of considerations drawn from folk wisdom. Prior to developments in eighteenth-century chemistry, no one ever judged something to be water on the basis of anything other than such folkish considerations. But it clearly does not follow from this alone that water is not a natural kind. For all Murphy's argument shows, the same is true of delusions as well. What is required is some reason to suppose that in the case of delusion, things really are different: that metaphysical issues about the nature of the kind, and epistemic issues about how we know about instances of the kind *ought* to be collapsed. But no such argument is forthcoming; and in the absence of such an argument, the present considerations simply beg the question against the NK thesis.

3.6.2 The cultural relativity of delusion

Still, there are various ways one might try to develop the view that delusions are response-dependent in a way that threatens the NK thesis. One obvious strategy turns on the widely noted fact that the content of delusions is highly sensitive to social context. Indeed, the diagnosis of delusions often turns heavily on whether the patient's belief is accepted by other members of their culture or subculture. By way of illustration, consider the case of religious delusions. If I believe that there is an all-powerful deity, I do not have a delusion. I merely subscribe to a widely held, socially sanctioned religious viewpoint. If I believe, however, that *I* am God, then I will likely be judged delusional. What makes for the difference? We might suppose that both beliefs are false, fixed, incompatible with the available evidence, and highly resistant to counter-argument. But what seems to make the difference is that in one case, the belief is socially sanctioned (within a particular culture) whilst in the other case it is not. Delusions would thus appear to be response-dependent at least to the extent that what is a delusion depends on what beliefs are socially prevalent. In which case, it would seem that the NK thesis is false.

Response: What the sensitivity of delusions to social context shows is that the nature of delusion, as such, cannot be characterized in terms of its contents. But the fact that what counts as a delusion varies from culture to culture need not undermine the natural kind status of delusions so long as there is some culturally *invariant* way to characterize the nature of this cultural sensitivity. Fortunately, there seems to be just such a characterization. In brief, what the cultural sensitivity of delusions appears to track is the insensitivity of delusions to an important source of epistemic warrant and epistemic defeat: *testimony*. Many of the beliefs that we adopt are held on the basis of testimony. That is, we adopt beliefs on the basis of reasons, evidence, or information provided by (putatively) authoritative sources. So, for example, we accept much on the basis of reading the newspaper, or consulting encyclopedias, or talking with local experts, or on the basis of the prevailing 'commonsense' or popular consensus – itself a species of testimony. Much the same applies to religious belief. When I believe that there is an all-powerful God, I do so in part on the basis of widespread access to testimony: (putative) experts – e.g. priests and rabbis – television shows, popular opinion, and so on. The belief may well be false, and such testimony may ultimately be subject to defeaters. But there is little doubt that testimony is a genuine source of warrant; and there is little doubt that in societies where theism is widespread, many such lines of testimony exist, and most of us are exposed to it from an early age. This contrasts strongly with the case of religious delusions – such as the belief that I am God. Here, there are no such lines of testimony since no one else holds the belief. Moreover, if testimony is to guide belief, then such a delusional belief would likely be defeated many times over by the testimony of others since no one else accepts the delusion as true. Of course, none of this makes much difference to the patient with a religious delusion. They are, it would seem, resistant to testimony, at least where the delusion itself is concerned. So the suggestion is this: the cultural relativity of delusions is not of the kind that threatens the NK thesis. What it shows is that delusions are resistant to testimony – a culturally invariant feature of delusion – and not that being a delusion is a response-dependent property.

3.6.3 The normativity of delusion

Let us now turn to what I take to be the most challenging version of the mind-dependence objection: one that focuses on the *normative* character of delusions. Delusions are the sorts of states that are normatively assessable. Indeed, one might suppose that they are *essentially*, negatively assessable. When one is deluded, there is necessarily something *wrong*. But the objection continues: the relevant norms are *social* norms. They are norms that depend on our cultural modes of thought. In which case, the existence of delusions, as such, is essentially dependent on cultural modes of thought. And if this is so, then delusions are not individuatively independent kinds and, hence, not natural kinds at all.

Response: For the present objection to the NK thesis to succeed, it needs to be the case both that some normative conditions are essential to being a delusion *and* that these very same normative conditions are social/cultural ones whose existence depends on our modes of thinking. But we have little reason to suppose that this is so. Though delusions are plausibly subject to *some* social norms, these social norms are not essential to being a delusion; and though there are some normative conditions that are plausibly essential to being a delusion, these norms are not plausibly social. Let me explain.

In order to appreciate the situation we need first to consider the question: What norms are delusions subject to? There are two plausible candidates: medical norms and norms of rationality. Medical norms are those that determine whether or not something is pathological: a disease, illness, or disorder. Norms of rationality are those norms that determine whether or not something is rational or reasonable. Let us consider these types of norm in turn.

Medical norms determine whether or not a given state is pathological: whether or not there is something medically *wrong* with the organism. Precisely how best to characterize such norms is, I suspect, a largely open matter; and it may be that they are not social norms at all. Even so, there is widespread consensus amongst those interested in the notions of disease and disorder that such norms are at least partially social in character. So, for example, even Jerome Wakefield – whose *harmful dysfunction* account of disorder is one of the least socially laden extant proposals – readily accepts that the notion of harm should be understood in sociocultural terms. Roughly, the relevant notion of harm is to be characterized in terms of a reduction in well-being, as defined by social values and meanings.

Suppose that this is true. Medical norms are at least partially social norms. Does this pose a problem for the NK thesis? Only if delusions are *necessarily* harmful or otherwise problematic relative to the relevant medical norms. But why suppose that this is true? As far as I can tell, there is no good reason to suppose that it is. Indeed, if our earlier discussion of the continuity objection ran along the right lines, then it seems quite possible for delusions not to be pathological. In saying this, I do not deny (of course) that delusions are *very typically* pathological. Rather, the point is a modal one: though delusions are very often pathological – we might even suppose that they are in fact invariably pathological – the connection between pathology and delusion is, for all that has been said so far, a contingent one. And without some reason to suppose that the connection is a necessary one, the (putative) social character of such norms poses no threat to the NK thesis.

Let us now consider the relationship between delusion and norms of rationality. First, are delusions essentially irrational or unreasonable? How best to answer this question is far from clear. To be sure, delusions are *very typically* irrational or unreasonable. We might even suppose that they are *invariably* irrational. But whether to treat the connection as a necessary one – as opposed to merely a contingent, though (highly) reliable one – is not at all obvious. Perhaps, the initial description that we associate with delusions – and use to identify them – partially characterizes them as irrational. This would, in fact, appear to be the case – at least to the extent that the standard account of delusion is the description we associate with delusions. For, it mentions two properties that impugn the (epistemic) rationality of delusions: their resistance to rational persuasion and their resistance to incompatible information. But, to repeat: the fact that irrationality is part of the description that we associate with (prototypical) delusions does not imply that irrationality is an *essential* property of delusions.

Still, let us suppose for the sake of argument that delusions are necessarily irrational or unreasonable. Would this pose a problem for the NK thesis? Not unless the relevant rational norms are *social* norms. The problem for the present version of the mind-dependence objection is that a social constructionist view of rational norms really is not plausible. This is a familiar topic that has been the subject of longstanding discussion; and we do not have time to discuss it in detail here. But let me mention just two considerations. First, a social norms conception of rationality appears to make it metaphysically impossible for a person to rationally criticize the prevailing epistemic and practical norms of their own society. But this does not seem at all impossible (Gibbard, 1990). Second, of the many extant theories of rationality currently entertained by philosophers, the vast proportion articulate rational norms in a way that does not reduce them to social norms. Consider, for example, Bayesian accounts of rationality (Howson and Urbach, 1993) or reliabilist accounts (Nozick, 1993), or pragmatic accounts (Stich, 1990). All render rationality in a manner that is not social in any sense that threatens the NK thesis. But if this is so, then the proponent of the present objection to the NK thesis needs to show that a social conception of rationality is preferable to such alternatives. I am pessimistic that such a position could be sustained.

3.7 **Heterogeneity objections**

As we saw earlier, if the NK thesis is true, there must be some underlying causal essence – e.g. mechanism, process, or structure – that explains the symptom cluster associated with delusions. In this section, I consider a range of objections that challenge this requirement on the grounds that there is no sufficiently heterogeneous kind of mechanism or process that can play this role.

3.7.1 **Causal heterogeneity**

A common view about delusions – often associated with the so-called biopsychosocial model – is that 'many factors are implicated in delusion development, and the contribution of each in individual cases varies' (Freeman and Garety, 2006). From this, it is common to conclude that they are unlikely to admit of unified explanation (*ibid.*); and from this, it may seem like only a small step to the conclusion that delusions are not a natural kind. For what the NK thesis demands is that delusions admit of some kind of explanatory unity.

But appearances are, at least on this occasion, misleading. The claim that something is an instance of a natural kind is wholly consistent with its being produced and maintained by *many* different causal factors. To take an obvious example, the development of an organism – a tiger, for example – depends on a huge array of causal factors: gravitational forces, appropriate levels of nutrients and oxygen, thermal conditions, the occurrence of appropriate patterns of gene expression and regulation, the presence of chemical gradients within the growing organism, and so on. The factors relevant to maintaining a (live) tiger are similarly numerous. But it surely does not follow from this alone that tigers are not a natural kind.

Why not? There are at least two reasons. First, in order to understand the role that the identification and citation of causal essences plays in scientific research, we need to respect the distinction between background causal conditions and explanatorily salient causal mechanism. There is nothing here that is peculiar to the case of delusion. All causal explanation presupposes such a distinction. So, for example, when I kick a ball, there are many enabling conditions that must obtain in order that my action succeeds. Oxygen must be present, gravitation must be in force, appropriate levels of ambient light must be available so that I can see the ball, and so on. Moreover, there are many prior conditions that must hold in order that can kick the ball. I must have been born, life on Earth must have evolved, the planet itself must have developed out of cosmic particles, and so on.[15] Nevertheless, a causal *explanation* of ball kicking need not cite all these factors. Rather, they are treated as background conditions that need to obtain, but are not central to explaining the specific phenomenon. The same is true of delusions. Though there may be many factors that contribute to their occurrence, this alone is not incompatible with the idea that they are all produced by some kind of mechanism since most of the causal factors responsible for delusions may be part of the background conditions as opposed to aspects of the mechanism itself.

Second, it is important to distinguish between different *levels* of explanation. The identification of a natural kind is typically made relative to a particular level of explanation. Sodium is a kind of chemistry. Quark is a kind of physics. Neuron is a kind of biology, and so on. The mere fact that there are many different causes of delusion poses no problem for the NK thesis if they are causes that obtain at different levels of explanation. This is because the causes need not be *distinct* causal factors so much as factors that bear various dependency relations to each other. So, for example, the fact that my behaviour can correctly be said to be caused both by my mental states and by neural states, is not by itself reason to suppose that my behaviour is caused by a multiplicity of *distinct* causal factors since in this case presumably mental activity is not independent of neural activity but rather metaphysically depends on – e.g. is identical to, realized by, or supervenes on – neural activity. In such cases, higher and lower level causes do not compete: they are not evidence of heterogeneity but of dependency.

3.7.2 Neural heterogeneity

So the mere fact that delusions have many different causes in no way undermines the claim that delusions are a natural kind. Nevertheless, the NK thesis is committed to the claim that delusions depend on the activity of some kind of mechanism (process or structure, etc.). And this leads to a new version of the heterogeneity argument. Since mental phenomena in general depend on neural activity, presumably delusions, *qua* mental phenomena, depend on neural mechanisms (process or structure, etc.). In which case, it may seem that the NK thesis mandates that there exist some kind of neural mechanism on which delusions depend. But this appears to pose a problem. For what neuroscientific research suggests is that different delusions depend on different neural states, processes, and mechanisms. For example, both the neuroanatomy and neurochemistry of Capgras delusion appear quite different from the neuroanatomy and neurochemistry of persecutory delusions or passivity phenomena. But if this is so, then it seems implausible to claim that the same neurobiological mechanism is responsible for all delusions. In which case, the NK thesis would appear to be false.

Response: So formulated, there is a general, and I think, plausible response to the present objection. Indeed, the response falls out of one of the most widespread (and

---

[15] Indeed, on the assumption that causal is transitive, every causal relation that links my kicking the ball to the big bang will be *a* cause of my kicking the ball!

plausible) assumptions of contemporary cognitive science and philosophy of mind: the *multiple realizability of the mental*. In brief, according to this thesis, psychological kinds (such as pain and belief) can be realized by many distinct physical kinds. Most importantly for our purposes, multiple realizability implies that a psychological kind can be realized by many different neural kinds. In such cases, there need be no one–one relation between a psychological kind and an underlying neural kind. Instead, the psychological kind will bear a *one–many* relation to neural kinds. Or, to put the point slightly more precisely, a psychological kind that is multiply, neurally realized, will participate in a *one-to-many* dependency relation with neural kinds, where these kinds are characterized in the terms of *biological neuroscience*: roughly, the chemistry, physiology, morphology, and anatomy of neurons and neuronal assemblies (Stoljar and Gold, 1998).[16]

The above characterization of multiple realizability, suggests a response to the present objection. If delusions are multiply realizable, then different delusions can be realized by quite different kinds of neural states and processes. In which case, it should be wholly unsurprising that neuroscience fails to identify a neat one–one correspondence between delusions and neurobiology. Instead, we should expect the emerging picture to be a complex one marked by a one–many relation between delusion and underlying neurobiology. But this alone does not show that delusions are not a natural kind of any sort. All it shows is that they are not a *neurobiological* natural kind – i.e. a kind that is (non-disjunctively) characterizable in the vocabulary of biological neuroscience. In which case, what follows from the NK thesis is that delusion will be a natural kind relative to some *other* level of explanation in much the same way that quarks and species are kinds relative to levels of explanation other than biological neuroscience.

But what might this level be? In the case of quarks and species, we seem to know the answer – fundamental physics and evolutionary biology, respectively. But what is the right level for the purposes of delusion? There is an obvious suggestion that surely merits further exploration. Historically, the multiple realizability of the mental was widely (and correctly) taken to suggest that a science of the mind requires levels of description and explanation more abstract than those afforded by biological neuroscience. Specifically, the multiple realizability thesis was central to motivating the view that psychological science requires computational/functional levels of description. Such levels of description have been central to contemporary cognitive science and cognitive neuroscience, among other reasons, because they permit stable mechanistic descriptions that abstract away from neurobiological heterogeneity. Such descriptions have proven hugely productive in understanding myriad psychological phenomena. Indeed, there has in recent years been considerable effort to apply this approach to the study of delusions. (See, for example, Birchwood *et al.*, 2000; Freeman *et al.*, 2002; Bell *et al.*, 2006b). This leads to a further positive moral.

---

[16] Multiple realizability has been the subject of intensive philosophical attention over the past three decades. For more detailed discussions see Pylyshyn, 1984; Kim, 1992; Block, 1997; and Shapiro, 2000.

Positive moral # 3: Delusions as a cognitive kind. If the NK thesis is true, then delusions are a multiply neurally realized kind. Moreover, given extant efforts to understand psychological phenomena that are multiply realized, it is plausible to adopt the working assumption that the relevant level of description is a computational-cum-functional one. In short, the most plausible version of the NK thesis is one that views delusions are a *cognitive kind*.

3.7.3 Cognitive heterogeneity

But there is a reformulation of the previous objection that requires our attention. According to the multiple realizability thesis, mental states of the same type – in the present case individual delusions – are realized by different neural kinds, where those kinds are individuated via the traditional methods of neurobiology – e.g. chemistry, anatomy, and physiology. But in the case of delusions, it seems not merely that delusions are multiply realized in this sense. Rather, it seems that they also depend on different kinds of *psychological* states and processes – where such types are individuated by their functional-cum-computational properties. So, for example, according to one familiar view – one that clearly will not generalize to all delusions – Capgras delusion depends crucially on states of the face-recognition system (Ellis and Lewis, 2001). Similarly, according to a prominent account of passivity phenomena – again, an account that clearly will not generalize to all delusions – delusions of control depend crucially on disruption to forward models within our motor systems (Blakemore *et al.*, 2003). For present purposes, the crucial point is that these differences are not merely neurobiological but also involve functional-cum-representational differences between the kinds on which delusions are supposed to depend. As a consequence, it would seem that we not only have plurality at the level of biological neuroscience but also at the level(s) of psychology. Even abstracting from the messy neurobiological details,delusions appear not to be a unified kind.

Response: How should an advocate of the NK thesis respond to the present point? One option would be to suggest that delusions are multiply realizable not only relative to neurobiological levels of description but also relative to psychological levels of description as well. But this response is unsatisfactory. Multiple realizability – at least as ordinarily construed – is a one–many, *inter*-level relation. When a kind K is multiply realized by a set of kinds K', K", . . . , there exists a one–many relationship between K at level L and the many kinds at L*. So, for example, corkscrews are plausibly multiply realizable in this sense because there is a one–many relation between the functional kind *corkscrews* and numerous arrangements of atoms that can be instances of the kind. With this in mind, the problem with claiming that delusions are multiply realizable relative to our psychology is that it is utterly unclear whether there is any other level of explanation relative to which they constitute a single kind. To the extent that delusions comprise a coherent kind, it is surely most plausible to maintain that they comprise a psychological kind of some sort. Indeed, delusions appear to a *paradigmatic* example of a psychological kind. But if delusions are multiply realizable relative to our psychology, then what would the level of unity be? Sociological? Historical? What? The problem is that there seems to be no plausible option other than psychology. In which case, if delusions constitute a unified kind at all, then it would seem that they have to constitute a psychological kind.

A second, more plausible response to the neural heterogeneity objection turns on the distinction between specific and generic natural kinds. By way of illustration, consider a case from chemistry. Magnesium is plausibly a natural kind. It is one of the chemical elements: one that exhibits a complex cluster of properties, and is subject to many robust empirical generalizations. But metals also constitute a natural kind, though it is a more generic kind that has magnesium (and iron and aluminum etc.) as subordinate kinds or species. The suggestion is that advocates of the NK thesis can respond to the present objection by claming that what goes for chemical kinds is true of psychiatric kinds as well. Again, this leads to a positive moral.

Positive moral # 4: If the NK thesis is true, then delusions are most plausibly construed as a generic kind – one that may well subsume many different subordinate or species kinds. Indeed, this seems to be the right result for proponents of the NK thesis to embrace. For there really does seem to be myriad different kinds of delusions; and an adequate version of the NK thesis is required to capture not merely the unity in the kind but also the theoretically salient dissimilarities as well. Precisely what these theoretically salient groupings are, should not, of course, be considered a matter for *a priori* speculation. Rather, if the NK thesis is true, then it is a matter to be determined by further empirical inquiry. This is, among other things, because the matter of how best to subdivide delusion will turn crucially on which sorts of mechanisms turn out to be responsible for different kinds of delusions. And this is clearly an empirical matter.

3.8 Conclusion: the unity problem

This chapter has been an extended exercise in philosophical ground clearing intended to clarify and defend the thesis that delusions constitute a natural kind. Specifically, I have argued that the main extant reasons for rejecting the NK thesis are unsatisfactory. The argument from anti-essentialism fails because natural kinds need not have sortal essences. Continuity arguments fail because, at most, they establish a continuity of symptoms wholly compatible with the NK thesis. The arguments for mind dependence fail because they do not show that delusions are individuatively dependent; and heterogeneity objections fail because they only impose constraints on the sort of natural kind that delusions would need to be, as opposed to showing that they are not a natural kind of any sort.

In addition to these negative conclusions, I have also argued that there are *prima facie* reasons for taking the NK thesis seriously; and laboured to identify both the general conception of natural kinds that should be relevant to the present discussion and those more specific properties that delusions would need to possess, if the NK thesis is true. Specifically, if the NK thesis is true, then delusions most likely constitute a multiply realizable, generic cognitive kind whose members characteristically, though not invariably, exhibit those properties enumerated by the standard account of delusion: falsity, entrenchment, doxastic isolation, resistance to rational persuasion, and resistance to available incompatible information. On this view, then, there may be many species of mechanisms responsible for the production of those properties characteristic of delusions. But these various species of mechanism will need to bear important similarities to each other. They will need to be mechanisms of the same generic kind.

This raises perhaps *the* fundamental explanatory challenge for any natural kinds approach to delusion; what I call the *unity problem*. If many different subtypes of mechanism are responsible for delusions, why treat delusions *as such* as a natural kind? It must be because these mechanisms are themselves of the same kind. For, by assumption, natural kinds are individuated by their causal essences. But what is it about these various mechanisms that make them sub-types of some more general mechanism type, as opposed to merely a heterogeneous collection of *different* mechanisms? This is the unity problem. An adequate answer must specify a unifying characterization of the relevant mechanism type; and moreover, must do so without merely deferring to the fact that they produce similar effects – i.e. those properties associated with delusion. With the ground clearing complete, it is this challenge that should form the focus of future naturalistic research on the nature of delusion.

Acknowledgements

I would like to thank Ben Caplan, Dominic Murphy, and Tim Schroeder for stimulating discussions of the issues covered in this chapter. I would also like to thank the editors for their helpful comments on an earlier draft.

References

Bell, V., Halligan, P. W., and Ellis, H. D. (2006a). Diagnosing delusions: a review of inter-rater reliability. *Schizophrenia Research*, **86**(1–3), 76–79.

Bell, V., Halligan, P., and Ellis, H. D. (2006b). Explaining delusions: a cognitive perspective. *Trends in Cognitive Sciences*, **10**(5), 219–226.

Birchwood, M., Iqbal, Z., Chadwick, P., and Trower, P. (2000). Cognitive approach to depression and suicidal thinking in psychosis: 1. Ontogeny of post-psychotic depression. *British Journal of Psychiatry*, **177**, 516–521.

Blakemore, S. J., Wolpert, D. M., and Frith, C. D. (2002). Abnormalities in the awareness of action. *Trends in Cognitive Sciences*, **6**(6), 237–242.

Blakemore, S. J., Oakley, D. A., and Frith, C. D. (2003). Delusions of alien control in the normal brain. *Neuropsychologia*, **41**, 1058–1067.

Block, N. (1997). Anti-reductionism slaps back. In *Philosophical Perspectives 11: Mind, Causation, and World* (ed. J. E. Tomberlin), pp. 107–133. Oxford, Blackwell.

Boyd, R. (1990). What realism implies and what it does not. *Dialectica*, **43**, 5–29.

Boyd, R. (1991). Realism, antifoundationalism, and the enthusiasm for natural kinds. *Philosophical Studies*, **61**, 127–148.

Buchanan, A. and Wessely, S. (2004). Delusions, action and insight. In *Insight and Psychosis* (eds. X. F. Aamdor and A. S. David), 2nd edn. Oxford, Oxford University Press.

Dennett, D. C. (1995). *Darwin's Dangerous Idea*. New York, Simon and Schuster.

Ellis, B. (2001). *Scientific Essentialism*. Cambridge, Cambridge University Press.

Ellis, H.D. and Lewis, M.B. (2001). Capgras delusion: a window on face recognition. *Trends in Cognitive Science*, **5**, 149–156.

Ereshefsky, M. (forthcoming) Natural kinds in biology In *Routledge Encyclopedia of Philosophy* (ed. E. Craig).

Freeman, D. (2007) Suspicious minds: the psychology of persecutory delusions. *Clinical Psychology Review*, **27**(4), 425–457.

Freeman, D. and Garety, P. A. (2006). Delusions. In *Practitioners' Guide to Evidence-Based Psychotherapy* (eds. E. Fisher and W. O'Donohue). New York, Springer Academic.

Freeman, D., Garety, P. A., Kuipers, E., Fowler, D., and Bebbington, P. E. (2002). A cognitive model of persecutory delusions. *British Journal of Clinical Psychology, 41*, 331–347.

Fulford, K. W. M. (1994). Insight, delusion and the intentionality of action: framework for a philosophical psychopathology. In *Philosophical Psychopathology* (eds. G. Graham and G. L. Stephens) Cambridge, MA, MIT Press.

Garety, P. A. and Hemsley, D. R. (1994). *Delusions: Investigations into the Psychology of Delusional Reasoning.* Oxford, Oxford University Press.

Gelman, S. and Hirschfeld, L. (1999). How biological is essentialism? In *Folkbiology* (eds. D. Medin and S. Atran). Cambridge, MA, MIT Press.

Ghaemi, S. N. (2004). The perils of belief: delusions reexamined. *Philosophy, Psychiatry, and Psychology, 11*(1), 49–54.

Gibbard, A. (1990). *Wise Choices, Apt Feelings.* Oxford, Oxford University Press.

Griffiths, P. E. (1997). *What Emotions Really Are.* Chicago, IL, University of Chicago Press, Chicago.

Hacking, I. (1991). A tradition of natural kinds. *Philosophical Studies, 61*, 109–126.

Howson, C. and Urbach, P. (1993). *Scientific Reasoning: The Bayesian Approach,* 2nd edn. Chicago, Open Court.

Johns, L. C. and van Os, J. (2001). The continuity of psychotic experiences in the general population. *Clinical Psychology Review, 21*, 1125–1141.

Kim, J. (1992). Multiple realization and the metaphysics of reduction. *Philosophy and Phenomenological Research, 52*, 1–26.

Kripke, S. (1972). Naming and necessity. In *Semantics of Natural Language* (eds. D. Davidson and G. Harman). The Netherlands, Reidel, Dordrecht.

Lewis, D. (1986). *On the Plurality of Worlds.* Oxford, Blackwell.

Machery, E. (2005). Concepts are not a natural kind. *Philosophy of Science, 72*, 444–467.

Murphy, D. (2006). *Psychiatry in the Scientific Image.* Cambridge, MA, MIT Press.

Nozick, R. (1993). *The Nature of Rationality.* Princeton, NJ, Princeton University Press.

Page, S. (2006). Mind-independence disambiguated: separating the meat from the straw in the realism/anti-realism debate. *Ratio XIX 3*, 321–335.

Putnam, H. (1975). The meaning of 'meaning'. In *Mind Language, and Reality* (ed. H. Putnam), pp. 215–271. Cambridge, Cambridge University Press.

Pylyshyn, Z. (1984). *Computation and Cognition.* Cambridge, MA, MIT Press.

Quine, W. V. O. (1969). Natural kinds. In *Ontological Relativity and Other Essays* (ed. W. V. O. Quine), pp. 114–138. New York, Columbia University Press.

Shapiro, L. (2000). Multiple realizations. *Journal of Philosophy, 97*, 635–654.

Soames, S. (Forthcoming) What are natural kinds? *Philosophical Topics.*

Sorensen, R. (2006). 'Epistemic paradoxes', 'Nothingness', and 'Vagueness.' In *Stanford Encyclopedia of Philosophy* (ed. E. Zalta). (http://plato.stanford.edu)

Stich, S. (1990). *The Fragmentation of Reason.* Cambridge, MA, MIT Press.

Stoljar, D. and Gold, I. (1998). On cognitive and biological neuroscience. *Mind and Language 13*(1), 110–131.

Unger, P. (1979). I do not exist. In *Perception and Identity* (ed. G. F. MacDonald). London, Macmillan.

van Os, J. (2003). Is there a continuum of psychotic experiences in the general population? *Epidemiologia e Psichiatria Sociale*, **12**, 242–252.

Verdoux, H., Maurice-Tison, S., Gay, B., Van Os, J., Salamon, R., and Bourgeois, M. L. (1998). A survey of delusional ideation in primary-care patients. *Psychological Medicine*, **28**(1), 127–134.

Verdoux, H., Van Os, J. (2002). Psychotic symptoms in non-clinical populations and the continuum of psychosis. *Schizophrenia research*, **54**(1–2), 59–65.

Wakefield, J. C. (1992). Disorder as harmful dysfunction: a conceptual critique of DSM-III-R's definition of mental disorder. *Psychological Review*, **99**, 232–247.

Weisberg, M. (2005). Water is not H$_2$O. In *Philosophy of Chemistry: Synthesis of a New Discipline* (eds. D. Baird, E. Scerri, and L. McIntyre), pp. 337–345. New York, Springer.

Zachar, P. (2000). Psychiatric disorders are not natural kinds. *Philosophy, Psychiatry, and Psychology*, **7**, 167–182.

Section 2

The nature of mental illness

Chapter 4

Mental illness is indeed a myth

Hanna Pickard

Abstract

This chapter offers a novel defence of Szasz's claim that mental illness is a myth by bringing to bear a standard type of thought experiment used in philosophical discussions of the meaning of natural kind concepts. This makes it possible to accept Szasz's conclusion that mental illness involves problems of living, some of which may be moral in nature, while bypassing the debate about the meaning of the concept of illness. The chapter then considers the nature of schizophrenia and the personality disorders (PDs) within this framework. It argues that neither is likely to constitute a scientifically valid category, but that nonetheless their symptoms can be scientifically explained. It concludes with a discussion of the way in which Cluster B or 'bad' PDs involve failures of virtue or character, and argues that this does not preclude them from being appropriately treated within contemporary, multidisciplinary, mental health services.

4.1 **Introduction**

Thomas Szasz is famous for his slogan that mental illness is a myth (Szasz, 1960, 1974). Its pithiness makes it ambiguous. Its shock content makes it politically serviceable. But nonetheless it summarizes an interesting and substantial philosophical position. Szasz's position is that the problems which psychiatry treats are not medical but moral. That is because mental illness is not actually an illness – properly understood.

The aim of this chapter is to explore what is right and what is wrong in this view. The chapter has three parts. In the first part, I outline Szasz's argument that mental illness is not actually an illness, together with some of the more common objections to it. I resolve this debate by bringing to bear a type of thought experiment which is standardly used in philosophical accounts of the meaning of natural kind concepts. This makes it possible to get beyond semantic disputes over the meaning of the concept of illness. Szasz's claim that mental illness is a myth can then be reconciled with the potential scientific validity of particular kinds of mental illnesses. In the second part,

I briefly examine the evidence against schizophrenia having this status. Although there is reason to be sceptical that schizophrenia constitutes a scientifically valid category, I suggest that this should not make us sceptical that its symptoms are open to scientific explanation, broadly conceived. In the third part, I turn to the Cluster B or 'bad' PDs. PDs are generally regarded as poorly defined and unlikely to be real illnesses or diseases. Louis Charland has argued that the Cluster B categories – narcissistic, histrionic, borderline, and antisocial – are by definition moral as opposed to clinical conditions (Charland, 2004, 2006). Hence the Cluster B PDs seem poised to vindicate Szasz's position. I argue that Charland's account of Cluster B PDs is overly simplistic. The Cluster B PDs do involve, among other traits, failures of virtue and character. However, it is possible to construct scientific explanations of the development of virtue and character – of how it progresses or fails. And this in turn helps us understand why one of the most effective treatments for PDs, namely, group psychotherapy, works. For these and other reasons, Cluster B PDs are appropriately treated in contemporary, multidisciplinary, mental health clinics. Taken together, these considerations make the question of whether or not the PDs are medical conditions idle. The chapter concludes by highlighting the relevance of these findings to Szasz's overall view.

4.2 Bodily illness, mental illness, and natural kinds

The aim of this section is to show that Szasz's positive conclusions about the nature of mental illness can be preserved even if his argument purporting to establish these conclusions is rejected. In outline, Szasz's argument for the claim that mental illness is a myth is as follows. Mental illness would appear from its name to be a kind of illness. But Szasz believes that our understanding of illness is fundamentally bodily: bodily illness is our basic paradigm or model of illness. We do not have two equal species of a single conceptual kind. Hence, only if mental illness meets the criteria for illness, as established by reflection on the paradigm or model of bodily illness, can it count as real. What then are the criteria for illness? Szasz holds that illness involves a deviation from the normal anatomical or physiological structure and functioning of the human body. Clearly, such deviations can be of great concern to us: illness has negative connotations, just as health has positive ones. But Szasz thinks we should aim to extract the scientific core of the concept of illness from its more evaluative connotations. The deviations are to be biologically defined as, for instance, lesions can be. Given this account of our concept of illness, we can now ask whether or not mental illness is indeed a real illness. The answer will depend on whether or not mental illness involves a deviation from the normal anatomical or physiological structure and functioning of the human body. And Szasz claims that the scientific evidence suggests that it does not. It involves instead a deviation from 'psychosocial, ethical, and legal' norms (Szasz, 1960, p.114).

Hence, according to Szasz, the term 'mental illness' is a misnomer. Mental illness is not illness. It is rather a form of cultural deviation – a failure, whether voluntary or not, to conform to normal physical and psychological behavioural expectations. The concept is used to refer to 'problems of living' so severe, wayward, or disturbing, for the individual or society, that they are not treated as falling within the more ordinary, acceptable miseries and difficulties of human life. These problems are of course perfectly real. Something is very much wrong. But they do not constitute an illness, according to Szasz, once that term has been properly understood.

Szasz has always claimed that, if science ultimately provides evidence for an organic, biological basis for mental illness, then it would count as a real illness. The most likely basis would of course involve a deviation from the normal structure and functioning of the human brain. Hence he concedes that if, for instance, a brain lesion was discovered which reliably correlated with schizophrenia, then schizophrenia would count as a real illness. Mental illness would not be a myth.

Critics often seize on this concession. On the one hand, neuroscience has progressed since Szasz first put forward this argument. Perhaps, there is now sufficient evidence for a correlation between abnormal structure and functioning of the brain and schizophrenia for it to count as a real illness. I shall discuss some of this evidence in the following section. But, even if the jury is still out on the current strength of the evidence, one might think that it is a good bet that strong evidence for a neural basis for mental illness will in the end be forthcoming. Scientific optimism in this respect may not seem irrational.

On the other hand, critics often seize on Szasz's account of bodily illness, for it is clearly open to counterexample. Athletic prowess, for instance, is a deviation from normal anatomical or physiological structure and functioning. But it is not an illness. Moreover, the account provides no measure for determining how much deviation is required for illness. When, for instance, does raised blood sugar truly become diabetes?[1] These gaps in Szasz's account have contributed to a growing literature attempting to analyse our concepts of illness and disease, and correspondingly, well-being and health. One powerful alternative account links illness or disease to evolutionary disadvantage: illness or disease is a dysfunction which is likely to reduce life or reproductive expectancy (Boorse, 1975; Kendell, 1975). Scientific evidence can then be mustered to argue that particular kinds of mental illnesses do or do not constitute this sort of dysfunction. There is evidence, for instance, that schizophrenia is correlated with reduced life expectancy and increased risk of suicide (Radomsky et al., 1999; Hannerz et al., 2001). Another alternative account links illness or disease to failures of action or 'ordinary doing' (Fulford, 1989). Many symptoms of mental illness are failures of action. For instance, arguably most of the negative symptoms of schizophrenia, such as athymia (flattening of emotional expressions and action), alogia (reduction in speech and poverty of speech content), and abulia (lack of personal grooming and general low energy), as well as some of the positive symptoms, such as delusions of control, involve disorders of action. Hence according to both these alternative accounts, mental illness again would not be a myth.

But Szasz should not have made his initial concession. Or, more precisely, it is possible to hold both of the following claims: first, that particular kinds of mental illnesses may prove to be valid scientific kinds, and second, that our concept of mental

---

[1] See Haslam, 2002 for an attempt to answer this kind of question through practical considerations.

illness, as an overarching or generic category, involves a deviation from 'psychosocial, ethical, and legal' norms and, in this sense, may be unlike our concept of bodily illness – however this is ultimately correctly understood. To see why this conjunction is possible, I want to bring to bear on this debate the standard type of thought experiment used in philosophy to establish whether or not a concept is a natural kind concept.

This type of philosophical thought experiment involves prying apart the superficial properties of a kind of thing from its underlying, scientific properties. This allows us to test our intuitions about the meaning of the concept of that kind: to determine which sorts of properties the concept tracks. Consider, for instance, a famous example from Hilary Putnam's early work on externalism about meaning (Putnam, 1973).[2] Water is a colourless, clear liquid which we drink and with which we clean. It is found in oceans, lakes, and rain clouds, as well as baths and bottles. It freezes and evaporates in certain circumstances. These are some of its superficial properties. We learn about these properties of water simply by living in the ordinary world, observing, and interacting with it. But water also has the chemical composition H_2O. We learn about this only by doing science. Now imagine that there is a planet called Twin Earth. On Twin Earth, there is a liquid which looks and behaves and is used just like water. It is even called 'water' by the natives. But it has a different chemical composition. We can call this XYZ. Is the liquid found on Twin Earth actually water? Putnam thinks that our intuitions are clear: it is not. Water is H_2O. This liquid is XYZ.

What we learn from this thought experiment is that our concept of water is not determined by superficial properties. It is rather determined by underlying, scientific properties, such as chemical composition. That is the essence of what water is. Only something that possesses the scientific property of having the chemical composition of H_2O can be water. That is why XYZ is not water despite having all the same superficial properties. Hence, our concept of water is a natural kind concept because its meaning is linked to underlying, scientific properties, as opposed to superficial properties. The concept tracks a kind of thing which exists in the natural world independently of us and our interactions with or conceptions of that thing.

Now imagine the following thought experiment about schizophrenia. Schizophrenia is currently defined by its symptoms. These are superficial or personal-level properties pertaining to psychological and physical functioning and behaviour, which are identified by psychiatrists through interview and observation. But now suppose that, as Szasz concedes is possible, we discover a brain lesion that correlates with schizophrenia. Suppose that this correlation is extremely reliable. It is so reliable, in fact, that the diagnostic procedure for schizophrenia changes. When psychiatrists see a new patient who, at first sight, has a clinical presentation which might indicate schizophrenia, rather than using interview and observation, they perform a brain scan in aid of diagnosis: they test in the first instance for the underlying scientific property, not for the superficial symptoms.

---

[2] See also Kripke, 1972 for a seminal discussion of these topics.

Now suppose that, in the course of routine brain scans, say, we discover a person who has this lesion, but none of the symptoms currently definitional of schizophrenia.[3] Her problems of living are perfectly ordinary. Nothing is terribly wrong. That is a conceptual possibility we seem to be able to coherently imagine once we have embarked on this thought experiment. It may also be a metaphysical possibility. Compare, for instance, prostate cancer. A man may have prostate cancer (because the cells in his prostate have mutated into cancer cells) without having any superficial symptoms which would have led to a diagnosis in absence of advance screening (such as a blood-test for increased prostate-specific antigen). But, for our needs, conceptual possibility is sufficient: our interest lies in probing the meaning of our concepts.

Does this woman have schizophrenia? We may be unsure, but, it seems at least possible that, given the conditions imagined in this thought experiment, our intuitions incline us to think that she does. For instance, we can easily imagine that she might be advised that the lesion should be operated on for preventative reason, lest it develop from 'latent' into 'full-blown' schizophrenia. But instead, suppose we ask: is this woman mentally ill? It seems our intuitions about this are entirely clear. She is not. We may in the end judge that she has schizophrenia, given the hypothesized discovery of its underlying, scientific property and its place in diagnostic procedures. But she is not mentally ill – any more than she is mentally disturbed, or mentally distressed, or mad, or crazy, or insane. She has no superficial or personal-level symptoms. She does not deviate from our 'psychosocial, ethical, and legal' norms.

Hence Szasz's claim that mental illness, considered as an overarching or generic category, is a myth is compatible with the claim that particular kinds of mental illnesses, like schizophrenia, are valid scientific kinds. If we pry apart the superficial and the underlying scientific properties, our concept of mental illness tracks the former, even if our concepts of particular kinds of mental illnesses track or come to track the latter.

The importance of this point is twofold. First, it is important because it means that Szasz need not concede that science may in the end prove him wrong. Practically, that helps safeguard the various positive clinical and political changes that have their origins partly in Szasz's ideas, such as the new focus on mental health service-user involvement and responsibility. Theoretically, that allows us to begin to set the potential interest and truth of Szasz's views about the moral nature of psychiatric problems within a developing psychiatric science. I shall discuss what this means in more detail in the following sections of this chapter.

Second, it is important because it allows us to bypass the ongoing debate about the meaning of our concepts of illness, disease, well-being, and health. For it is reasonable to be sceptical that this debate will prove fruitful if conducted as an analytic enterprise. On the one hand, just as there were counterexamples to Szasz's account of bodily illness, so too there are counterexamples to evolutionary and action accounts. For instance, evolutionary accounts typically count homosexuality as an illness or disease, whilst failing to count conditions like non-erythrodermic psoriasis. Action accounts

---

[3] To aid the imagination, we can hypothesize if we wish that her cognitive reserve is extraordinarily high.

have difficulty accommodating illnesses whose symptoms involve not dysfunctions of movement, but abnormal subjective experiences and pain, for instance, mild tooth decay, or the common cold. On the other hand, all these accounts face the problem of how much these concepts involve phenomenological as opposed to scientific criteria; and, relatedly, how much they involve the idea that illness and disease are bad, health and well-being good.[4]

We can, of course, choose to stipulate what we shall take these concepts to mean. It might be helpful, for instance, both for political and theoretical purposes, to reserve the concept of disease for evolutionary dysfunction, and to use the concept of illness to cover more subjective, experiential properties of poor health.[5] But that would constitute a decision, not an analysis. Our concepts of illness, disease, well-being, and health – whether mental or physical – lie at the interface of science and common sense, of fact and value, as well as exhibiting a large degree of cultural and historical development and variation.[6] It is thus highly unlikely that they are the right kind of concepts to admit of the kind of analytical definition which is needed to ground philosophical arguments of the sort Szasz and his critics alike envisage. Of course, that is not to say that their exploration is not of considerable interest. But it should be undertaken firmly as a social and historical explanatory endeavour, not as a question of semantic analysis.

Hence, no matter how the concept of illness is properly understood, and whether or not mental illness conforms to it, we can yet draw two conclusions. First, Szasz is correct that our concept of mental illness and its cognates involve 'deviation from psychosocial, ethical, and legal norms'. These concepts refer to problems of living which are certainly personal, and possibly moral. Second, particular kinds of mental illnesses may yet constitute valid scientific kinds. The next section looks at the status of schizophrenia in this regard.

4.3 **The scientific status of schizophrenia**

The paradigm example of a kind of mental illness which might count as a real illness is schizophrenia. But scepticism about the prospects of analyzing illness and related concepts should make us wary of focusing too narrowly on the question of whether or not schizophrenia is an illness. Instead, we can ask a related though distinct question, namely, whether or not it constitutes a valid scientific kind or category. This is because, a positive answer to that question might be sufficient – given the clinical features of schizophrenia, which are not in dispute – for schizophrenia to then count as a real illness, whatever that ultimately does or should mean.

Is schizophrenia a valid scientific kind or category? Sometimes philosophers intend something very modest by this idea. They mean only that a category is in fact scientifically studied and supports explanations and inductive inferences (Dupre, 1993; Cooper, 2007).

---

[4] See Carel, 2008 for an account that emphasizes the phenomenological aspects of health and illness.

[5] Arguably this is how Boorse, 1975 should be read.

[6] See, for instance, Foucault, 1971 and 1976; Kleinman, 1980; Thagard, 1997; Porter, 2002.

But if that is all that is meant, then PDs are as scientifically valid as schizophrenia. For there is a wealth of scientific research on, for instance, borderline PD, and it is clear that knowing that a person is borderline allows one to offer explanations and make inductive inferences which are potentially as reliable as any psychological inferences can be (e.g. if someone is borderline, then perceptions of abandonment will cause immoderate fear and anger responses). In the next section, I shall explore the extent to which the Cluster B PDs may indeed be open to scientific explanation. But it is clear that those who appeal to schizophrenia as a scientifically valid category of mental illness would wish to distinguish it from the more amorphous PDs. So this modest understanding cannot be sufficient to capture the scientific hope for schizophrenia.

The potential scientific validity of schizophrenia instead typically involves two ideas. The first is that schizophrenia is a category which carves the world at its joints: it accurately picks out a real and independently existing kind of thing, objectively distinct from other, perhaps superficially comparable, kinds of things. Indeed, this is explicitly recognized in DSM-IV which states that psychiatric categories succeed when 'there are clear boundaries between classes, and when the different classes are mutually exclusive' (APA, 1994, p. xxii). The second is that an underlying, scientific basis for schizophrenia will be found which is correlated with and potentially explanatory of the development and nature of its superficial symptoms.

It is now widely accepted within schizophrenia research that there is strong evidence for questioning whether schizophrenia is a scientifically valid category thus understood. The evidence involves the difficulty distinguishing it from other mental illnesses and, in particular, the other major Axis I psychosis, bipolar disorder, together with the presence of minor psychotic symptoms in the general and prodrome population. Broadly speaking, there are at least six major considerations.[7]

Genetics and brain structure. The most likely underlying, scientific correlate for schizophrenia is genes or brain structure. With respect to genetics, it is well known that mental illness runs in families. There is some evidence that certain specific psychotic symptoms, like thought disorder, may do as well (Wahlberg *et al.*, 1997). However, other symptoms, like paranoid tendencies and delusions, probably do not (Coolidge *et al.*, 2001). But it is clear that genetic factors are only one element in a causal explanation of schizophrenia. Analysis of twin and adoptive studies, for instance, seems to point to the importance of non-genetic factors in the development of schizophrenia (Bentall, 2003). Prenatal development, substance abuse, stress, anxiety, and mood disorders, and social and environmental factors such as urban life, migration, poverty, family dysfunction, and isolation, are all thought to be contributors (Broome *et al.*, 2005). Many of these factors, of course, are known to contribute to the development of other kinds of mental illnesses too. Finally, the genes that seem to be correlated with schizophrenia are non-specific: they are also correlated with bipolar disorder (Craddock *et al.*, 2006).

With respect to brain structure, there is ample evidence for structural and functional brain abnormalities in schizophrenia (Shenton *et al.*, 2001). However, there is

---

[7] See Bentall, 2003 for a good survey of this and related evidence.

some evidence that some of these abnormalities may be caused by medication (Molina *et al.*, 2005). And there are relatively few studies of brain abnormalities in other mental illnesses, in particular, bipolar disorder, so comparative studies are not readily available. Finally, until we have a fuller and more precise understanding of how the brain abnormalities in schizophrenia cause superficial symptoms, we cannot rule out the possibility that they are caused by them.

Reliability of diagnoses. The reliability of diagnoses for mental illness is not high. A reliability study of diagnosis of schizophrenia and bipolar disorder for DSM-III where conditions were idealized, places the reliability of diagnoses at 0.6 (Williams *et al.*, 1992). A more recent study in non-idealized conditions places it at 0.65 (McGorry *et al.*, 1995). Meanwhile, the further criteria and complications introduced in DSM-IV make the categories of mental illness themselves appear increasingly gerrymandered (Kutchins and Kirk, 1997). Of course, lack of reliability is not conclusive evidence. Clinical training and procedures vary. Humans are fallible. However, reliability is nonetheless a general indication or guide to stable and objective categories. When a category is scientifically valid and a procedure for identifying the category standard, it is reasonable to expect reliability to be good.

Exclusion rules and co-morbidity. A salient form of gerrymandering is the use of exclusion rules to ensure the uniqueness of diagnosis in DSM-IV. For instance, a person cannot be diagnosed with schizophrenia if he or she meets the criteria for schizoaffective disorder, major depression, or mania. Similarly, a patient cannot be diagnosed with bipolar disorder if his or her symptoms fit a different diagnosis better. In a large-scale study funded by the American National Institute for Mental Health involving over 18 000 patients, it was found that 60% of people who met the criteria for one disorder equally met the criteria for another disorder if the exclusion rules were suspended (Robins *et al.*, 1991). This level of co-morbidity is higher than chance. It is also higher than we might expect even taking into account the potential causal interaction between different categories of mental illness. It seems likely that it reflects a failure of the DSM-IV categories to capture objectively real and distinct scientific kinds.

Discriminant function analysis. Studies using discriminant function analysis seem to indicate a continuum between schizophrenia and bipolar disorder. The basic idea behind this sort of analysis is simple. Patients are not diagnosed but are instead assigned scores according to the extent to which their individual symptoms are schizophrenic, and the extent to which their individual symptoms are bipolar. If schizophrenia and bipolar disorder are real and distinct kinds, the majority of the patients' scores should cluster at one or either pole. Instead, the opposite appears to be the case: most patients' scores are intermediate (Kendell and Gourlay, 1970; Brockington *et al.*, 1991).

Psychotic symptoms in the general and prodrome population. Isolated and transient psychotic phenomena are present in the general population. One study suggests that 25% of the general population report hallucinations or delusions (Poulton *et al.*, 2000). Some of the risk factors associated with schizophrenia are also associated with such minor psychotic phenomena (van Os *et al.*, 2000). Hence there is evidence that minor symptoms in the general population are related to the psychotic symptoms of schizophrenia. There are also prodromal patients who seem to develop along a trajectory: from cognitive dysfunction, to decreased motivation and social-ization, to positive psychotic symptoms but without sufficient intensity and longevity to meet the criteria for schizophrenia (Broome *et al.*, 2005). Some of these patients go on to develop symptoms which do meet the criteria, but others do not. This combined evidence suggests that schizophrenic-type symptoms are not unique to schizophrenia, but rather exist along a continuum.

The history and sociology of psychiatry. This topic is too large to be adequately addressed within the scope of this chapter. However, it is worth emphasizing that psychiatry has had a complicated history, and has been more subject, than many disciplines, to political, social, and legal pressures. Decisions about how to demarcate psychiatric categories have clear practical human import, in a way that decisions about how to demarcate sub-atomic particles do not. It is also worth remembering that mental illnesses befall people who then come to think of themselves as a particular kind of person, with a particular sort of problem. Ways of conceptualizing symptoms can then become less tractable, and can also spread through cultural transmission. Although this may be less applicable to schizophrenia than to identity, eating, and personality disorders, an awareness of the historical and social context of psychiatry is still essential.[8]

Taken together, this evidence suggests that schizophrenia is not a category that carves the world at its joints. As yet, scientists have not discovered an underlying, scientific property, whether genetic or neurological, with which it is distinctively cor-related. Meanwhile, evidence stemming from studies of reliability, co-morbidity, dis-criminant function analysis, psychotic symptoms in the general and prodrome population, and the history and sociology of psychiatry, suggests that the category as currently defined, by superficial properties, is unlikely to be tracking a unified and distinct kind of thing. Hence the possibility that schizophrenia picks out real symp-toms without tracking a scientifically valid kind is genuine.[9] Importantly, this does not mean that the symptoms of schizophrenia cannot be scientifically explained.

Suppose that, rather than conceive of our current categories of mental illnesses as falling into real and distinct kinds, we conceive of them as positioned along a continuum or spectrum: there are various dimensions along which all patients vary. It may none-theless be possible to carve up the continuum or spectrum in a scientifically objective way. Factor analyses attempt to do just this. They attempt scientifically to establish how symptoms cluster together. There is growing evidence, for instance, that schizophrenia divides into three clusters: positive symptoms (e.g. hallucinations and delusions), negative

---

[8] For discussion of some of these themes, see, for instance, Hacking, 1995, 1998, and 1999; Bentall, 2003; Fulford *et al.*, 2006; Radden, 2006.

[9] It is possible to accept this point while yet holding that schizophrenia is nonetheless a kind and not just a collection of symptoms. Haslam, 2002, suggests that we need to allow for many 'kinds of kinds': psychiatric illnesses may not be natural kinds, but they may nonetheless be practical, fuzzy, or discrete kinds.

symptoms (e.g. apathy, athymia, and asociality), and cognitive disorganization (e.g. disturbed speech and problems of attention) (Liddle, 1987; Andreasen *et al.*, 1995). There is also some evidence that these clusters may be valid not only for schizophrenia, but also for major depression and bipolar disorder (Toomey *et al.*, 1998). There are substantive questions about the validity of factor analysis, involving selection of symptoms, patients, and methods of calculation. But importantly, if the division of symptoms into clusters can be validated, the process of discovering an underlying, scientific property, which is not only correlated with the cluster, but potentially explanatory of it, can begin. Cognitive models for clusters of symptoms can be constructed. Bridges to neuroscience can then be built. And causal and development conditions can be explored. A focus on clusters of symptoms opens the door to scientific explanation, in a way that a focus on categories of mental illness currently does not.[10]

If schizophrenia is not a scientifically valid kind, then the prospects of any of our current categories of mental illness proving to be so are dim. But nonetheless, we have a model of how the symptoms of schizophrenia – Szasz's 'problems of living' – can potentially be scientifically explained. In the next and final section of this paper, I consider the Cluster B PDs, and whether or not this is equally true of them.

4.4 **The 'bad' personality disorders: moral or medical conditions?**

PDs are not generally regarded as mental illnesses, although few would deny that people with PD experience high levels of mental distress and disturbance. They are defined as 'an enduring pattern of inner experience and behaviour that departs markedly from the individual's culture, is pervasive and inflexible, has an onset in adolescence or early adulthood, is stable over time, and leads to distress and impairment' (APA, 1994, p. 629). Classifications of PDs have shifted over time. DSM-IV groups them into three clusters. Cluster A includes paranoid, schizoid, and schizotypal; Cluster B includes antisocial, borderline, histrionic, and narcissistic; Cluster C includes avoidant, dependent, and obsessive–compulsive. These are colloquially called the 'mad', 'bad', and 'sad' clusters respectively. Although precise percentages are disputed, there appear to be high levels of co-morbidity between PDs, and between PDs and Axis I disorders, as well as high levels of PD in the population at large. Patients with PDs have a reputation of being difficult to treat, and being disliked by clinicians.

Louis Charland has argued that Cluster B PDs are empirically valid categories, in that they represent genuine behavioural syndromes and capture regularities in human behaviour, but that they are not clinically valid categories (Charland, 2004, 2006). Charland does not define what a clinically valid category is. But the reason he gives is that, in contrast with the other types of PDs, he takes Cluster B PDs to be moral conditions: they are defined by moral failings. He points out that the criteria for antisocial PD include lying and conning. Narcissistic PD is partly defined by a lack of empathy. And he takes the

---

[10] For a paradigm example of this approach, see Frith, 1992. Frith explains schizophrenic disorders of thought and action as stemming from a failure of self-monitoring. Although I am sympathetic to the spirit of this kind of account, I question the adequacy of some of its details in my 'Schizophrenia and the epistemology of self-knowledge' (under review).

inappropriate sexual behaviour characteristic of histrionic PD, and the intense anger, impulsivity, and instability of personal relationships characteristic of borderline PD, to imply 'moral deficits in empathy and regard for others' (Charland, 2006, p. 122). Hence, he concludes that Cluster B PDs are not clinical but rather moral conditions. For this reason, recovery from a Cluster B PD involves something more akin to 'moral conversion' than medical treatment or therapy (*ibid.*). And there is no reason to think that psychiatrists, psychologists, or psychotherapists of virtually any bent are well placed to effect this.

Charland's argument is problematic in at least two regards. On the one hand, the supposed moral dimension of narcissistic, histrionic, and borderline PD is only one aspect of these categories. The criteria for diagnosis are polythetic: they are various, and a patient need only meet a required number for diagnosis, not all. So it is possible, for instance, to meet the threshold for diagnosis with narcissistic PD without lacking empathy. A person could instead suffer from grandiosity and a need for admiration on a sufficiently large scale. Similarly, severe and persistent self-harming behaviour is as central to borderline PD as intense anger towards others. Antisocial PD is perhaps different: here a pervasive disregard for and violation of the rights of others is more central to the syndrome. But, in general, the fact that certain categories of PD have a supposedly moral dimension does not on its own make them moral as opposed to clinical conditions. That would be to ignore all the other, standard clinical, dimensions of the category.

On the other hand, it is not clear that the dimensions of histrionic and borderline PD that concern Charland are properly described as moral deficits. Bernard Williams has suggested that morality proper is fundamentally to do with rights and obligations (Williams, 1985; 1993). Even if this seems too narrow, it does seem important to distinguish our concept of the moral from a broader, ethical perspective, which is concerned more generally with human virtue and goodness. Engaging in inappropriate sexual behaviour, as the histrionic person may, or failing to control intense anger and to lash out at others, as the borderline person may, certainly count as failings, but they are not obviously failures of morality. They are failures of character. These are not the kinds of things that the virtuous do. I work in a NHS Therapeutic Community for people with PD. Most of the patients meet the threshold for diagnosis with one or more Cluster B PD. Compared with people whose personalities are not diagnosable, these patients often seem to lack the virtues of, for instance, temperance and moderation, fairness and generosity to others, humility, trust, patience, and love and respect for self and others. Hence Charland has put his finger on something important, even if he has oversimplified his case. The Cluster B PDs do seem to represent an instance where Szasz's position is correct to this extent: psychiatry here treats problems which clearly pertain to questions, if not exactly of morality, then certainly of virtue and character. This raises two questions. First, can the 'bad' PDs nonetheless be scientifically explained? Second, are they medical conditions? In particular, should they be treated by psychiatrists within contemporary, multidisciplinary mental health clinics?

Consider first the question of scientific explanation. Charland claims that the Cluster B PDs are empirically valid categories in the modest sense of capturing regularities in behaviour and so supporting explanations and inductive inferences. This is clearly correct. But the more demanding question is whether it is possible to construct, at least in principle, a scientific explanation of how they develop. Part of the difficulty in answering this question is that, on the whole, there is little to go by. On the one hand, psychoanaltyic theory has offered developmental explanations for many of the features associated with PDs.[11] This body of theory can be clinically helpful. And some of its ideas are, once clarified, potentially important and testable. But as it stands as a theoretical corpus, its scientific status is dim. Academic psychology, on the other hand, has not tended to address itself explicitly to questions of the development of the virtues and the formation of character. For instance, Lawrence Kohlberg has developed a justly famous, clear, rigourous, and empirically validated theory of the stages of moral development (Kohlberg, 1981). But Kohlberg's theory – and the literature surrounding it – is concerned with moral reasoning, with a particular emphasis on justice. It does not address questions of virtue and character.

Indeed, arguably our best account of the development of the virtues and the formation of character is still Aristotle's.[12] Unlike many moral philosophers, Aristotle emphasizes the development of the good person over time. The acquisition of virtue and character is a long process, each phase consequent on what has come before. Simplifying somewhat, we can see Aristotle as dividing this process into three stages.

The first stage involves a good upbringing and a habituation to virtue. Desires and feelings start to shape patterns of motivation and response – start to shape character traits – well before children become reasonable and reflective beings. Children need to be brought up in an environment which allows virtuous ways of being to become their second nature. The virtues need to become habits, flowing more or less readily and easily, as opposed to involving deliberation or ambivalence. For this to happen, children need guidance. But the nature of this guidance is very distinctive. It is not only that the child must be guided so that he or she acquires the right habits. The child must also be guided so that, in acquiring these habits, he or she is able to come to see that they are good.

This is the second stage of development. What Aristotle means by the claim that the child must see that the virtues are good is not simple to spell out, but, roughly speaking, it involves knowing that behaving virtuously is good not simply because that is what one has been told, but for oneself. And Aristotle holds that one comes to this knowledge through pleasure and enjoyment of virtuous ways of being: one comes to see that virtue is good because one is guided in one's doing of virtuous actions so that one finds pleasure or enjoyment in the doing. This pleasure, and the knowledge that it produces, serves to transform childhood habits into stable states of character.

The third and final stage, which can only occur once the child has grown up and become a fully mature human being, is the acquisition, through reason and reflection, of the knowledge of why virtue is good. For Aristotle, such knowledge is only available to the person who already knows that it is.

---

[11] See, for instance, McWilliams, 1994, for a survey of the contribution of psychoanalysis to understanding personality and character.

[12] I owe my understanding of Aristotle's position to Myles Burnyeat's seminal paper 'Aristotle on learning to be good' (Burnyeat, 1980).

To make this more concrete, let us take as an example of the development of the capacity to share. Children need to be told that they must share. They need to be made to do it, so that it becomes a natural expectation that they have – a habit. But this guidance must not proceed by brute force. It must allow them to come to enjoy sharing, to find the pleasure in giving, and so to learn for themselves that sharing is good. Now it is a serious question what such guidance in fact involves. It is natural to conjecture that it should be, for instance, firm but not punishing; conscious of and open about the genuine struggle of sharing for the child, as well as praising of his or her successes; lastly, it should ensure that the child is also the recipient of sharing – that he or she gets a chance to experience how nice it is to be shared with. But whatever the precise nature of the guidance must be, the point is that it must allow the child to feel the pleasure in sharing. This pleasure then serves to cement the capacity to share in children – to make it a stable part of their character. Later, once they are grown, they can then reflect on why sharing is good. For instance, perhaps it is a requirement of kindness, or alternatively, of the principles of equality and justice.

The importance of Aristotle's account is that it provides us with a general and clear theory about how character traits form and develop over time – an abstract schema. And that schema is something that can be scientifically explored, both quite generally, and in the case of particular character traits.

Consider, for instance, the intense anger and impulsivity which is characteristic of borderline PD. This trait is essentially a failure of moderation and control of anger. No doubt one component of the explanation of possession of this trait is genetic predisposition. But most borderline patients have suffered terrible childhoods, with high levels of emotional, sexual, or physical abuse or neglect. They have not had the sort of upbringing and guidance Aristotle suggests the virtues require. Meanwhile, we are beginning to understand more about the development of the brain structure and functioning underpinning the control and moderation of anger. There is evidence that the orbitofrontal cortex is the part of the brain which, among other functions, is responsible for managing one's own emotions and responding to the emotions of others (O'Doherty et al., 2003; Schore, 2003). It can hold back strong and basic fear and anger responses, for instance, which originate in the evolutionarily more primitive amygdala and hypothalamus. But the proper development of the orbitofrontal cortex is experience-dependent. On the one hand, there is evidence that severe neglect in infancy is correlated with a lack of orbitofrontal development in later years (Chugani et al., 2001). On the other hand, there is evidence that positive attention – smiles, warmth, and praise – from carers produces a biochemical response with two effects: it is pleasurable and it helps the neurons in the obritofrontal cortex grow (Schore, 1994). The evidence about possible orbitofrontal abnormality among patients with borderline PD is limited, although there is some indication of hypometabolism and reduced volume (De La Fuente et al., 1997; Lyoo et al., 1998). However, an initial study comparing borderline PD patients with patients with damage to their obitofrontal cortex concludes that both categories of patients, in contrast with normal controls, were similar in the extent of their heightened anger and impulsivity, whilst differing in most other clinical respects (Berlin et al., 2005). Synthesizing this research suggests a simple hypothesis: the anger and impulsivity characteristic of borderline PD can be explained by abnormal development of the obitofrontal cortex because of early childhood neglect and abuse, perhaps in conjunction with genetic predisposition.

Of course, this hypothesis is only a beginning. It may prove wrong. And even if it proves true, there are many details left to flesh out. Can we say more about how and why the right sort of guidance facilitates orbitofrontal growth and the wrong sort of guidance impedes it? Can we say more about what the right or wrong sort of guidance is? How exactly does the orbitofrontal cortex control or fail to control these emotions? The point is that this hypothesis represents a kind of scientific explanation which should, in principle, be available for character traits quite generally – traits which we consider virtues, and traits which we consider vices. Aristotle has provided us with a general schema for thinking about the development of character. And the integration of research from genetics, psychology, psychiatry, neuroscience, and the social sciences can provide a way of explaining the genesis of particular traits within this schema.

It is possible that pursuing this sort of research will validate the categories of PD by revealing how each behavioural syndrome, with its polythetic criteria, has a coherent, unified scientific underlying and developmental explanation. More likely, perhaps, it will pry apart the different character traits within each category, explaining each individually, and suggesting how they naturally, although not inevitably, cluster together. The point is that the failings of virtue and character typical of PDs can be scientifically explained. Just as we can potentially explain the symptoms of schizophrenia and how they cluster, so too we can potentially explain the character traits typical of PDs and how they cluster. These explanations do not depend on either schizophrenia or the PDs being scientifically valid kinds.

Consider now the second question. Are Cluster B PDs medical conditions despite the fact that they involve failures of virtue and character? The fact that Cluster B PDs can potentially be scientifically explained does not entail that they should be properly treated through, broadly speaking, medical means. Indeed, according to an austere understanding of our concept of medicine, which links it strongly to our concept of illness, they should not. Nonetheless, there is good reason to hold that PDs are properly treated in contemporary, multidisciplinary, mental health clinics, involving psychiatrists, psychologists, and psychotherapists of various bents. At least in this respect, they are medical conditions.

There are three reasons for this. Two are practical. First, there are high levels of co-morbidity between PDs, and between PDs and Axis I disorders. Patients who possess traits which count as failings of virtue or character are likely also to possess traits and symptoms which do not. Many of these patients will have been placed on medication, like antipsychotics, antidepressants, and mood stabilizers which require medical monitoring. They may also need to be treated in conjunction with other services, for instance, those specializing in substance abuse or eating disorders. Hence, the bulk of their treatment is unlikely to be a form of 'moral conversion' – to use Charland's phrase – even if a part of their treatment is.

Second, the most effective treatment specifically targeting PDs themselves is psychotherapy (Fonagy *et al.*, 2006). Indeed, it is now widely held that recovery is possible. Of course, there is a long-standing question about whether psychotherapy itself should be conceived of as a medical treatment, and, relatedly, whether only medically trained clinicians should practice it. What seems clear, however, is that, again, treatment within contemporary, multidisciplinary, mental health clinics is appropriate.

The third reason is theoretical. Suppose we accept that psychotherapy counts as a medical treatment if this is modestly construed as meaning that treatment by mental health services is appropriate. We still face the question: why does this treatment work? Charland likens recovery from Cluster B PDs to 'moral conversion'. He is therefore inclined to believe that psychotherapy works because it harbours specifically moral imperatives and interventions. For instance, he suggests that the therapeutic aim with borderline patients is 'to convince the client to try and be more honest, more truthful, less manipulative, and less resentful and vindictive. These are deeply human matters, where success probably hinges largely, if not entirely, on the therapist's ability as a moral being rather than a professional clinician' (Charland, 2006, p. 124). There is ample evidence suggesting that a major factor in therapeutic success is the human relationship between patient and therapist (Yalom, 1970). But this characterization makes psychotherapy look as if it presents the patient with a series of moral demands with which he or she can then choose to comply – and hopefully will, if only the psychotherapist argues convincingly enough. That would certainly count as a form of 'moral conversion'. Indeed, this conception of the nature of psychotherapy is presumably part of why Charland is sympathetic to the idea that PDs do not excuse moral failings – that judgements of responsibility must be distinguished from questions of character (Charland, 2006, p. 116).

But if Aristotle's schema is correct, then this cannot be the right view of why psychotherapy works as a treatment for PDs quite generally, let alone when we consider Cluster B categories. For, the basic insight of his account is that virtue and character develop over time, becoming more and more cemented and stable within a person. A borderline patient does not become convinced through therapy that it is right to moderate and control their anger. Indeed, it is likely that borderline patients will only embark on therapy in the first place if they hold this belief. It is rather that therapy provides borderline patients with the skills needed to moderate and control their anger: they learn to be less impulsive, more considered. Similarly, narcissistic patients may develop the capacity to be empathetic: through therapy, they come to acquire a new skill. More generally, the success of psychotherapy as a treatment for PDs – of whichever cluster – would seem not to depend on 'moral conversion' but rather on its potential for changing a person's character.

The Therapeutic Community where I work requires patients to commit to an 18-month, full-time programme of various kinds of group therapy, including, for instance, cognitive behavioural therapy, analytic group work, medication and self-diagnostic groups, psychodrama, and art therapy. The patients are also required to cook, clean, and generally participate in the running of the programme and the life of the community. The programme offers many different routes to change. But broadly speaking, these fall into two major kinds. The first is the chance to form new habits. This involves at least four components. First, therapists and more senior patients in the community both model and actively guide the behaviour of new patients. Second, therapy groups offer patients the opportunity to try new kinds of social behaviour in a safe environment. Third, the community actively supports new behaviour, allowing patients the chance to experience its rewards – to find pleasure in it. Fourth, patients are given the opportunity to practice this behaviour – to try to solidify newly acquired traits. These routes to change can be seen as mirroring the processes Aristotle identifies as the first and second stages of a good upbringing.

The second kind of route to change is the acquisition of knowledge of the self. Through group therapy, patients come to know what they are like as a person, and how they developed that particular combination of traits. This knowledge is acquired through reflection on their behaviour within the group, and the exploration of its link to past experience (including the chance to re-live some of those experiences). It serves greatly to expand a patient's freedom and sense of self-esteem. Knowledge increases freedom because it allows mastery of and choice in behaviour that was previously automatic.[13] Knowledge increases self-esteem because an understanding of the nature and development of one's character offers the possibility of more realistic self-assessment. These routes to change do not explicitly mirror Aristotle's third stage of moral development, because they do not overtly address the question of why the virtues are good. They rather address the question of who one is and how one got there. However, they are likely to involve reflection on who one would like to become. An answer to this question usually requires exploring the nature of human virtue and goodness.

Cluster B PDs involve failures of virtue and character. There is potential for a scientific explanation of these disorders through a multilevel account of the development and formation of virtue and character. Meanwhile, psychotherapy works as a treatment because it can effect a change in character. Hence, there is a coherent and unified account of the nature, explanation, and treatment of Cluster B PDs. Finally, the treatment is most practically delivered within multidisciplinary, mental health clinics. So are Cluster B PDs medical conditions? At this point, it is difficult to see what knowledge can be gained by pressing this question: it is idle. For, it seems only to express a demand for an analysis of the meaning of our concept of medicine which goes beyond a modest construal that links it to contemporary health services. But, it is difficult to see how to pursue this demand without drawing on an analysis of our concepts of illness and disease, health and well-being. For instance, it is natural to suggest that medicine involves the diagnosis and treatment of illnesses or diseases, with the aim of restoring health or improving well-being. But now, we shall need an analysis of these concepts. As we saw ealier, this is not a need we should aim to meet. These concepts, and, relatedly, the concept of medicine, lie at the interface of science and common sense, of fact and value, as well as exhibiting cultural and historical development and variation. We can undertake a social and historical explanation, or we can make a decision about what we want them to mean. But we should not pretend that analysis can lead us to discover what a medical condition is, and, correspondingly, whether or not Cluster B PDs count as such.

---

[13] For a discussion of how this is possible, see Hampshire, 1974.

4.5 **Conclusion**

Szasz got mired in questions of the meaning of terms. But his conclusions were nonetheless in many ways correct. He believed that psychiatry could be a science, and that psychotherapy could be an effective means of change. What we must do is 'recast and redefine the problem of "mental illness" so that it may be encompassed in a morally explicit science of man' (Szasz, 1974, p. 263). Cluster B PDs involve failures of virtue and character. From a Szaszian perspective, they are especially striking because of how clearly they are defined, at least in past, by deviations from 'psychosocial, ethical, and legal' norms. But they can nonetheless be scientifically explained and effectively treated within contemporary health services. There need be no antithesis between science and morality within psychiatry. Mental illness is a myth that science can explain.

Acknowledgements

I thank my colleagues at the Complex Needs Service as well as Lisa Bortolotti, Matthew Broome, Neil Levy, Ian Phillips, Maja Spener, and Nick Shea for extremely helpful comments on this chapter and discussion of its ideas.

References

American Psychiatric Association (APA) (1994). *Diagnostic and Statistical Manual of Mental Disorders*, 4th edn. Washington DC, American Psychiatric Association.

Andreasen, N. C., Roy, M. A., and Flaum, M. (1995). Positive and negative symptoms. In *Schizophrenia* (eds. S. R. Hirsch, and D. R. Weinberger). Oxford, Blackwell

Bentall, R. (2003). *Madness Explained*. London, Penguin Books.

Berlin, H. A., Rolls, E. T., and Iversen, S. D. (2005). Borderline personality disorder, impulsivity, and the orbitofrontal cortex. *American Journal of Psychiatry*, **162**, 2360–2373.

Boorse, C. (1975). On the distinction between disease and illness. *Philosophy and Public Affairs*, **5**, 49–68.

Brockington, I., Roper, A., and Buckley, M. *et al.*, (1991). Bipolar disorder, cycloid psychosis and schizophrenia: a study using 'lifetime' psychopathology ratings, factor analysis and canonical variate analysis. *European Journal of Psychiatry*, **6**, 223–236.

Broome, M. R., Woolley, J. B., and Tabraham, P. *et al.*, (2005). What causes the onset of psychosis? *Schizophrenia Research*, **79**, 23–24.

Burnyeat, M. (1980). Aristotle on learning to be good. In *Essays on Aristotle's Ethics* (ed. A. E. Rorty). Berkeley, CA, University of California Press.

Carel, H. (2008). *Illness*. London, Acumen Publishing Ltd.

Charland, L. (2004). Moral treatment and the personality disorders. In *The Philosophy of Psychiatry: A Companion* (ed. J. Radden). Oxford, Oxford University Press.

Charland, L. (2006). Moral nature of the DSM-IV Cluster B personality disorders. *Journal of Personality Disorders*, **20**, 116–125.

Chugani, H., Behen, M., Muzik, O., Juhász, C., Nagy, F., and Chugani, D. C. (2001). Local brain functional activity following early deprivation: a study of post-institutionalised Romanian orphans. *Neuroimage*, **14**, 1290–1301.

Coolidge, F. L., Thede, L. L., and Jang, K. L. (2001). Heritability of personality disorders in childhood: a preliminary investigation. *Journal of Personality Disorders*, **15**, 33–40.

Cooper, R. (2007). *Psychiatry and Philosophy of Science*. London, Acumen Publishing Ltd.

Craddock, N., O'Donovan, M. C., and Owen, M. J. (2006). Genes for schizophrenia and bipolar disorder? Implications for psychiatric nosology. *Schizophrenia Bulletin*, **32**, 9–16.

De La Fuenta, J. M., Goldman, S., and Stanus, E. *et al.*, (1997). Brain glucose metabolism in borderline personality disorder. *Journal of Psychiatric Research*, **31**, 531–541.

Dupre, J. (1993). *The Disorder of Things*. Cambridge, MA, Harvard University Press.

Fonagy, P. and Bateman, A.W. (2006). Progress in the treatment of borderline personality disorder. *British Journal of Psychiatry*, **188**, 1–3.

Foucault, M. (1971). *Madness and Civilisation*. London, Tavistock.

Foucault, M. (1976). *The Birth of the Clinic*. London, Tavistock.

Frith, C. D. (1992). *The Cognitive Neuropsychology of Schizophrenia*. Hove, UK, Erlbaum UK Taylor & Francis.

Fulford, K. W. M. (1989). *Moral Theory and Medical Practice*. Cambridge, Cambridge University Press.

Fulford, K. W. M., Thornton, T., and Graham, G. (2006). *Oxford Textbook of Philosophy and Psychiatry*. Oxford, Oxford University Press.

Hacking, I. (1995). *Rewriting the Soul*. Cambridge MA, Harvard University Press.

Hacking, I. (1998). *Mad Travellers*. Charlottesville VA, University of Virginia Press.

Hacking, I. (1999). *The Social Construction of What?* Cambridge MA, Harvard University Press.

Hampshire, S. (1974). Disposition and memory. In *Freud* (ed. R. Wollheim). New York, Anchor Books.

Hannerz, H., Borga, P., and Borritz, M. (2001). Life expectations for individuals with psychiatric diagnoses. *Public Health*, **115**, 328–337.

Haslam, N. (2002). Kinds of kinds: a conceptual taxonomy of psychiatric categories. *Philosophy, Psychiatry, and Psychology*, **9**, 203–217.

Kendell, R. E. (1975). The concept of disease and its implications for psychiatry. *British Journal of Psychiatry*, **127**, 305–15.

Kendell, R. E. and Gourlay, J. A. (1970). The clinical distinction between the affective psychoses and schizophrenia. *British Journal of Psychiatry*, **117**, 261–266.

Kleinman, A. (1980). *Patients and Healers in the Context of Culture: An Exploration of the Borderland between Anthropology, Medicine, and Psychiatry*. Berkeley, CA, University of California Press.

Kohlberg, L. (1981). *Essays on Moral Development, Vol. I: The Philosophy of Moral Development*. New York, Harper & Row.

Kripke, S. (1972). *Naming and Necessity*. Oxford, Blackwell.

Kutchins, H. and Kirk, S. A. (1997). *Making us Crazy: DSM – The Psychiatric Bible and the Creation of Mental Disorders*. New York, Free Press.

Liddle, P. F. (1987). The symptoms of chronic schizophrenia: a reexamination of the positive–negative dichotomy. *British Journal of Psychiatry*, **151**, 145–151.

Lyoo, I. K., Han, M. H., and Cho, D. Y. (1998). A brain MRI study in subjects with borderline personality disorder. *Journal of Affective Disorders*, **50**, 235–243.

McGorry, P. D., Mihalopoulos, C., Henry, L., *et al.* (1995). Spurious precision: procedural validity of diagnostic assessment in psychotic disorders. *American Journal of Psychiatry*, **152**, 220–223.

McWilliams, N. (1994). *Psychoanaltyic Diagnosis: Understanding Personality Structure in the Clinical Process*. New York, The Guildford Press.

Molina, V., Reig, S., Sanz, J., *et al.* (2005). Increase in gray matter and decrease in white matter volumes in the cortex during treatment with atypical neuroleptics in schizophrenia. *Schizophrenia Research*, **80**, 61–71.

O'Doherty, J., Critchley, H., Deichmann, R., and Dolan, R. J. (2003). Dissociating valence of outcome from behavioural control in human orbital and ventral prefrontal cortices. *Journal of Neuroscience*, **23**, 7931–7939.

Pickard, H. (under review). Schizophrenia and the Epistemology of Self-knowledge.

Poulton, R., Caspi, A., Moffitt, T. E., Cannon, M., Murray, R., and Harrington, H. (2000). Children's self-reported psychotic symptoms and adult schizophreniform disorder: a 15-year longitudinal study. *Archives of General Psychiatry*, **57**, 1053–1058.

Porter, R. (2002). *Madness: A Brief History*. Oxford, Oxford University Press.

Putnam, H. (1973). Meaning and reference. *Journal of Philosophy*, **70**, 699–711.

Radden, J. (ed.) (2004). *The Philosophy of Psychiatry: A Companion*. Oxford, Oxford University Press.

Radomsky, E. D., Haas G. L., Mann, J. J., and Sweeny, J. A. (1999). Suicide behaviour in patients with schizophrenia and other psychiatric disorders. *American Journal of Psychiatry*, **156**, 1590–1595.

Robins, L. N., Locke, B. Z., and Reiger, D. A. (1991). An overview of psychiatric disorders in America. In *Psychiatric Disorders in America* (eds. L. N. Robins, and B. Z. Locke). New York, Free Press.

Schore, A. (1994). *Affect Regulation and the Origin of the Self*. Hillsdale NJ, Lawrence Erlbaum Associates Inc.

Schore, A. (2003). *Affect Dysregulation and Disorders of the Self*. New York, Norton.

Shenton, M. E., Chandlee, C. D., Frumin, M. McCarley, R. W. (2001). A review of MRI findings in schizophrenia. *Schizophrenia Research*, **49**, 1–52.

Szasz, T. (1960). The myth of mental illness. *American Psychologist*, **15**, 113–118.

Szasz, T. (1974). *The Myth of Mental Illness*. London, Palladin.

Thagard, P. (1996). The concept of disease: structure and change. *Communication and Cognition*, **29**, 445–478.

Toomey, R., Faraone, S. V., Simpson, J. C., Tsung, M. T. (1998). Negative, positive and disorganized symptom dimension in schizophrenia, major depression, and bipolar disorder. *Journal of Nervous and Mental Disease*, **186**, 470–476.

Van Os, J., Hanssen, M., Bijl, R. V., and Ravelli, A. (2000). Strauss (1969) revisted: a psychosis continuum in the general population? *Schizophrenia Research*, **45**, 11–20.

Walhberg, K. E., Wynne, L. C., and Oja, H. *et al.*, (1997). Gene–environment interaction in vulnerability to schizophrenia: findings from the Finnish Adoptive Family Study of Schizophrenia. *American Journal of Psychiatry*, **154**, 355–362.

Williams, B. A. O. (1985). *Ethics and the Limits of Philosophy*. London, HarperCollins.

Williams, B. A. O. (1993). *Morality*. Cambridge, Cambridge University Press.

Williams, J. B., Gibbon, M., and First, M. B. *et al.*, (1992). The structured clinical interview for DSM-III-R (SCID): II. Multi-site test-retest reliability. *Archives of General Psychiatry*, **49**, 630–636.

Yalom, I. D. (1970). *The Theory and Practice of Group Psychotherapy*. NewYork, HarperCollins.

Chapter 5

Psychiatry and the concept of disease as pathology

Dominic Murphy

Abstract

I argue that contemporary biological psychiatry is moving away from the concept of disease as natural history towards the concept of disease as a destructive physical process underlying signs and symptoms. This lets us see psychiatric explanations as sharing features with other biomedical explanations and also with forms of theoretical justification derived from model organisms.

5.1 Introduction

People writing about psychiatry these days all agree that the field has adopted the 'medical model', but it is hard to find out exactly what that means. How do we know, for instance, when a piece of psychiatric theorizing departs from, adheres to, or adapts the medical model, and what difference does it make? In this chapter, I distinguish two ways to understand the medical model, which I call the minimal and strong interpretations. A minimal interpretation thinks of diseases as collections of symptoms that occur together and unfold in characteristic ways, but it makes no commitments about the underlying causes of mental illness. A strong interpretation of the medical model, on the other hand, does make commitments about causes. The strong interpretation argues that mental illnesses are caused by distinctive pathophysiological processes in the brain. Having made the distinction between strong and weak interpretations, I try to show what difference it makes to psychiatry if we choose one or the other.

I will try to clarify the distinction by recounting a little history. The point of the history is heuristic: I think that the story I tell can help in understanding the two inter-pretations of the medical model by seeing something about their origins. Minimalists, I will say, are best thought of as using a concept of disease that dates back to Sydenham in the seventeenth century. It treats a disease as a collection of symptoms that unfold together in a characteristic way, and it is agnostic about the specific disease mechanisms or causes. Kraepelin applied this concept of disease to psychiatry as the basis for differential diagnosis, for example, between hebephrenia and dementia praecox (schizophrenia) (Kraepelin, 1899, pp. 173–175).

This syndrome-driven approach to mental illness, together with a commitment to scientific methods of collecting and testing data, is the core of the minimal interpretation. But in medicine more generally, the syndrome-based view of disease was supplanted in the nineteenth century by the concept of diseases as destructive processes in bodily organs, which 'divert part of the substance of the individual from the actions which are natural to the species to another kind of action' (Snow, 1853, p. 155; cf. Whitbeck, 1977; Carter, 2003; Broome, 2006). The strong interpretation holds that mental illnesses are diseases of this type. They are not just sets of co-occurring systems, but destructive processes taking place in biological systems.

This strong interpretation goes beyond a neo-Kraepelinian conception of mental disorder, and makes much more specific and falsifiable claims. But the conceptual differences between the minimal and strong interpretations can be hard to detect, since both are continuous with much medical practice. Either interpretation is consistent with the collection of laboratory data on patients, for example, or the use of follow-up studies to adjudicate between competing treatments.

But what difference does it make? It may be that different interpretations of the medical model are currently in play, but we want to know how it makes a difference to psychiatry. This is the second question I take up.

The issue I attend to is the implications of the strong interpretation for the nature of psychiatric explanation. Suppose we agree that diseases are destructive processes. What, if any, constraints does that put on the classification and explanation of mental illness? I argue first, that the strong interpretation can underwrite the goal of a nosology based on causes. Second, I rebut some contemporary theorists who argue that a strong medical model implies reductive explanations of mental disorder in terms of molecular genetics or some other low-level neuroscience. This reductionism does not follow from the medical model. It confuses a commitment to causal explanation (which is certainly present in the medical model) with a commitment to explanation at a particular level (which is not). The medical model directs us to look for causal explanation in terms of brain systems, but those systems can be understood at many different levels.

5.2 **The medical model**

Many statements of the medical model provide little content. A typical textbook treatment informs us that the medical model 'is simply the consistent application, in psychiatry, of modern medical thinking and methods' (Black, 2005, p. 3). But what are these methods? The textbook goes on (p. 5) to list three core assumptions:

> First, the same approach should be used for mental illness as for other illnesses. One corollary of this assumption is that there exist different psychiatric illnesses with different causes, courses and optimal treatments. Second, empiric proof is the best way to test a medical theory. In other words, the scientific method should be medicine's approach to knowledge. A third assumption of medical model psychiatry is that an increased understanding of the physiology of the brain will eventually improve the care of patients with mental illness.

Black's three assumptions are characteristic of manifestos for the medical model, but they do not actually commit its adherents to anything very specific. We have a claim that psychiatry uses the methods of medicine, but no details on what they are, a claim that theories should be tested empirically, and a claim that neurophysiology is important. The problem with getting a clear view of the medical model is that two theorists can agree with all three positions but understand them in quite different ways, including ways that are sometimes thought of as opposed to the medical model. The methods of medicine could be understood to include very many different phenomena. The claim that mental illness could be illuminated by more knowledge of neurophysiology seems acceptable to anyone who agrees that at least some mental illnesses are real phenomena and is also a materialist who thinks that the brain is the basis of the mind. Most psychoanalysts, for example, would agree with that claim, since Freud always intended his theory to be a materialist one. Disagreement between camps is likely to appear when we ask how much illumination will come from neuroscience as opposed to other sciences, and from which parts of neuroscience.

It appears too that theorists from many different backgrounds could agree that theories should be tested empirically. You could certainly be a psychoanalyst and believe that. The disagreements are likely to come about what counts as a test. Much of the controversy surrounding Grunbaum's (1984) sceptical assessment of psychoanalysis, for instance, concerned not just his denigration of clinical, as opposed to experimental evidence, but what he counted as clinical evidence in the first place.

Outside psychoanalysis, there are many therapists who believe in the experimental assessment of, for example, cognitive behaviour therapy, but who pay little attention to neuroscience rather than psychology (Dawes, 1994). Some clinicians regard the medical model as overstressing neurobiological rather than cultural and cognitive variables, but are nonetheless materialists who are fully committed to empirical testing.

Even if we stick to professed believers in the medical model, we find disagreements about how Black's core commitments should be understood. For instance, Guze (1992, p. 129) likewise defines the medical model as 'using in psychiatry the intellectual traditions, basic concepts, and clinical as well as research strategies that have evolved in general medicine.' And Black's third claim, that the physiology of the brain is important, echoes Guze's insistence that mental illness 'represents the manifestations of disturbed function' in the brain (1992, p. 44). So far, Guze is fully in agreement with Black, and so is Nancy Andreasen when she says that psychiatry is a form of neuroscience (1997).

But disagreements emerge when we look closer. Andreasen means that psychiatry is a form of cognitive neuroscience, and thinks that we should aim for causal explanations of disease in terms of failures of information processing systems in the brain. But when Guze calls psychiatry a branch of medicine, all he means is that disorders can be distinguished by their characteristic symptoms and courses. He does not think of diseases as specific pathologies, but as conventional labels for groups of patients. They are associated with biological markers but not identified with causal processes in the brain. Similarly, the *Diagnostic and Statistical Manual of Mental Disorders* (DSM) (American Psychiatric Association, 2000) aims to classify mental illnesses based on course and symptoms but not specific causes. Andreasen (2001, pp. 172–176), on the other hand, argues that we are presently identifying the specific pathophysiologies that cause mental illnesses. Her account sees the medical model in a different way. It is not just a matter of using empirical methods to understand the nature and treatment of syndromes, but a matter of applying cognitive neuroscience to the causal-explanatory strategies of modern medicine.

Andreasen, as a partisan of the strong interpretation, seeks explanations that cite pathogenic processes in brain systems, just as bodily diseases are explained by processes in other organs. The process at issue need not be destructive in the sense that it completely destroys the system: it may be enough to put the system into a stable but suboptimal state. Bolton and Hill (2004, p. 252) point out that many mental illnesses appear to be manifestations of chronically dysregulated systems. But, as they say, the same is true of general medical conditions like hypertension.

However, Bolton and Hill resist the medical model because they argue that it can only explain disorders in which 'intentionality has run out' (2004, p. 256). They think this because they understand the medical model in exclusively biological terms; that means it cannot deal with intentional processes. But the brain is a cognitive organ – and, indeed, a social one. Many disciplines study the effects of healthy cognition on behaviour, and there is no reason to expect that cognition will suddenly become irrelevant when we study mental illness.

Most biological systems do not process information. Therefore, when general medicine explains pathologies in those systems in terms of their characteristic biological role, the explanation does not involve cognitive variables. It does not follow that cognition is thereby removed from the scope of the medical model. The medical model can easily accommodate cognitive processes, since it tries to understand the causes of disease in terms of the failure of a system to carry out its normal function. In that extended sense, intentional phenomena are just part of the biology of the human organism, just as digestive or reproductive phenomena are part of human biology.[1]

To find the specific causes of disease we need a background theory of normal function relative to which pathology can be identified. Cognitive neuroscience is the obvious background theory in the sense that it provides a general framework for understanding mental life as the upshot of information processing systems in the nervous system, just as medicine in general derives from theories of normal organ function. In this sense, cognitive neuroscience is a synthesis of several approaches, not just a theory pitched at a particular level of explanation.

However, some thinkers have argued that the background theory for psychiatry is molecular biology (Kandel, 2005, chapter 2). But there is no need to interpret the medical model in a reductive fashion, as Kandel does. In the first place, as a matter of logic the medical model privileges explanations of a certain form rather than a particular level of explanation; second, as a matter of fact, psychiatric explanations employ multiple levels of explanation. Biologists study gene expression but they also study the social dynamics of primate societies, and there is no reason to think that biological

---

[1] Finding a malfunction does not establish the existence of a disease on its own. The overwhelming consensus is that the concept of disease involves not just biological abnormalities but also obstacles to human flourishing (Boorse, 1976; Richman, 2004 ; Murphy, 2006; Horwitz and Wakefield, 2007.).

psychiatry has to commit itself to just one level of the hierarchy, especially since the mentally ill do in fact live in primate societies, just like the rest of us.

I will now defend this picture in more detail. I shall provide a historical characterization of the strong interpretation of the medical model and then argue for the primacy of causal explanation and classification in medicine.

5.3 Causal explanation in the medical model

It is a familiar idea that DSM-IV's syndrome-based conception of mental illnesses stands in the tradition of Kraepelin, who argued that '*only the overall picture of a medical case from the beginning to the end of its development* can provide justification for its being linked with other observations of the same kind' (1899, p. 3). This familiar neo-Krapelinian picture is of mental illnesses as collections of signs and symptoms that doubtless depend on physical processes but are not defined or classified in terms of those physical processes.

I mentioned above that we can think of this idea, as it has developed in contemporary psychiatry, as resonating with one strand in the history of medical conceptions of disease. It dates back to the careful observational medicine of Sydenham in the seventeenth century, which eschews causal explanations in favour of thinking of diseases as syndromes with characteristic natural histories: it is observable phenomena, not hidden causes, which make up the taxa of medicine.

Historically, this approach to syndromes is compatible with seeing great variability in their causes: what matters is the syndrome, not its causal antecedents, since the latter do not form part of the definition of the disease. Indeed, different instances of the same disease, on this picture, might have radically different aetiologies. Carter (2003, p. 11) gives examples of this thinking, including the following list of the causes of diabetes, from a medical encyclopedia published in 1845:

> frequent exposure to sudden alterations of heat and cold, indulgence in copious draughts of cold fluid when the system has been over-heated by labour or exercise, intemperate use of spirituous liquors, poor living, sleeping out the whole of the night in the open air in a state of intoxication, checking perspiration suddenly, and mental anxiety and distress [. . .].
>
> (Carter, 2003, p. 11)

If you understand diseases in terms of their symptoms, you can admit a great variety of causes provided they produce the same effects. Carter suggests that for the early nineteenth-century medical profession, the notion of *the* cause of a disease was meaningless.

Carter argues via a series of case histories that this picture was supplanted in the mid-nineteenth century by what he calls the aetiological standpoint. From a literature in which medical writings simply deny that the notion of cause is any use at all, we move to a situation in which experimentalists and epidemiologists look for the cause of a disease. The movement reaches its culmination in Koch's germ theory. The aetiological standpoint, thinks Carter, sees the causes of diseases as phenomena that are natural (i.e. diseases are not just a matter of transgressing norms), universal (i.e. the cause is common to every instance of the disease), and necessary (the disease does not occur in the absence of the cause (Carter, 2003, p. 1).

Carter thinks this a revolutionary break in the whole of Western medicine prior to this. To really make that the case, we might want to add a fourth condition, which is that the cause is usually categorically different from normal natural processes. This distinguishes the explanations offered by Pasteur and Koch from the long tradition in classical and Renaissance medicine of seeing disease as caused by unbalanced mixtures of normally occurring humours or temperaments.

Whether or not Carter's larger claims about a scientific revolution are correct, there really was a new conception of cause associated with mid-nineteenth century medicine. For the first time, researchers began to think of every disease in terms of a unique cause that was necessary and sufficient for the disease and could explain all the signs and symptoms associated with it. Conceptually, this shift in thinking of causes meant that diseases came to be defined in terms of their causes, and seen not as collections of symptoms but as pathophysiological processes. Thus the same observable phenomena could be seen as belonging to different diseases, since it is the underlying cause, not the outward show, which constitutes the disorder.

I suggest that we can see this shift from syndromes to causes as akin to a shift from minimal to strong interpretations of the medical model. I am not arguing for any direct historical influence of these debates, or suggesting that contemporary psychiatrists see themselves as belonging to historically conditioned camps. I do, however, want to suggest that we can see the strong and minimalist camps as divided on issues of causation and the nature of disease.

Sometimes this division shows up in the same piece of theorizing. McHugh and Slavney, for instance, say that a disease 'is a construct that conceptualizes a constellation of signs and symptoms as due to an underlying biological pathology, mechanism and cause' (1998, p. 302). McHugh and Slavney assert (p. 48) that a disease is a syndrome that we use as a starting point for investigating physical processes. They explicitly name Sydenham (p. 46) as a forerunner of this view, but Sydenham, though a pioneer of classification, was not interested in underlying causes, only in observable phenomena.

However, although they think mental illness is due to material causes, McHugh and Slavney deny that a disease is a physical process – 'its essence is conceptual and inferential' (p. 48). But as Carter (2003) and Whitbeck (1977) have argued, the nineteenth century left medicine with a conception of diseases as physical processes – morbid entities that unfold within the body of the patient. Whitbeck also notes (p. 626) that it is very difficult to draw a clear distinction between the clinical and pathological levels, as the minimal medical model tries to do with its sharp separation of syndromes and associated biological markers (as we saw in McHugh and Slavney, above, and earlier in Guze). A high temperature, for example, can be seen as both a clinical sign and a pathological process, such as a cause of further biological damage. Whitbeck concludes that we should think of a disease as a complex of biological processes that can be identified by different clinical or pathological manifestations. In medicine, generally we employ both causes and syndrome in classification. Ischaemic heart disease is a pathology, but it commonly leads to syndromes of angina pectoris or myocardial infarction.

Let me recap. I have endorsed philosophical accounts that argue for a definite shift in thinking about disease that dates from the middle of the nineteenth century. The shift moved away from thinking about diseases as collections of symptoms associated with diverse causes. It moved towards thinking of diseases as destructive processes that are manifested in symptoms. Along with this goes a shift from thinking of diseases as constructs designed to capture the observable similarities across a group of people to thinking of them as discrete underlying biological processes occurring in those people. The former is a dominant idea in contemporary psychiatry, but at odds with modern medicine. This tension between embracing medicine and avoiding causal mechanisms reflects the equivocation in psychiatry between the minimal and strong interpretations of the medical model. The strong interpretation amounts to the embrace by psychiatry not just of medical thinking and empirical methods in some general sense, but more the adoption specifically of the conception of disease bequeathed to us by the nineteenth century.

Interestingly, Spaulding, Sullivan, and Poland contend that the shift from psychoanalysis to biological and pharmacological psychiatry 'was accomplished without changes in the key premises of the underlying medical model' (2003, p. 8). Given the comparative neglect of classification in psychoanalysis relative to more recent psychiatry, this claim requires some qualification. But there is something right about it. They see the medical model in minimal terms as a combination of materialism, commitment to empirical method, and a view of disorders as syndromes. Those core commitments can be shared by otherwise different outlooks, as I noted earlier.

Both ways of thinking about disease, as syndromes or as pathological processes, are in some sense medical and can be supported by empirical methods. But they have different conceptual implications which make a difference to the way the empirical work is understood. One obvious location of this difference is the issue of classification.

5.4 **Classification and the medical model**

As sciences mature, they tend to move to a classification based on causal properties. Psychiatrists who embrace the strong interpretation of the medical model look forward to a nosology based on pathological processes in brain systems (e.g. Andreasen 2001, pp. 172–176). This development fits the pattern suggested by Hempel (1965), who expected psychiatry to develop specific causal hypotheses involving causal mechanisms posited by either neurobiological or matured psychodynamic theories that could be used as a basis for a revised classification.

Successful prediction often depends on knowledge of causal structure because if one member of a kind has a property, it does so in virtue of the mechanisms that distinguish that kind and usually, although not inevitably, cause the members of the kind to have their characteristic properties. In that sense prediction, as Strevens (2007) points out, is the inverse of categorization. Putting things into categories involves betting that entities belong to the same kind if they have the same properties. The bet is worth making because the presence of shared properties is evidence that the entities also share causal mechanisms that are responsible for their being the kind of things they are. It is these relations between causal relations, mechanisms, categorization, and prediction that support the argument that psychiatric nosology should be based on causes (Murphy, 2006). But the official taxonomies used by psychiatry at the moment are deliberately designed to eschew causes.

Psychiatry's squeamishness about including causal information in taxonomies is often called a neo-Kraepelinian approach to nosology. But the label is misleading. Kraepelin (1899, p. 2) believed that 'pathological anatomy promises to provide the safest foundation' for classification of mental illness. He assumed that the correct taxonomy would be one in which clinical description, aetiology, and pathophysiology coincided: his goal was a situation in which 'cases arising from the same causes would always have to present the same symptoms and the same post-mortem result' (p. 3).

Kraepelin saw classification by clinical description as an interim measure designed to satisfy the practical requirements of contemporary physicians. More importantly, it could also provide a fruitful heuristic for subsequent pathological and aetiological inquiry: 'the value of every diagnosis is thus rated essentially by the extent to which it opens up reliable prospects for the future' (1899, p. 4).

There is a substantial difference between thinking of clinically based, syndromic classification in this way and thinking of it in the DSM's way. The DSM classification is designed (DSM-IV-TR, p. xxiii) to improve communication across clinical specialties and underwrite clinical education, but not to serve as a spur towards an eventual system based on causal information. DSM-IV-TR is certainly intended to reflect and foster extensive empirical investigation, but the investigation is guided by the existing, acausal categories. It is not designed to revise those categories in the direction of a causal taxonomy, and it defines mental illness (p. xxxi) as a clinically significant syndrome rather than a destructive process. Unlike Kraepelin, the *DSM-IV* does not even envisage a causal taxonomy as a goal. This reflects a minimal interpretation of the medical model; it can guide empirical research but not uncover portions of the causal structure of the world.

The DSM leaves itself open to the charge of arbitrariness. It is a classification that rests on grouping together observable phenomena. We already know from other areas of medicine that what looks like the same phenomenon – a cough, say, or a sore throat, or chest pain – can reflect different casual pathways on the inside and hence different conditions. Any taxonomy that rests content with surface features risks lumping different conditions together.

In an important recent book, Horwitz and Wakefield (2007) argue that exactly this is the picture that has developed with respect to depression. True to its clinical basis, the DSM-IV-TR (p. 356) defines depression in terms of symptoms: more exactly, it requires that, to receive a diagnosis of major depressive episode, one must suffer five of the following nine symptoms over a two-week period (including either or both of depressed mood or diminished interest or pleasure in almost all activities):

   i. depressed mood;

   ii. diminished interest;

   iii. weight gain or loss (without dieting) or change in appetite;

   iv. insomnia or excessive sleep;

   v. observable psychomotor agitation or retardation;

   vi. fatigue or loss of energy;

   vii. feeling worthless or excessively guilty;

viii. diminished ability to think or concentrate, or indecisiveness; and

ix. recurrent thoughts of death or suicide or a planned or attempted suicide

Now, it is clear that, since being alive involves a series of disappointments, many of the ordinary episodes in a person's life can cause behaviours or feelings from this list. We can be depressed, inattentive, tired, and sleepless after losing a loved one, receiving a major professional setback, or a terminal medical diagnosis, or being jilted, or after many other trials. These vicissitudes of life were recognized and allowed for by the traditional concept of melancholy or depression, which has a continuous history going back to classical antiquity (Radden, 2000): we have always recognized that some people become melancholic because of life's misfortunes whereas others slip into depression without any apparently significant cause. The tradition sees pathology only in the latter case, consistently holding that 'pathological depression is an exaggerated form of a normal human emotional response' (Horwitz and Wakefield, 2007, p. 71). All of us are downcast by misfortune (even when we deserve it), but some people become melancholy without any apparent justification.

The DSM, however, ignores this tradition. Anyone who fits the syndrome receives the diagnosis – with one exception: grief following bereavement does not count towards diagnosis of major depressive disorder (the bereaved person gets two months to grieve after which time a diagnosis of clinical depression may be made.) Not even that qualification, however, is permitted if one shows depressive symptoms after one's spouse abandons one by emptying the bank account and running off with a lover, rather than dying.

Horwitz and Wakefield make a very compelling negative case, to wit that DSM-IV fails to respect common sense or previous psychiatric consensus about depression. It diagnoses many people as depressed when they are just miserable for ordinary human reasons. They conclude that the concept of depression defined by this diagnostic syndrome represents a major conceptual break with both past psychiatry and common-sense thought about human nature. This leads to needless alarmism about an epidemic of depression and has unfortunate consequences for many individuals who are diagnosed erroneously.

Horwitz and Wakefield's positive proposal is less convincing. They argue that evolved human nature includes a system that is adapted to respond to loss. The operations of this system explain why we get sad in those situations where we expect people to be sad. They argue that the traditional distinction between sadness and morbid melancholy tracks the normal and abnormal workings of the loss-response system. It causes normal sadness in response to serious loss or misfortune, for it is 'biologically designed to produce such responses at appropriate times' (p. 25). Conversely, it is the failure of this system to operate normally that explains major depression. The system kicks in for no reason, or it produces excessive responses to trivial misfortunes. (It also appears to follow that the system has malfunctioned in cases where we expect people to become depressed and they do not, although they do not talk about that.)

The existence of a loss-response mechanism is not supported by much evidence, unless 'loss-response mechanism' just means 'something in our brain that makes us sad when things go badly', in which case it is trivially true. Furthermore, even if there is a system that explains normal sadness, it does not follow that the system is not mal-functioning in those cases. It is possible that even normal cases of bad luck do something destructive to the mind/brain, rather than trigger an adaptive response. However, these questions cannot even be raised if we stick with the DSM concept of depression, which has no way to justify itself by appealing to facts about underlying systems or causes.

It is certainly possible to collect data using the DSM concept of depression, especially information about epidemiology and natural history: in that sense, we can indeed employ normal medical reasoning. But that reasoning does not rebut the charge that Horwitz and Wakefield make with great intuitive force: the DSM concept of depression lumps together different psychological and behavioural types in the same category because of observable similarities that may nonetheless reflect diverse aetiologies. There is no way to answer this charge, or to arrive at a satisfactory taxon-omy that mirrors that of general medicine, unless we adopt a causal foundation for nosology. Doing that involves not just the empirical study of mental disorder, but a strong interpretation of the medical model, with its commitment to a view of disease as not just a syndrome but a destructive process.

Yet, what kind of destructive process? And don't lots of mental illnesses, emphati-cally including depression, have myriad causes? I noted above that the causal explanations of nineteenth-century physicians assumed that a disease has a universal and necessary cause. I contrasted this to the earlier view which the aetiological program superseded. According to that earlier view, two people could share a diagno-sis even though their symptoms had very different causes. But you might still think there is an impediment to embracing the medical model even if the foregoing is true, namely that many mental illnesses appear to have numerous causes. This seems to depart from the strong medical model's idea namely that each disease has one necessary cause. I will conclude by taking up these issues.

I argue that we are better off thinking of diseases as being realized in biological systems rather than caused by them, and this permits strong medical thinking to acknowledge that a realization which is shared across patients might have a variety of specific, peculiar causes.

5.5 **Explanation**

Donald Gillies raises the objection I just mentioned as a more general problem for Carter's analysis. He wonders (2007, p. 370) whether it is not true that

> the modern concept of causality looks rather like the early 19th century plurivalent approach to causality which Pasteur and Koch rejected. Consider a modern account of heart disease for example. It would be quite legitimate to say that heart disease can be caused by smoking and/or by eating fast food. Yet these two causes are neither necessary nor sufficient. There might well be a patient who gets heart disease from smoking 60 cigarettes a day without consuming even a mouthful of fast food; while another might succumb as a result of eating hamburgers and fries twice a day without smoking even once.
>
> (Gillies, 2007, p. 370)

There are two responses one can make to this, both of which are relevant to thinking about causal explanation. Indeed, they complement each other, although it would take a bit more time than I have at the moment to fully explain why. First, as Gillies himself goes on to note (p. 371), the modern conception of causation in the life sciences is not really the same as the early nineteenth-century one that was elbowed out of the way by the medical revolutionaries. The difference lies in the way modern thinking has incorporated statistical methods to give much greater empirical content to the claim that different risk factors cause the same disease. For instance, Kendler and Prescott (2006, p. 148ff) found that 'stressful life events' are among the chief causes of depression, and that they are especially depressogenic if they involve experiences of humiliation (pp. 160) (Kendler and Prescott, 2006). Constructs like these can be operationalized and their probabilistic relationships to each other studied in order to reach a much clearer understanding of the ways in which different causes interact so as to produce a case of depression.

Second, we can distinguish between more remote and more proximate causes, or talk, as Kraepelin did, of aetiology and pathology. Many factors can interact to produce the pathology that is common to all cases of a condition. On this view, all the people who share a diagnosis do so in virtue of having a common destructive process in their mind/brain: indeed, the diagnosis names that process: as Gillies (p. 371) says, an example is one variety of heart disease, atherosclerosis, which does have a necessary cause, *viz.* tangled arterial plaques (atheromata). Such factors as overdoing the fried food and cigarettes are more remote causes, or risk factors, that bear a probabilistic relation to the pathology depending on other factors.

We might prefer to say that the neuropathology realizes the disease, rather than causes it. A particular destructive process is the way the disease occurs in humans. It can happen in many ways via combinations of risk factors operating in concert. On that view, atherogenesis is simply identical to a biochemical process of plaque formation and its sequelae, which can be caused in many ways. For instance, it can happen in blood vessels whose narrowing is of no physiological consequence, and hence not a disease process. Similarly, one might think that major depression is the same thing as a specific, as yet unknown, cognitive and/or neurological process (or, perhaps, a family of specific processes). The process, depression, can be triggered in diverse ways that depend on one's genetic inheritance, acquired psychology, and contingent biography.

If mental illness is realized by pathological brain systems we must understand those systems in terms of their normal function. Any conception of normal neurological functioning must take information processing into account, because processing information is what brains are for. Nothing in the strong interpretation of the medical model rules out explanations that cite cognitive processes in brains, because it tells us to look for the process that realizes the disease. But it leaves open whether the pathology is to be understood in terms of gene expression, systems neuroscience, adverse learning, or something else. The medical model sees mental illness as pathogenic processes taking place in brain systems but does not force us to choose reductive explanations as a matter of logic. The medical model privileges explanations that cite underlying processes as the realization of a disease entity. It does not require one to identify processes at any particular level of explanation. No part of biology or psychology has proprietary rights to psychiatric explanation.

It may be that reductive, molecular explanations of a given pathology will carry the day. But if psychiatry should adopt a multilevel explanatory structure, it will be in no way exceptional among the life sciences. Existing medical and biological practice already uses cross-level explanations (Schaffner, 1994). There is, as I said, no objection in principle to adding an intentional level to the mix since cognition is just another biological property of humans, as is living within a culture.

I do not suggest that all explanations will involve cognitive levels of explanation as opposed to other levels of brain function. But cognitive neuroscience provides a general framework for understanding mental life as the upshot of information processing in the nervous system. Psychiatry can exploit this knowledge of normal function in our cognitive organs just as medicine in general identifies departures from normal organ function via theories of how the systems behave when they are healthy. One of the disadvantages of the minimal medical model has been that its neglect of underlying systems has divorced psychiatry from the wider sciences of the mind that aim to understand those systems in their normal state.[2]

Since pathological processes are supposed to be common to all the people who share a diagnosis, the big explanatory challenge is to identify the *robust processes* (Sterelny 2003, pp. 131–132, 207–208) that are repeatable or systematic in various ways across individuals, rather than the actual processes that occur as a disorder unfolds in one person. We want to know what common process is that which accounts for the form of the disease entity abstracted away from individual variation. Throughout the history of psychiatry, theorists have drawn attention to this issue, urging that a disorder is an ideal type that can be realized differently in different individuals. It is the common processes which the different subjects share that we must identify and explain. Charcot (1887–1888), for instance, distinguished *archetypes* – or the basic forms of a disorder – from *formes frustes*, in which the disorder appeared in individual subjects with some of its characteristic components absent or altered. Birnbaum (1923) argued along similar lines that a psychotic disorder inevitably contains both *pathogenic* features, which define its essential structure, and *pathoplastic* features, which depend on the personal circumstances of a given patient.

Although clinicians dealing with particular cases may be more interested in the pathoplastic features of their patients, it is the ideal form of a disorder that we need to explain. I have argued that we should do this by constructing and trying to explain exemplars of disorders (Murphy, 2006).

An exemplar is best thought of as an imaginary patient who has the ideal textbook form – the symptoms and natural history – of a disorder, and only that disorder. (Or, we can think of an actual patient as an exemplar of a disorder enriched with a set of real-world facts.) Thus, the exemplar for major depression might include lowered affect, serotonin imbalances, negative (but complicated) self-assessment, disturbed sleep, and lethargy and lack of motivation. As well as information about the

---

[2] Of course, what counts as normal or healthy cognition depends on whether, and how far, science can achieve a big picture of how people are, and why they are that way. The very possibility of this is contested. I discuss the issues at length in Murphy, 2006 (chapters 3 and 5).

presentation of a patient at a time, exemplars include information about the natural history of disorders.

We can apply the same process of exemplar construction to individual symptoms. The stereotypical features of hopelessness, a symptom of depression, might include a cognitive process that produces chronic, wide-ranging, negative self-evaluations. The overall goal is to vindicate the strong interpretation of the medical model by explaining the failure of the exemplars to exhibit the normal or healthy relations that exist within and between neuropsychological systems.

Psychiatry, like the rest of medicine, faces a familiar scientific trade-off. We confront both great variation in reality and the need to render that reality empirically tractable. We typically seek, as I said, to isolate the robust processes: features of a condition that recur across individuals but are often masked by the diversity of the phenomena. A disease process may take a unique form in an individual, but it is still an instance of a disease, and we need to identify and explain what is common across instances. The traditional scientific response to the trade-off between variation and tractability is idealization.

The role of an idealization in medicine is to let us classify real systems according to their departure from the ideal and explain those departures in terms of failures in the ideal system. This approach is a standard medical heuristic. As Wachbroit (1994) argued, when we say that an organ is normal, we employ a biomedical concept of normality that is neither normative nor statistical. Rather, it is an idealized description of a component of a biological system in an unperturbed state. Actual systems may never attain the ideal. But it is the idealized organ that gets into the physiology textbook. It draws its authority from its predictive and explanatory utility: against the background of idealized normal heart function, for example, we account for variation in actual hearts (a particular rhythm, say). We cite the textbook rhythmic pattern (which may be very unusual statistically) and identify other patterns as arrhythmic. Likewise, psychiatrists and neuropsychologists need a theory of normal function of ideal cognitive brain systems. Then we can try to explain exemplary mental disorders in those terms. In doing so, we can realize the medical model fully. We can align psychiatry more closely with the causal and explanatory practices of modern medicine. At the same time, we can knit it together with the cognitive and biological sciences. They provide the background theory of normal function against which pathology can be identified and understood.

References

American Psychiatric Association (2000). *Diagnostic and Statistical Manual of Mental Disorders*, 4th edn., textual revision. Washington, DC, American Psychiatric Association.

Andreasen, N. C. (1997). Linking mind and brain in the study of mental illnesses: a project for a scientific psychopathology. *Science*, 275, 1586–1593.

Andreasen, N. C. (2001). *Brave New Brain*. New York, Oxford University Press.

Birnbaum, K. (1923). The making of a psychosis. Tr. H. Marshall, In *Themes and Variations in European Psychiatry* (eds. S. R. Hirsch, and M. Shepherd), pp. 197–238. Bristol, John Wright (1974).

Black, K. (2005). Psychiatry and the medical model. In *Adult Psychiatry* (eds. E. Rubin and C. Zorumski), 2nd edn, pp. 3–15. Malden, MA, Blackwell.

Bolton, D. and Hill, J. (2005). *Mind, Meaning and Mental Disorder: The Nature of Causal Explanation in Psychiatry*, 2nd edn. New York, Oxford University Press.

Boorse, C. (1976). What a theory of mental health should be. *Journal for the Theory of Social Behavior*, **6**, 61–84.

Broome, M. (2006). Taxonomy and ontology in psychiatry: a survey of recent literature. *Philosophy, Psychiatry and Psychology*, **13**, 303–319.

Carter, K. C. (2003). *The Rise of Causal Concepts of Disease*. Aldershot, Ashgate.

Charcot, J-M. (1987). *Charcot, the Clinician: The Tuesday Lessons*. (Tr C. G. Goetz). Philadelphia, PA, Lippincott, Williams and Wilkins.

Dawes, R. (1994). *House of Cards: Psychology and Psychotherapy Built on Myth*. New York, Free Press.

Gillies, D. (2007). Review of Carter (2003). *British Journal for the Philosophy of Science*, **58**, 365–377.

Grunbaum, A. (1984). *The Foundations of Psychoanalysis*. Berkeley, CA, University of California Press.

Guze, S. B. (1992). *Why Psychiatry Is a Branch of Medicine*. New York, Oxford University Press.

Hempel, C. (1965). Fundamentals of taxonomy. In *Aspects of Scientific Explanation* (ed. C. Hempel), pp. 137–154. New York, The Free Press.

Horwitz, A. and Wakefield, J. (2007). *The Loss of Sadness*. New York, Oxford University Press.

Kandel, E. (2005). *Psychiatry, Psychoanalysis and the New Biology of Mind*. Arlington, VA, American Psychiatric Publishing.

Kendler, K. S. and Prescott, C. A. (2006). *Genes, Environment, and Psychopathology: Understanding the Causes of Psychiatric and Substance Use Disorders*. New York, Guilford Press.

Kraepelin, E. (1899). *Psychiatry: A Textbook for Students and Physicians*, vol. 2. (Tr. S. Ayed). Science History Publications, 1990.

McHugh, P. and Slavney, P. (1998). *The Perspectives of Psychiatry*, 2nd edn. Baltimore, MD, Johns Hopkins University Press.

Murphy, D. (2006). *Psychiatry in the Scientific Image*. Cambridge, MA, MIT Press.

Radden, J. (2000). *The Nature of Melancholy: From Aristotle to Kristeva*. New York, Oxford University Press.

Richman, K. (2004). *Ethics and the Metaphysics of Medicine*. Cambridge, MA, MIT Press.

Schaffner, K. F. (1994). Reductionistic approaches to schizophrenia. In *Philosophical Perspectives on Psychiatric Diagnostic Classification* (eds. J. Sadler, O. Wiggins, and M. Schwartz), pp. 279–294. Baltimore, MD, Johns Hopkins University Press.

Snow, J. (1853).On continuous molecular changes, more particularly in their relation to epidemic diseases. In *Snow on Cholera* (ed. W. H. Frost), pp. 147–175. NewYork, Hafner (1965.)

Spaulding, W., Sullivan, M., and Poland, J. (2003). *Treatment and Rehabilitation of Severe Mental Illness*. New York, Guilford Press.

Sterelny, K. (2003). *The Evolution of Agency and Other Essays*. Cambridge, MA, Cambridge University Press.

Strevens, M. (2007). Why represent causal relations? In *Causal Learning: Psychology, Philosophy, Computation* (eds. A. Gopnik, and L. Schulz). New York, Oxford University Press.

Wachbroit, R. (1994). Normality as a biological concept. *Philosophy of Science*, **61**, 579–591.

Whitbeck, C. (1977). Causation in medicine: the disease entity model. *Philosophy of Science*, **44**, 619–637.

Section 3

Reconciling paradigms

Chapter 6

On the interface problem in philosophy and psychiatry

Tim Thornton

Abstract

A significant family of antireductionist approaches to the philosophy of mind argues that mental states answer to distinct normative and rational constitutive principles which have no echo in physical theory. The mind is, in Bermúdez's phrase, autonomous. But, at the same time, human actions are part of the natural world and thus susceptible to explanations at a variety of levels, from that of whole persons down, via cognitive psychology and neurology, to the basic biology, chemistry, and physics of the cellular level. But if the mind is autonomous, how can person-level explanation interface with lower-level explanations? This is the interface problem and it has been regarded by some philosophers, such as Sellars, as *the* framing problem for philosophy as a whole. In this chapter, I argue that the interface problem is sustained as a global problem for *a priori* philosophy by a tension between the antireductionism of normative properties to nomological science and a construal of nomological science as a metaphysical benchmark. It is this which leads to a dualism of norm and nature which neither an appeal to supervenience nor the 'stance stance' popularized by Dennett can bridge. But, I suggest, the dualism can be at least partially and progressively dismantled by marshalling recent ideas which question the metaphysical pretensions of nomological science, its completeness and explanatory basicness. This gives way to a conception of the interface problem as a substantial but merely local matter for psychiatry and other sciences of the mind rather than the framing problem for philosophy or philosophy of psychiatry.

6.1 Introduction to the interface problem

The interface problem, in José Bermúdez's phrase, is a practical problem for the philosophy of psychiatry (Bermúdez, 2005). The call by the World Psychiatric Association for the development of a comprehensive or integrative model of diagnosis, as part of its institutional program on psychiatry for the person, is a call to combine distinct elements into a single diagnosis. Juan Mezzich, for example, sets out the aim as:

> understanding and formulating what is important in the mind, the body and the context of the person who presents for care. This is attempted by addressing the various aspects of ill- and positive-health, by interactively engaging clinicians, patient and family, and by employing categorical, dimensional and narrative descriptive approaches in multilevel schemas.
>
> (Mezzich, 2005, p. 91)

But this might be a call to attempt to combine immiscible elements in an uneasy mixture rather than elements that interact to shed genuine light on subjects' experiences. Assuming that there is an important role for a normative, person-level description, or narrative, within psychiatry and assuming that it cannot be reduced to, or be analysed in, the terms of a natural science, how can natural scientific descriptions and explanations interface with person-level narratives? This is the interface problem.

In an overview of the philosophy of psychology, José Bermúdez uses the interface problem to draw up a framework for philosophical approaches to the mind: autonomous, functional, representational, and neurocomputational. He states the problem as follows:

> How does commonsense psychological explanation interface with explanations of cognition and mental operations given scientific psychology, cognitive science, cognitive neuroscience and the other levels in the explanatory hierarchy?
>
> (Bermúdez, 2005, p. 35)

What kind of answer should be given to this problem? It has been seen as at the heart of philosophy, *the* central problem of philosophy, calling for a global philosophical answer. Wilfrid Sellars (1912–89), for example, argues that the central task for philosophy is to reconcile the *manifest* image of man in the world with the *scientific* image, in a synoptic or stereoscopic view.

Sellars suggests that light can be shed on the scientific image through what he describes as a 'historical and a methodological fiction' – but a useful fiction – of thinking of science in abstraction from actual historical processes as a matter of correlating phenomena and postulating explanatory mechanisms. The scientific image is thus 'the image derived from the fruits of postulational theory construction' (Sellars, 1963, p. 19).

The manifest image is more complex. Sellars says:

> The 'manifest' image of man-in-the-world . . . is . . . the framework in terms of which man came to be aware of himself as man-in-the-world . . . [A]nything which can properly be called conceptual thinking can occur only within a framework of conceptual thinking in terms of which it can be criticized, supported, refuted, in short, evaluated. To be able to think is to be able to measure one's thoughts by standards of correctness, of relevance, of evidence . . .
>
> [T]he transition from pre-conceptual patterns of behaviour to conceptual thinking was a holistic one, a jump to a level of awareness which is irreducibly new, a jump which was the coming into being of man.
>
> (Sellars, 1963 p. 6)

This summary of the manifest image has three important aspects:

1 The manifest image is closely connected to the ability to exercise conceptual thought.

2 Conceptual thought depends essentially on critical evaluation.

3 There is a fundamental discontinuity between, on the one hand, conceptually structured thought and action and, on the other, preconceptual behaviour.

These three elements mark an important contrast with the elements that make up a scientific image of man.

Sellars is not alone in assuming that there is a key distinction between person-level descriptions and underlying natural scientific accounts. Building on Sellars' work, John McDowell, for example, contrasts the logical space of reasons with the realm of law or of natural science (McDowell, 1994). Donald Davidson argues for the 'constitutive ideal of rationality' which has 'no echo in physical theory' (Davidson, 1980, pp. 223, 231). What all three authors share, is an assumption about the central importance of the normativity of person-level descriptions. Normativity cannot be accounted for in natural scientific descriptions of the world.

The fact that it is possible to conceptualize aspects of the world in these two distinct ways, prompts the question: how are they related? Sellars suggests both that this is a central philosophical question and that it should be given a single unifying philosophical answer:

> [T]he most fruitful way of approaching the problem of integrating theoretical science with the framework of sophisticated common sense into one comprehensive synoptic vision is to view it not as a piecemeal task . . . but rather as a matter of articulating two whole ways of seeing the sum of things, two images of man-in-the-world and attempting to bring them together in a 'stereoscopic' view.
>
> (Sellars, 1963, p. 19)

What are the prospects for a synoptic or stereoscopic view? The prospects will seem dimmer the more one takes the distinction between the manifest and scientific images of man to be a fundamental distinction of kind. The more it approaches a dualism, the less the possibility of combining the two images into one. By contrast, the less the dualism seems to be a distinction of kind, and the more the manifest image can be reduced to the scientific image (few hold out hopes for the reciprocal reduction), the easier it will seem. Thus reductionists can escape the threat of dualism and answer the interface problem. But the cost of this is providing an analysis of the normative notions of the manifest image in non-normative terms. Despite valiant attempts, this seems to me to be a hopeless task and I will ignore it in what follows (see Thornton, 1998).

Antireductionists can respect the distinct logic of normative and non-normative language, but, apparently at least, only at a cost of subscribing to a dualism of two kinds of properties and thus having no solution to the interface problem.

Is there a third way? In the next section of this chapter I will sketch out two familiar middle ground attempts at a synoptic view and will argue that, for fairly familiar reasons, they cannot succeed. Then, in the third and final section, I will indicate what

I think is a more promising approach: undermining the felt need for a global, philosophical solution and looking instead for a variety of local solutions.

6.2 A third way between reductionism and antireductionism?

6.2.1 The 'stance stance'

The idea that distinct and irreducible conceptualizations reflect distinct interpretative 'stances' is most closely associated with Daniel Dennett although W. V. O. Quine's invocation of 'radical translation' and Donald Davidson's 'radical interpretation' have similarities. Dennett attempts to shed light on mental and intentional phenomena by stepping back and describing the 'intentional stance' that brings them into focus. To do this, he contrasts three stances: physical, design, and intentional. Briskly, their internal logic is as follows:

Physical: To predict the behaviour of a system, determine its physical constitution, physical impingements, and physical laws.

Design: To predict the behaviour of a designed system, ignore its physical details and predict that it will behave as it is designed to do.

Intentional: For rational systems, determine what beliefs and desires it ought to have given its position in the world and determine what behaviour would further its ends and predict that it will behave like that.

The underlying suggestion is that the normative properties of Sellars' manifest image can be made to seem less mysterious if the particular interpretative stance that is their home is described. Following Fred Dretske, I will call this general approach the 'stance stance' (Dretske, 1988).

The stance stance promises a solution, to the interface problem, which is neither reductionist nor dualist. It is not reductionist because there need be no prospect of any reduction or mapping of terms within the intentional (or, for that matter, the design) stance to the physical stance. But it is not dualist – or so it is hoped – because, although the concepts used in different stances are incommensurable, they mark merely internal aspects of different approaches taken towards the same world. The properties articulated are internal to the stance in the following sense: there is no further question as to whether they are really instantiated in the world over and above whether the stance can usefully be adopted.

The problem with this as an attempted middle-ground response to the interface problem is that the stance stance only provides a synoptic view if the stances can be described without appeal to the properties that they deploy or if, in other words, they do not describe independently existing phenomena. If not, shifting philosophical attention from the normative phenomena of the manifest image to the interpretative stance that weaves them together changes nothing. Understanding the content of the stance is just the same as understanding the problematic properties and thus, if there is a problem in relating the manifest and scientific images, a parallel problem will exist in relating the intentional and physical stances, understood as the stances that describe intentional and physical properties respectively.

In earlier papers, Dennett advocates the kind of pragmatic reading of the intentional stance that might promise a solution to the interface problem. He says, for example:

> Lingering doubts about whether the chess playing computer really has beliefs and desires are misplaced; for the definition of intentional systems I have given does not say that intentional systems really have beliefs and desires, but that one can explain and predict the behaviour by ascribing beliefs and desires to them . . . The decision to adopt the strategy is pragmatic, and is not intrinsically right or wrong.
>
> (Dennett, 1978, p. 7)

On the assumption that pragmatic advantage can be explained without appeal to the idea of getting the normative or intentional properties right, Dennett implies that the stance stance sheds light on intentional properties by deflating them. They are aspects of a stance rather than puzzling extra-theoretic features.

Sadly, however, in later papers Dennett himself is forced to retreat from this view in the face of the worry that pragmatic advantage is perspectival. The worry is illustrated by the idea of Martian neuroscientists who, armed with an advanced physical stance theory of the human brain, might be able to be make sufficiently exact predictions of human behaviour that the adoption of the intentional stance would not have pragmatic advantage for them (Dennett, 1987, p. 23). This is made worse by another example Dennett gives: predicting the behaviour of a lectern through the ascription of balanced intentional states that would motivate it to remain still (*ibid.*, p. 25). In the case of the lectern, Dennett assures us, there is no pragmatic advantage in moving from the physical to the intentional stance and so we do not have to ascribe mental states to it. The same consideration seems now to apply to Martians theorizing about human behaviour.

Against this idea, Dennett argues that the Martians would, nevertheless, miss something if they did not adopt the intentional stance. They would miss the real intentional patterns in human affairs. But whilst this move protects the ascription of intentional states against the charge of perspectivalism, it undermines it as a deflationary solution to the interface problem. The intentional stance seems to inflate under critical scrutiny into a dualism of manifest and scientific properties.

It may still seem that Dennett's account is immune from such inflation. After all, in specifying the intentional stance, he places no constraints on what instantiates or implements the functions it describes. Further, using the example of man-made devices, such as chess-playing computer programmes, to exemplify intentional systems emphasizes their unmysterious status (whilst permitting multiple instantiation). Nevertheless, this aspect of what instantiates mental properties does nothing to address the natural status of those higher order properties themselves (see, e.g., Bilgrami, 2004). Without some such argument, Dennett's later realism about patterns undermines the use of the stance stance to address the interface problem.

Dennett's early pragmatism may not be the only motivation for prioritizing the stance over its content in the order of explanation. In moral philosophy, there is a more or less honourable tradition of attempting to explain moral judgements as resulting from a projective error. The phenomenology of moral judgement, the sense that our judgements answer to something worldly, is explained through the idea that we mistakenly project our moral sentiments onto the world. In fact, there are no worldly moral features for judgements to answer to. Given this view, the moral stance cannot be explained in terms of its content. It is the other way round. Could a similar error theory be applied to the use of the intentional stance?

Clearly, yes. Eliminativists argue that the kind of interpretation that Dennett articulates in the intentional stance is in error in the way that a theory of combustion based on phlogiston was. Presumably, therefore, it is subject to the same kind of explanation as false theories – not by invoking its responsiveness to the non-existent features it purportedly describes.

But in the context of deflationary responses to the interface problem this will not do. Eliminativism is an extreme form of reductionism in which the modifications to the reduced theory that characterize most reductions are taken to the limit and the reduced theory is simply eliminated in favour of the reducing theory. Eliminativism does not aim at a synoptic or stereoscopic view of both the manifest and scientific image. It aims to eliminate the manifest image in favour of the scientific image.

6.2.2 Supervenience

The second global deflationary solution to the interface problem is to claim that the manifest image supervenes on the scientific image. Since so much has been written about supervenience, I will merely introduce it and sketch an objection in the context of the interface problem.

The idea of supervenience was originally articulated by G. E. Moore (1873–1958) to relate moral properties to physical properties given the assumption that moral properties cannot be analysed into physical descriptions.

> [I]f a given thing possesses any kind of intrinsic value in a certain degree, then not only must that same thing possess it, under all circumstances, in the same degree, but also anything *exactly like it*, must, under all circumstances, possess it in exactly the same degree ... it is not *possible* that of two exactly similar things one should possess it and the other not, or that one should possess it in one degree, and the other in a different one.
>
> (Moore, 1922, p. 261)

More recently, it has been used most often in the philosophy of mind. It claims that determining the physical properties of a system determines its mental properties but not vice versa. It was most famously asserted by Davidson to further characterize his token identity theory which claims that every mental event is a physical event (Davidson, 1980, pp. 207–227). But as John Haugeland pointed out, it need not be associated with a position even apparently as weakly reductionist as a token identity theory (Haugeland, 1982). It could be used to characterize a yet weaker relation between mental and physical descriptions as a whole even where there is no claim that the same individuals (entities or events) can be identified in both. Haugeland calls this 'weak supervenience' (although that ambiguous label is also used for modally constrained versions of supervenience).

Supervenience promises to provide a global solution to the interface problem. It is designed to accommodate two intuitions. On the one hand, the manifest and scientific images answer to distinct constitutive principles. But on the other, they describe two aspects of the same natural world. The properties of the manifest image cannot float free of those described in the scientific image. They are asymmetrically determined by them.

Nevertheless as I will explain, supervenience cannot ease the interface problem. It is easier to set out this objection in the case of a supervenience claim combined with a token identity theory and then generalize it.

A key motivation for advocating a merely token identity theory of mental and physical properties is doubt about the plausibility of a stronger form of reduction of the mental to the physical. In Davidson's case, this doubt centres on the idea that the mental is governed by a constitutive principle of rationality which cannot be accounted for in physical terms. It is because of this that the prospect of defining the normative or rational pattern of the manifest image in non-normative natural scientific terms seems dim. Thus the attempt to reduce mental types to physical types looks unpromising.

A token identity theory can escape this problem because it does not aim at reductionist explanation of content. It does not set out to explain normative concepts in non-normative terms as reductionist identity theories do. A token identity theory identifies an instance of being in a particular or token mental state at a particular time with being in a particular or token physical state at that time. It does not owe an account of which causal dispositions, in physical terms, correspond to mental features because it does not attempt to define the content of the mental state or disposition in physical terms. Nevertheless, even a non-reductive, merely token, identity theory falls to a related criticism of a reductionist approach.

The problem is this (cf. Child, 1994, pp. 80–89). If the dispositions of physical states described in causal terms do not *define* or *set* the normative standard, then they must instead *conform* to that standard. Thus, if a token mental state is identified with a token physical state, the causal role of that mental state, when physically described, must match its normative role when described in intentional terms. Because they have abandoned the responsibility for attempting to *explain* how the content of a state arises in physical terms, token identity theories have instead the duty of explaining how the physical and mental properties of states keep in step. But they lack any resources for doing this.

The same kind of argument applies even if one weakens the relation between manifest and scientific images to supervenience without token identities. In this context, the problem is: what explains why the rational normative pattern of the former keeps in step with the nomological pattern of the latter? Giving up a full-blooded attempt at reduction makes this merely a mysterious pre-established harmony.

This problem suggests that non-reductionist supervenience physicalism is not a stable middle point between a form of dualism that eschews supervenience or a reductionist physicalism that can also explain supervenience. That in turn suggests that supervenience cannot, any more than the stance stance, provide a deflationary resolution to the interface problem.

6.3 **Towards a global dissolution and local solutions**

Both the stance stance and supervenience seem, at first sight, to be promising ways to attempt to accommodate a significant distinction between the manifest and scientific image of man in the world whilst at the same time addressing the question of how distinct explanations might interface with one another. They attempt to provide accounts of how different kinds of explanation might relate to each other without attempting to reduce one explanation to another. Neither, however, succeed.

One might, in response to this, reconsider the prospects of reduction. After all, the objection to supervenience turned on the fact that it postulated a harmony for which, in the absence of a reductionist account, it had no explanation. But given the significant difficulties of reducing the normative concepts of the manifest image to non-normative nomological terms, that remains unattractive.

A third option questions the terms of the distinction in a different way – not with the aim of blurring the boundaries but, rather, with the aim of questioning their significance. The aim is to reduce the stakes of the debate to leave the possibility that the interface problem is best answered not in a global way by philosophy but rather locally.

In this final section, I will outline three familiar thoughts that should help shake the felt need to offer a global solution to the interface problem. The threefold strategy is to:

1 undermine the metaphysical status of physicalism;

2 question the content and truth of physicalism; and

3 recognize that explanations are contextual.

6.3.1 **The metaphysical significance of physicalism**

One widespread assumption of contemporary philosophy is that nature is exhausted by the description that will eventually be offered by a completed physics. In a book on meaning, the assumption that all natural phenomena are really physical is shaped into an explicit argument by the philosopher Jerry Fodor, which is worth quoting at length:

> I suppose that sooner or later the physicists will complete the catalogue they've been compiling of the ultimate and irreducible properties of things. When they do, the likes of *spin*, *charm* and *charge* will perhaps appear upon their list. But *aboutness* surely won't; intentionality simply doesn't go that deep. It's hard to see, in face of this consideration, how one can be a Realist about intentionality without also being, to some extent or other, a Reductionist. If the semantic and intentional are real properties of things, it must be in virtue of their identity with (or maybe of their supervenience on?) properties that are *neither* intentional *nor* semantic. If aboutness is real, it must be really something else.
>
> (Fodor, 1987, p. 97)

Fodor's argument takes it for granted that a complete catalogue of physical properties is a complete catalogue of nature. With this assumption in place, a necessary condition for a property to be a genuine or real feature of the world is either that it is found in that catalogue of physical properties or that it can, at least, be related to properties found there.

If, by contrast, no such relation obtains, then the problematic concepts cannot describe genuine features of the world.

This meta-*physical* view gives rise to a characteristic meta-*philosophical* view. Philosophy should aim to 'naturalize' problematic concepts, ideas, or phenomena by relating them back to the more basic vocabulary of natural science or physics that serves as a standard or benchmark. Showing how a philosophically puzzling phenomenon can be reduced to (or constructed from) something more basic and not puzzling should ease philosophical confusion. Naturalism so understood is a form of reductionism.

Whilst the quotation from Fodor expresses an argument for reduction to basic physics, there are other approaches to less basic science. Teleosemantics, for example, aims to reduce mental content to biological or proper functions. Ruth Millikan asserts that 'an appeal to teleology, to function, is what is needed to fly a naturalist theory of content' (Millikan, 1989, p. 282). But because 'teleology' in this context is to be explained as a biological function and that is regarded as a feature of causal explanation in biology, the account is still naturalistic in the reductionist sense and in accord with Fodor's argument.

But neither this view of naturalism nor this assessment of the strength of the argument are mandatory. Consider again the significance of a failure to reduce a concept to those found in basic physics. This might show that it is not the concept of a genuine property, a property that is really real. But it might also reveal that an assumption has been made about the nature of reality which is overly restrictive. Why should we take it that nature or reality is exhausted by what is charted in physics? Furthermore, without that assumption, naturalism as a philosophical aim might take a different form – not the attempt to reduce problematic concepts to those of basic physics but rather show in some other way why they need not be regarded as problematic. An alternative approach to the aim of naturalizing normativity is thus not by reducing norms to the nomological structures of nature (where there is no echo of them) but rather by questioning the assumptions that disbar nature from containing norms.

This alternative view of both the nature of nature and the nature of philosophy has been promoted by John McDowell. He suggests that although the assumption, that what is real is exhausted by the natural sciences, seems at present to be a natural one, it is by no means compulsory.

> What is at work here is a conception of nature that can seem sheer common sense, though it was not always so; the conception I mean was made available only by a hard-won achievement of human thought at a specific time, the time of the rise of modern science. Modern science understands its subject matter in a way that threatens, at least, to leave it disenchanted.
>
> (McDowell, 1994, p. 70)

One reason for saying that science leaves its subject matter 'disenchanted' is that the mediaeval idea that nature comprised of a book of moral lessons has been rightly rejected. But in addition, McDowell suggests that it threatens to limit what is real to the realm of law. This contrasts with those phenomena that have to be fitted within a different pattern of intelligibility – the space of reasons that describes the rational pattern of intentional states. He suggests that nature should not be equated just with the realm of law but should also be taken to include the space of reasons.

By suggesting that nature includes more than just what lies within the realm of law, McDowell does not aim to slight the success of science. Nor does he suggest that there should be no place for a disenchanted view of nature within scientific method:

> But it is one thing to recognise that the impersonal stance of scientific investigation is a methodological necessity for the achievement of a valuable mode of understanding reality; it is quite another thing to take the dawning grasp of this, in the modern era, for a metaphysical insight into the notion of objectivity as such, so that objective correctness in any mode of thought must be anchored in this kind of access to the real. . . .[It] is not the educated common sense it represents itself as being; it is shallow metaphysics.
>
> (McDowell, 1998, p. 182)

The moral that McDowell draws is that there is more to nature than can be described within the natural sciences. Nature is broader than that. This is not to advance an anti-scientific claim. Science has been very successful in explaining a range of phenomena by subsuming them under general laws. But that need not imply that phenomena that cannot be so set out are not real.

6.3.2 The truth of physicalism

One reason for attributing a metaphysical significance to the physical would be commitment to the truth of physicalism. This is, roughly, the claim that everything is physical. But in the light of apparent self-contradiction in saying that things which are usually contrasted with the physical really are physical (and the quotation from Fodor in section 6.3.1), it is more usual to say that everything either is or supervenes on the physical. If supervenience physicalism were true, that would help to provide some support for the metaphysical significance of the physical, and the physical would be the most general account of the world. But it is not obviously true.

The challenge for supervenience physicalists is to produce a non-question-begging argument for their position. One such approach is to start from the completeness of physics defined, roughly, as the claim that the chances of every event can be set out in physical terms or none at all. Taken together with an assumption that the world is not generally causally overdetermined, this can be used to frame an argument for mental supervenience (Papineau, 1990). When events can be explained by invoking mental causes, then by the completeness of physics, they can also be explained by their physical causes. If the world is not causally overdetermined, then the physical causes must determine the mental causes. Because the mental is not causally complete, the opposite is not true. Hence the physical determines the mental but not vice versa. Hence supervenience is true.

But as Tim Crane argued in the early 1990s, the completeness of physics so defined is just as contentious as supervenience physicalism itself (Crane, 1991). If one doubts the latter, one will claim that some effects are determined by mental as well as physical causes. Such effects are *not* determined by physics alone and thus completeness of physics is not true. The challenge is thus to find a way to define 'physics' such that the claim that physics is complete is both substantial and true without merely assuming supervenience. This leads to a dilemma:

If 'physics' were simply (and insubstantially) defined as whatever would be included in an explanatorily complete science, that need not rule out psychology as an essential part of a future complete science.

If, by contrast, 'physics' is substantially defined by reference to the microsciences, one could claim that by determining the microfeatures of a situation, one determines the macrofeatures. The motivation for this claim is the thought that, at heart, physics deals with the fundamental particles which make up matter and whose behaviour ultimately determines what happens in the universe. But if one simply assumes that microlevel phenomena determine what happens at the macroscopic level, and thus that the physical determines the non-physical, this comes to the same thing as assuming that there will be no macroscopic difference without microscopic difference. And this assumption is just supervenience again. One will, in other words, have simply assumed supervenience in the argument which was supposed to give it independent support.

This is, of course, just to present a challenge for the defence of supervenience physicalism rather than to argue that it is false. But the empirical data need not be seen as supporting its truth either. Nancy Cartwright suggests that close examination of the way that fundamental physical explanations are offered favours a view of the world in which the world itself is gappy. That is, there are gaps in principle in what can be explained by natural laws. To contrast the usual assumption of the completeness of physics and drawing on her interpretation of the practice of science, she says:

> I imagine that natural objects are much like people in societies. Their behaviour is constrained by some specific laws and by a handful of general principles, but it is not determined in detail even statistically. What happens on most occasions is dictated by no law at all. This is not a metaphysical picture that I urge. My claim is that this picture is as plausible as the alternative. God may have written just a few laws and grown tired.
>
> (Cartwright, 1983, p. 49)

This gives rise to a picture which contrasts the usual hierarchy of levels:

> The laws that describe this world are a patchwork, not a pyramid. They do not take after the simple, elegant and abstract structure of a system of axioms and theorems. Rather they look like – and steadfastly stick to looking like – science as we know it: apportioned into disciplines, apparently arbitrarily grown up; governing different sets of properties at different levels of abstraction; pockets of great precision; large parcels of qualitative maxims resisting precise formulation; erratic overlaps; here and there, once in a while, corners that line up, but mostly ragged edges; and always the cover of law just loosely attached to the jumbled world of material things.
>
> (Cartwright, 1999, p.1)

The idea sketched here does not seem to be impossible in principle. Cartwright's claim is, further, that it is better empirically supported than the usual assumption about science which helps drive the quest for an *a priori* solution to the interface problem.

6.3.3 **Physicalism and explanation**

A second reason for asserting the metaphysical significance of the physical would be a claim about the basic role of physical explanation. Two familiar considerations seem to support this. One is the idea that physical explanations 'trump' other higher-level explanations. The other is the idea, motivated by a nomological theory of causation, that causal explanations are underpinned by laws and only physics can provide the right kind of laws. I will consider these, again very briefly, in turn.

If one already has reason to subscribe to the metaphysical significance of the physical or supervenience physicalism, then it can seem obvious that physical explanations must trump higher-level explanations. This is because such explanations seem to chart the underlying mechanism that drives higher level phenomena. But if the latter consideration is supposed to support the former, and the former is not assumed, it is by no means clear that it can.

Hilary Putnam gives the example of an everyday explanation for why a square peg will not fit into a round hole (Putnam, 1975, pp. 295–298). An explanation pitched at the level of the rigidity of the peg and hole and their relative cross-sections is complete. It does not need further augmentation in microphysical terms.

Putnam's example is a physical explanation albeit one at the level of everyday objects. But his point can be broadened by consideration of the autonomy of explanation of human behaviour couched in the terms of Sellars' manifest image, or Dennett's intentional stance. Following Cartwright's suggestion that one looks to actual explanatory practice (albeit more broadly than just within the physical sciences), person-level explanation is in perfect order as it stands and requires no lower-level underpinning.

Whilst appearances themselves do not support the fundamental status of physical explanation, an underlying argument for that claim could be deployed based on considerations Davidson offers (Davidson, 1980, pp. 149–162). In the tradition of Humean analyses, Davidson assumes that wherever there is a causal relation between events, those events must be subsumable under a strict law. But, he argues, such strict laws are only available at the level of basic physics. Thus wherever there is a causal relation describable at a higher level, and perhaps charted in a higher level explanation, it is also describable in low-level physical terms. This in turn suggests that where there is a high-level causal explanation, there is a lower-level explanation in physical terms that subsumes it.

This is not the place to attempt to undermine a nomological account of causation. But it is worth flagging the fact that although it may support the metaphysical significance of physics, it is an optional philosophical commitment. If, historically, the main argument for a nomological account is Hume's failure to reduce the idea of a singular or one-off necessary connection then, akin to the response to Fodor I suggested earlier, one might instead regard this not as undermining that idea but rather casting doubt on the reductionist programme. A nomological account of causation is part of a package of ideas that helps sustain the idea that the interface problem is *the* framing problem for philosophy as a whole. The cost of escaping the need for an *a priori* solution may be the principled rejection of all elements that make it up.

6.3.4 **Local solutions to the interface problem**

My point in setting out these three objections to the usual picture is not to attempt to solve the interface problem. I think that it is a mistake to try to solve that problem by attempting a global stereoscopic or synoptic view. What is needed, instead, is to find local accommodations once at least some of the assumptions that make it seem more pressing than it need have been, are undermined. To illustrate this, I will consider one example drawn from psychiatry.

In 1978, the sociologist George Brown and psychologist Tirril Harris published the results of a study of aetiological factors for depression based on a study of 458 women in Camberwell in South London. They outlined a causal model of clinical depression based on three broad groups of factors:

> the provoking agents, the vulnerability factors, and the symptom-formation factors. These . . . relate in differing ways to a central experience of hopelessness which develops out of the appraisal of particular circumstances, usually involving loss.
>
> (Brown and Harris, 1978, p. 233)

Brown and Harris followed a longstanding tradition in taking depression to be the result of an experience of loss. But loss might comprise a variety of different kinds of events. Thus they construe it in a very general way as 'deprivation of sources of value or reward' (*ibid.*, p. 233). Loss, however, is not the specific determinant of depression. One might, for example, feel that one had coped well with a loss and that might, in fact, help protect against depression. Instead, they argue that 'hopelessness is the key factor in the genesis of clinical depression and loss is probably the most likely cause of profound hopelessness' (*ibid.*, p. 234).

Many people experience loss without developing a feeling of hopelessness and hence, based on the model, depression. Why is this? Brown and Harris suggest that prior low self-esteem and a prior feeling of not being in control of one's life or broader events is what is key for turning the experience of loss into a general sense of hopelessness. This general claim is realized in distinct vulnerability factors which comprise:

> an odd assortment: loss of mother before eleven, presence at home of three or more children under fourteen, absence of a confiding relationship, particularly with a husband, and lack of a full- or part-time job.
>
> (*ibid.*, pp. 235–236)

Thus the model (Fig. 6.1) is one in which contingent factors in the past comprise vulnerability factors which lead to ongoing low self-esteem. Then, in the face of an experience of loss, which leads to a feeling of specific hopelessness about this, the vulnerability factors cause this feeling to escalate to one of general hopelessness and then in turn to the onset of clinical depression.

The model traces a causal connection between concepts which belong to each of Sellars' manifest and scientific images without offering any general synoptic view. The outcome, the causal effect, is depression which involves 'profound bodily changes' (*ibid.*, p. 235). But the causes include two sets of heterogeneous events. Brown and Harris offer a small list of vulnerability factors – early maternal loss, lack of a confiding relationship, more than three children under the age of 14 at home,

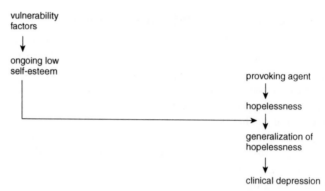

Fig. 6.1 Reproduced with permission from Brown and Harris (1978, p. 238).

and unemployment – identified through empirical research. The more immediate cause is unified at one level – a sense of hopelessness. That, in turn, is explained as the result of a loss but what the specific loss is in each case is left open-ended. Thus identifying new cases that fit the underlying model requires an interpretative judgement that such and such an event is a case of loss of personal value. Nevertheless, according to the model, these stand in a causal relationship to eventual depression. They are not a reason for the subject for her depression. This helps to exemplify the way in which the model crosses levels.

It is an empirical question whether this model is accurate and really does chart a complex causal dependence. But if it is and does, it manages to do this without solving the interface problem generally. It is a local matter that this particular set of mental and physical states and events can be reliably identified and can reliably stand in the relations set out. Little follows for the development of other cross-boundary causal models. But it is at least an indication of the kind of local solutions that may be found, not through *a priori* philosophy, but piecemeal empirical research.

Where does this leave the World Psychiatric Association's Institutional Program on Psychiatry for the Person? A key idea is the development of a comprehensive model of diagnosis:

> This comprehensive concept of diagnosis is implemented through the articulation of two diagnostic levels. The first is a standardised multi-axial diagnostic formulation, which describes the patient's illness and clinical condition through standardised typologies and scales. . . .The second is an idiographic diagnostic formulation, which complements the standardised formulation with a personalised and flexible statement.
>
> (IDGA Workgroup, WPA 2003, p. 55)

If the model is to be a genuinely successful contribution to psychiatric understanding, then it will have to be the case that the features described through standardized typologies and scales interact with those described through personalized and flexible statements. One indication of this would be the development of a causal or otherwise explanatory model with aspects from both elements. Another indication would be the genuine contribution of the comprehensive model to guide treatment and management, a contribution over and above conventional diagnosis. The purpose of this chapter, however, has been to suggest the potential independence of that issue from the broader goal of solving the interface problem generally.

In meeting the challenge raised by person-centred psychiatry, there seem to be four broad options. There might be a global reduction of the normative person-level elements of the manifest image or the space of reasons to the scientific image or realm of law. Or, there might be some other *a priori* and global reconciliation of the two elements which also recognizes their fundamental distinctiveness. Although I have provided no fresh argument for pessimism about the first in this chapter, neither seems to be a very likely outcome.

A third option is that psychiatry might increasingly see itself as confined to cognitive neuroscience. That is, it might limit itself to what Sellars describes as postulational theory construction. If so then, inferring from past developments, there are likely to be increasing technological developments to underpin prediction, treatment, and management of psychiatric illness. But it will cut itself off from an account or description of the context of these states. This is significant because what constitutes underlying mechanisms as pathological turns on the effects of those mechanisms at the level of the manifest image (see, e.g., Thornton, 2007, pp. 39–48). (Mere deviation from the norm at a neurological level need not amount to a pathology, for example.) In some areas of medicine, there is sufficient agreement about what constitutes a healthy heart, for example, that this person-level context can be taken for granted. But because psychiatry charts such potentially broad problems of living, it would be a mistake to rule out debate within psychiatric theory itself of what constitutes mental health and illness (Fulford, 1989).

This leaves the fourth option, which I have sketched above. Provided the apparent need for a global account of the interface between higher and lower levels can be eased, there is space for local accounts of how descriptions at the level of the whole person can interact with underlying cognitive neuroscience. That is not, of course, to make the task of charting such connections through psychiatric research any easier.

References

Bermúdez, J. L. (2005). *Philosophy of Psychology*. London, Routledge.

Bilgrami, A. (2004). Intentionality and norms. In *Naturalism in Question* (eds. M. de Caro, and D. MacArthur). Cambridge, MA, Harvard University Press.

Brown, G. W. and Harris, T. (1978). *Social Origins of Depression*. London, Free Press and New York, Tavistock Press.

Cartwright, N. (1983). *How the Laws of Physics Lie*. Oxford, Oxford University Press.

Cartwright, N. (1999). *The Dappled World: A Study of the Boundaries of Science*. Cambridge, Cambridge University Press.

Child, W. (1994). *Causality, Interpretation and the Mind*. Oxford, Oxford University Press.

Crane, T. (1991). Why indeed? Papineau on supervenience. *Analysis*, **51**, 32–37.

Davidson, D. (1980). *Essays on Actions and Events*. Oxford, Oxford University Press.

Dennett, D. (1978). *Brainstorms*. Montgomery, VT, Bradford Books.

Dennett, D. (1987). *The Intentional Stance*. Cambridge, MA, MIT Press.

Dretske, F. (1988). The stance stance. *Behavioral and Brain Sciences*, **11**, 511–512.

Fodor, J. A. (1987). *Psychosemantics: The problem of Meaning in the Philosophy of Mind.* Cambridge, MA, MIT Press.

Fulford, K. W. M. (1989). *Moral Theory and Medical Practice.* Cambridge, Cambridge University Press.

Haugeland, J. (1982). Weak supervenience. *American Philosophical Quarterly,* **19**, 93–103.

IDGA Workgroup, WPA (2003). IGDA 8: Idiographic (personalised) diagnostic formulation. *British Journal of Psychiatry,* **18**(45), 55–57.

McDowell, J. (1994). *Mind and World.* Cambridge, MA, Harvard University Press.

McDowell, J. (1998). *Mind Value and Reality.* Cambridge, MA, Harvard University Press.

Mezzich, J. E. (2005). Values and comprehensive diagnosis. *World Psychiatry,* **4**, 91–92.

Millikan, R. G. (1989). Biosemantics. *Journal of Philosophy,* **86**, 281–297.

Moore, G. E. (1922). *Philosophical Studies.* London, Routledge.

Papineau, D. (1990). Why supervenience? *Analysis,* **50**, 66–71.

Putnam, H. (1975). *Mind, Language and Reality: Philosophical Papers,* vol. 2. Cambridge, Cambridge University Press.

Sellars, W. (1963). Philosophy and the scientific image of man. In *Science, Perception and Reality,* pp. 1–40. London, Routledge and Kegan Paul.

Thornton, T. (1998). *Wittgenstein on Language and Thought.* Edinburgh, Edinburgh University Press.

Thornton, T. (2007). *Essential Philosophy of Psychiatry.* Oxford, Oxford University Press.

Chapter 7

What does rationality have to do with psychological causation? Propositional attitudes as mechanisms and as control variables

John Campbell

Abstract

How are we to decide what variables to use in characterizing the causal structure of a complex system? I'll argue that one central component is the search for 'control variables'. We want to be able to characterize the space of possible outcomes of interventions on the system in such a way that we can find 'control variables' – variables that have large, systematic, and specific effects on those outcomes. I look at the implications of this approach for a number of questions concerning causation in psychiatry.

7.1 Introduction

I contrast two causal roles for propositional attitudes. One is that they play a role in our conception of a psychological mechanism: we think of rationally connected propositional attitudes as constituting psychological mechanisms. The second, more fundamental role for propositional attitudes is that they function as control variables in the psychological lives of subjects. These two roles for propositional attitudes come apart dramatically in the case of deluded subjects. We have propositional attitudes as control variables. But they do not figure in rational connections.

Separating these two roles for propositional attitudes makes a difference to how we think of the relation between ordinary propositional-attitude psychology and cognitive-neuroscience approaches to mental illness. Suppose the only causal connections between propositional attitudes are rational connections. Then consider what happens in a case, such as a case of delusion, in which we do not seem to have ordinary rationality. Then, one possibility is that, as Young suggests, the subject's propositional states are after all broadly rational reactions to sensory states whose occurrence can be explained by cognitive neuroscience (de Clérambault, 1924/2002; Maher, 1974; Young, 2000). Or else we could abandon the appeal to propositional attitudes altogether, and explain the subject's reactions purely in terms of cognitive neuroscience, as Churchland (2002) recommends.

Suppose, however, we think that there can be causal relations between propositional attitudes that are not rational connections. We can think there are causal relations between propositional states in this sense – that an intervention on one state would have made a difference to the other. A causal connection in this sense need not be a rational connection. There is still a question, though, about the mechanism linking the two states. And here we might find a role for cognitive neuroscience, in explaining what that mechanism is. This is a role for cognitive neuroscience in explaining the mediation between two propositional attitudes that are not themselves rationally linked. In this chapter I will try only to set out the issue a bit more fully.

7.2 **Rational connections as mechanisms**

Suppose you are an epidemiologist investigating the impact of environmental factors on the risk of contracting some disease. Suppose, for example, that you are looking at whether contaminated water is a risk factor for cholera. You may do observational studies that suggest it is a risk factor, as John Snow observed that cholera cases in Soho were centred round the water pump (Snow, 1855). The critical test for a causal link comes when you intervene on the water supply, for example, by removing the handle on the pump. If that makes a difference to the contraction of cholera, then there is a causal link between the water supply and cholera. Even though that is all it takes to establish a causal connection, there is a further question – that is, how to characterize the mechanism that links the water supply to the disease? It would seem a kind of madness if someone were to acknowledge that there is a causal link, but propose that there may be no mechanism linking the two. The notion of mechanism thus seems essential to describing how science proceeds in many cases. We cannot simply dispense with the notion, as we would then have no way of saying what was missing in the water–cholera case. But it is notoriously difficult to give any general characterization of what a mechanism is. Case by case, what is meant is often plain enough. In the case of cholera, for instance, once we have in place the germ theory of disease, it gives us a general template for a detailed description of the link between water contamination and cholera. But it is not easy to give a description of what it takes to describe a 'mechanism' in general. Consider the case of poverty and mental illness. There has long been known to be a correlation between the two. But what is the direction of causation, and what is the mechanism by which causal influence is transmitted? Recently, there was a 'natural experiment' in a population of American Indians and others living side by side. A casino opened on the reservation, and there was an income supplement for the American Indians which increased annually. Psychiatrists were at the time engaged in a longitudinal study of the whole population. So, they could look at the impact of this intervention on poverty on levels of mental illness in the American Indian population, using the rest of population as controls. They found that poverty was indeed a cause of mental illness; as a result of the intervention on income, levels of certain types of mental illness fell in the American Indian population. But, the compelling question is, what was the mechanism by which this happened? The question here is formally the same as in the case of cholera; but here the germ theory of disease hardly seems to the point. The investigators proposed that a principal mechanism here – not the only one, no doubt – was that the relief of poverty made it possible for there to be more parental supervision of children, in particular teenage children (Costello, *et al.*, 2003). Of course, this is not a definitive answer, but it is a reasonable conjecture. What is the general notion of 'mechanism' that covers both the water–cholera case and this case? It is not obvious that we know how to characterize this notion, essential though it is.

One approach is to do without a fully general description of the notion of mechanism, and instead to try to characterize certain prototypical or basic cases of mechanisms. We might then think that insofar as we have a fully general notion of 'mechanism' it is achieved only by a kind of extension or analogy with these basic cases. In the physical case, we might think about examples like the following. Suppose you flip a switch and the light comes on. What is the mechanism? There must be one, even if you are not very sure what it is. Suppose, in contrast, that one billiard ball hits another and the second one moves on. What is the mechanism by which movement was transmitted from one billiard ball to the other? There is no immediate need here to postulate hidden strings or pulleys. The transmission of motion by impulse is one of our prototypical mechanisms. We do not need to postulate some mechanism other than the impact of one ball on the other to explain how it happens that the movement of the first ball causes the second to move. When you move to the level of microphysical analysis, you might give a further breakdown of how this mechanism works. But you are not giving a description of some different mechanism; rather, you are re-describing the communication of motion by impulse.

There is a still simpler case. Suppose I light an oil heater while outdoors. Then, a bit later, I carry the heater indoors. The lighting of the heater happened outdoors. It is now hotter indoors. How did that happen? What is the mechanism by which causal influence was transmitted from place to place? We obviously do not need to postulate hidden strings and pulleys here. The movement of the heater from one place to another was the mechanism by which causal influence was transmitted from the one place to the other. Once the movement of the object is reckoned into account, there is no need to look for further mechanisms. This is a quite general point: the movement of an object from one place to another is the principal mechanism by which causal influence is transmitted from one place to another. This is one of the simplest cases of 'mechanism', because unlike the case of billiard-ball collisions, there is only one object here. (Of course I come in as lighting the heater and as carrying the heater, but these are, as it were, supporting roles; the mechanism for the transmission of causal influence from place to place is the movement of the object.)

There is much to be said about these cases, but in this chapter I want to focus on the psychological case. What can we make of the notion of a psychological mechanism? We have already glimpsed the kind of question and answer that might be given here, in the case of the casino on the reservation. But let us look at some much simpler cases. Suppose you say to me, 'I think Sally would be a good person for this post.' I say,

'What makes you think that?' Your reply is, 'I saw a sparrow on the lawn last night.' It cannot stop there. How did you get from one to the other? What was the mechanism? How did seeing a sparrow on the lawn cause you to have this belief about Sally? If there is no answer, if the causation here was genuinely without any further rational filling-in, then we have here a kind of spooky 'action-at-a-distance' between your belief and your perception. Suppose, in contrast, you say, 'I saw Martha, whose judgement I believe to be flawless, and she said we should give Sally the post. So I think we should give Sally the post.' Here there is no causal question as to how your seeing Martha caused your belief. We do not here have spooky 'action-at-a-distance'. You and I might of course have an argument about normative questions – whether you should give such weight to Martha's views, and so on. But there is, on the face of it, nothing similarly puzzling about the *causation* here. It is like the case of movement of the heater from one place to another. To grasp the rationality of the transition is already to grasp the cognitive mechanism by which one psychological state caused the other.

Let me sum up. The notion of a mechanism is essential to much, perhaps most scientific research. At the same time, it is hard to see how to give a general characterization of it. It is hard because in particular, there are both psychological and physical mechanisms. A cognitive psychologist asking whether traumatic experiences cause depression, for example, might naturally want to pursue the cognitive mechanisms involved. But it is hard to see how to give a characterization of 'mechanism' that would cover both this case and the cholera case. So we can instead try to characterize the prototypical psychological and physical mechanisms. I am proposing that we can use the notion of rationality to characterize the prototypical psychological mechanisms. When we have a rational causal sequence of psychological states, we do not need to look for the cognitive mechanism by which our subject got from one state to the other: we have it already. You might say that there must be brain sequences here, which we can try to characterize. But that is not a matter of trying to find a different mechanism here, some different strings and pulleys. Just so, when I move the heater from outdoors to indoors, the mechanism by which causal influence is transmitted from place to place is evident. You might indeed look at the microstructural analysis of the heater. But that is not a matter of you providing a different mechanism, another route by which causal influence is transmitted from outside to inside. You might say that you feel uneasy about the weight that is being put on these judgements about when we do and do not need to find a mechanism. I have a certain sympathy with that uneasiness, but I have to point out to you that you are deeply out of tune with the science of the past 400 years. Science is driven by these judgements about when we have found a mechanism and when we have still to find a mechanism. All I have done so far is suggest that we look at the application of the notion of mechanism to the very simplest cases, and see how it works there. This is a cautious step. Throwing out the notion of mechanism altogether is a radical move we might yet make – but not yet.

The role I have proposed for the notion of rationality is related to, but not the same as, the place that is usually accorded to the notion in analyses of propositional-attitude psychology. The classical view in philosophy of mind is that the ascription of propositional attitudes depends on an assumption that the subject is broadly rational.

Davidson thought that the ascription of propositional attitudes depends on a background assumption of the rationality of the agent. Ascribing propositional attitudes is a way of making sense of the agent, and making sense of the agent requires that we discern rationality in the agent. In fact, there is something paradoxical about the very idea that we might find an agent without rationality. We cannot find propositional attitudes without finding rationality.

> When thought takes thought as its subject matter, the observer can only identify what he is studying by finding it rational – that is, in accord with his own standards of rationality.
>
> (Davidson, 2004, p. 98)

Now it seems to me that this view has some difficulty with cases of mental illness. Consider the following report of the beliefs of a schizophrenic patient:

> A 22-year-old woman had the delusion that thoughts and feelings emanating from her mother's unconscious were being carried in raindrops that fell on her air conditioner. When the raindrops hit the air conditioner they made a noise, and simultaneously these thoughts and feelings merged with her own unconscious. This merging had resulted in her own mental illness.
>
> (Spitzer *et al.*, 1993, p. 882)

It is possible to argue that even the schizophrenic displaying symptoms is fully rational, and simply illustrates Davidson's point. But it does stretch credulity that the figure of the schizophrenic could be used to explain what Davidson meant by 'rational'. The trouble is not even that patient is not rational. We have no idea what a rational way of going on would be, once one has accepted that thoughts are being inserted into one's mind. How must the world be, for that to happen? Would it make sense to argue with this patient that, by her own lights, it is not the raindrops and the air conditioning that should be blamed, but rather the electrical sockets all around? We have departed so far from the ordinary world that we have no idea what stands fast and what has to go. We do not know what a reasonable way of arguing would look like. (For further argument that deluded subjects cannot be regarded as rational, see Bortolotti, 2005a, b.)

On the other hand, you could argue that the schizophrenic does not have propositional attitudes. (For a sophisticated form of this view, see Currie, 2000. For resistance see Bayne and Pacherie, 2005.) The attitude usually expressed by the phrase, 'a crazy person', is something like: we do not have to reckon this person's propositional attitudes into account. In the present context, though, we do (see Bayne and Pacherie again). The patient does have propositional attitudes, even though there is little rationality exhibited. That ought to be impossible, in Davidson's view. Dennett provides a blunter expression of the same idea. Would you like to know how to ascribe beliefs and desires to people?

> Here is how it works: first you decide to treat the object whose behavior is to be predicted as a rational agent; then you figure out what beliefs that agent ought to have, given its place in the world and its purpose. Then you figure out what desires it ought to have, on the same considerations, and finally you predict that this rational agent will act to further

its goals in the light of its beliefs. A little practical reasoning from the chosen set of beliefs and desires will in most instances yield a decision about what the agent ought to do; that is what you predict the agent will do.

(Dennett, 1987, p. 17)

This strategy would not allow us to ascribe propositional attitudes to many of the mentally ill. The trouble is that despite the deficiencies in rationality, many mental patients seem plainly to have propositional attitudes. I will pursue this point in a moment.

On the approach I am recommending, though, there is something highly puzzling about these patients. They do have propositional attitudes, and there are causal relations among their propositional attitudes. But so long as we lack insight into how these relations among propositional attitudes can be seen as rational, we lack insight into the psychological mechanisms involved in the formation of their delusions. There is no contradiction, though, in the idea that the causal patterns in the world may be such that there are no mechanisms to be found to underpin them.

On this analysis, there is an analogy between:

1 the idea that propositional-attitude ascriptions depends on the ascription of rationality to the subject, and

2 the idea that all causal interactions between pieces of matter must be comprehensible in mechanistic terms.

Both ideas express an insight – that we find it extremely puzzling when we encounter causal relations among propositional attitudes that are not broadly rational, just as we find it extremely puzzling when we encounter causal interactions between physical objects that are not mechanistic, and that involve spooky 'action-at-a-distance'. Both ideas express a natural impulse of philosophers – to elevate this kind of point into a kind of synthetic *a priori* demand that reason makes on the world. This impulse has to be resisted. Delusional patients provide a dramatic example where it looks as though we have causal relations among propositional attitudes that are not rational. Quantum-mechanical phenomena provide dramatic cases where it looks as though we have causal interactions between pieces of matter that require spooky action-at-a-distance.

In the case of delusion as in the case of quantum mechanics, the detailed analysis of the phenomena is not a matter to be settled quickly. I make no attempt to settle either quickly here. The point I am making is that we should not try to settle these cases in advance by appealing to *a priori* constraints on how the world must be. We should not appeal to the idea that there are *a priori* constraints on causal relations among propositional attitudes. We have to accept that the propositional attitudes are one thing and the causal relations among them are another. If the propositional attitudes do not conform to rationality, that is puzzling. But we cannot legislate in advance that this cannot happen. Similarly in the case of matter, we should not appeal to the idea that there are *a priori* constraints on how matter must be. If matter does not conform to mechanistic constraints, that is puzzling. But we cannot legislate in advance that the world cannot be so, that spooky action-at-a-distance is impossible.

7.3 **Interventions**

One role for propositional attitudes in psychological causation is through their implication in rational sequences, the psychological mechanisms by which causal influence is transmitted. But there is another element to causal role. In an interventionist analysis of causation, for X to be a cause of Y is for intervening on X to be a way of manipulating Y. (An 'intervention' on X with respect to Y will have to meet the conditions of an ideal experiment, such as a randomized controlled trial (RCT). For discussion and details see Woodward, 2003; Woodward and Hitchcock, 2003; Campbell, 2007.)

This analysis makes no appeal to any notion of mechanism. It says only that for X to be a cause of Y is for the values of X and Y to be correlated under interventions on X. So in this analysis, for one belief to be a cause of another is for intervening on the first belief to be a way of changing the second. Suppose you believe:

1 that this man is stroking his chin, and

2 that this man believes you need to shave.

(For more on such 'delusions of reference' see Startup and Startup, 2005.) What is it for the first belief to be a cause of the second? On the interventionist analysis, it is for intervention on the first belief to be a way of changing whether you have the second belief. So if some external force changed your belief that this man is stroking his chin, you would no longer believe that he believes you need to shave. There is no appeal to rationality here, no appeal to mechanisms.

Someone who suffers from delusions of reference in this way is not rational, and we naturally look for some explanation as to why it can happen that belief (1) causes belief (2). This is where cognitive neuroscience accounts might be expected to play some role; but the role is to explain a causal connection that we know already to exist. We want to find the background against which these kinds of causal connections can occur. Let me give another example:

> A 22-year-old Rastafarian man of Jamaican parents was admitted from casualty, having superficially stabbed himself in the chest with broken glass. He had become acutely distressed over the past 2-3 days, feeling anxious and depressed and believing that his movements were watched by TV cameras, that signals about him were passed between shopkeepers and that people in shops were talking about him. In addition, he was particularly distressed by the scaly appearance of his skin, which he believed was caused by a lizard growing inside his body, the lizard's skin being evident on his arms and legs. He gave the growth of the lizard inside his chest as the reason for stabbing himself. He related this to an incident 10 years before when, in Jamaica, a lizard had run across his face. He believed the lizard had 'left its mark' and that a curse then had produced his skin lesions.
>
> (Browning and Jones, 1988, p. 766)

You might try to argue that we have here a 'background of rationality' against which the delusions make sense. The trouble is that the delusion is so far-reaching in its implications for the patient's other beliefs that it is hard to see what significant 'background of rationality' there is left, once we subtract the delusion. It is sometimes suggested that delusions are broadly rational reactions to unusual experiences that the patient has. This kind of approach is typically proposed only for monothematic delusions, and the present case brings out something of the reason for the restriction (cf. Davies and Coltheart, 2000). The problem is that in this case we seem to know what experience the patient is reacting to. He is reacting to the scaly appearance of his skin. It is hard to see how his reaction can be regarded as broadly rational. This remains true even if we emphasize that the reaction is being said to be only 'broadly' rational, and that there may be reasoning biases. This patient is not just unusually suspicious or inclined to jump to conclusions. Nevertheless, there are causal links here between his propositional attitudes. It may well be that this patient is predisposed to form some delusion or other anyhow. But there is a question about the causes of the specific content of the delusion the patient actually forms. What is causing the patient to form a belief about lizard invasion, rather than any other kind of delusion, is his belief that his skin is scaly, and his memory of a lizard running across his face 10 years ago.

Whatever procedure we are using when we ascribe propositional attitudes to this subject, it does not seem that it can be this procedure: 'first you decide to treat the object whose behavior is to be predicted as a rational agent; then you figure out what beliefs that agent ought to have, given its place in the world and its purpose. Then you figure out what desires it ought to have, on the same considerations, and finally you predict that this rational agent will act to further its goals in the light of its beliefs' (Dennett, 1987, p. 17). It is difficult to see how use of this procedure could allow you to predict that this patient would stab himself.

I am suggesting that what it comes to that there is a causal link between the propositional attitudes is this: that were there to be an intervention on the cause, there would be a difference in the outcome (cf. e.g. Woodward, 2003). In this account, the existence of causal links between propositional attitudes does not depend on the existence of rational connections between them, and it does not depend on the existence of any mechanism at all to connect them. Scientists will always search for a mechanism, and that is what cognitive neuroscience aims to do. But the causal link is one thing, and the mechanism is another. Suppose we consider the epidemiological case again. Suppose you are asking whether some environment risk factor is a cause of a particular disease. Suppose, as before, that you are asking whether infected water is a cause of cholera. The decisive answer in this kind of case would usually be taken to be provided by a RCT. Here, there is an intervention on the level of consumption of infected water, and we observe whether consumption and cholera are correlated under the intervention. In any particular case, you might ask whether the RCT was carried out correctly. But it hardly makes sense to suppose that the RCT was methodologically unproblematic but there was no causal connection. The causal link is established without any need to find mechanisms linking cause and effect. Whether there is a causal link is one thing and whether there is a mechanism linking cause and effect is another. Similarly, to establish that there is a causal connection between one propositional attitude and another is one thing, and to establish that there is a rational connection or mechanism linking the two is another.

7.4 **Control variables**

In the case of psychological states and mental illness, there is a question that comes up with some urgency. This is the question whether we are identifying candidate causes and effects 'at the right level'. After all, you might say, are not all the phenomena of psychiatry fundamentally biological? Are not psychological variables 'at the wrong level' to identify the causes of mental illness and its symptoms? One motivation for such an approach is provided by the idea that it is *a priori* that the 'mechanisms' of causation here must be biological and that the 'right level' of variable must always be found to relate to the 'biological mechanism'. There are problems with this idea. It is not *a priori* that the mechanisms of causation here must be entirely biological. Recall the case I mentioned earlier, of the impact of poverty on mental illness. It is by no means obvious that there is a biological mechanism to be found that links poverty to mental illness. As I remarked, the researchers in this case conjectured that one mechanism linking poverty to illness is that relief from poverty provides the possibility of greater parental supervision. This is not a biological mechanism. There may nonetheless be a causal link between poverty and mental illness. Second, even in cases in which there is a 'biological mechanism' linking cause and effect, it does not follow that cause and effect must themselves be identified in biological terms. Smoking is a cause of cancer. The mechanism is biological. 'Smoking' is not itself a variable defined at the biological level. It does not follow from this that we are using a variable 'at the wrong level' when we say that smoking is a cause of cancer. Similarly, propositional-attitude variables could be causes of psychological outcomes even if the mechanisms linking cause and effect were biological.

How are we to determine the 'right level' of variable to use in characterizing mental illnesses? Suppose we had a scanner that would give a complete microphysical description of a human body. This is not even a description at the level of cell biology, it is much finer-grained than that. And suppose we scan thousands of subjects at various stages of their lives, over a period of years. And we observe which of those subjects develop schizophrenia and which do not. We will be able to form a big disjunctive characterization of total microphysical states that are nomically sufficient for schizophrenia. This will not be an exhaustive disjunction – there may well be total microphysical states not on the list that would lead to the onset of the disease. But for all that, it will be informative. Would such a list tell us anything at all about the causes of schizophrenia?

There are a number of problems with this strategy for finding the causes of schizophrenia. In general, when we characterize the correlation between potential interventions on a 'cause' variable and the values of an outcome variable, we are describing a function from one state space to another. What we have in the present case is a function from one complex variable – total microphysical condition – to another: risk of schizophrenia. Notice first that this is likely to be a 'function' only in the formal sense of 'a set of ordered pairs', the first element of which specifies total microphysical conditions and the second element of which specifies risk of schizophrenia. However, the function here is likely to be 'pathological' in the sense that it defies concise mathematical expression in familiar terms. In effect, we will have a complex or 'gerrymandered' function from one state space to the other. In general, when we look for the causes of a phenomenon, we are looking for variables which do have a 'dose–response' relation to the outcome, in that we can find a relatively concise mathematical expression, in familiar terms, of the relation between the state space of the cause variable and the state space of the outcome variable. Similarly, when we try to track the impact of particular genetic variants on risk of schizophrenia, we are looking at relatively simple functions from genetic structure to risk. Even complex models on which multiple genes have weak interlinked effects on risk for schizophrenia have nothing of the unsurveyable complexity of a microphysical approach.

Relatedly, we want our characterization of causes to be a characterization of variables that can be affected by local processes. The total microphysical state of the individual is not a variable that can be systematically affected by any local process. In contrast, variables such as those relating to genetic structure can be affected by local processes. They are, therefore, better candidates for cause variables.

Second, we want changes in the 'cause' variable to be correlated with changes in the 'effect' variable. To take a simple example, suppose our outcome variable is 'the state of H_2O', as solid/liquid/gas, within ordinary temperature ranges. You might suppose that the cause variable here is temperature. But that seems to give us too fine-grained a way of characterizing the cause. If we ask why H_2O is frozen, one answer is 'because its temperature is $-23°C$'. But it does not matter whether H_2O is at that particular temperature. The variable we want here is simpler. It has just three values: at or below $0°C$, between $0°C$ and $100°C$, and at or over $100°C$. Then we say that the cause of the particular state of H_2O is the variable having some particular one of those three values. In this sense, we want the 'cause' variable to be 'specific' to the outcome variable. The sense of 'specificity' here is not that the cause variable has an impact only on the outcome variable; any variable will participate in multiple causal processes and have multiple effects. Rather, the point is that we want changes in the cause variable to be correlated, as much as possible, with changes in the outcome variable. And we also have to describe the state space of the cause variable in a sufficiently fine-grained way that we can draw all the distinctions that do make a difference to the outcome variable. So we do not want to say that the cause of the state of H_2O is 'whether the substance is above or below $0°C$', because that does not allow us to draw all the distinctions we need to explain the various states of the substance (cf. Woodward, in press).

Suppose we now go back to the examples I was discussing earlier. These are cases in which there are causal connections between propositional attitudes even though those propositional attitudes are not rationally connected. For example, we have delusions of reference, where a belief that someone is stroking his chin causes me to believe that he thinks I need to shave, or the case in which perception of a skin disorder causes me to believe that I am being invaded by a lizard. For the propositional attitudes to be 'cause' variables in these cases, I suggest there should be: (1) systematic relations between the cause variables and the subsequent delusions. Relatedly, local action on the cause variables should be possible, and (2) correlation between change in the cause variables and change in the outcome variables. That is, an intervention on whether one sees the other person scratch his chin, or on whether one believes one has the skin disorder, should make a systematic difference to the content of the delusion.

It seems evident that these conditions for causation could be met, whether or not there are rational connections between the propositional-attitude variables. But still, you might say, the role I am envisaging here for causal relations among propositional-attitude variables is peripheral. It has to do only with the specific content of one's delusions. It does not explain why one has a tendency to form delusions in the first place.

That is of course correct, and I am not trying to construct a detailed general theory of the causation of psychosis. My point is rather about the role of ordinary beliefs and desires and so on in such an account. The classical philosophical approach has been to regard propositional attitudes as part of a 'conceptual scheme' that we bring to bear in describing the ordinary world. This conceptual scheme is taken to have strong *a priori* constraints on its applicability. In particular, as we have seen, rationality is taken to be a norm with which the scheme has to comply. In this view, we are at 'at the right level' to use psychological predicates only when we can ascribe propositional attitudes in such a way as to find the other person 'consistent, a believer of truth, and a lover of the good (all by our own lights, it goes without saying)' (Davidson, 2001). In this view, cognitive neuroscience steps in when we cannot find rationality, and eliminates the propositional attitudes in favour of notions internal to cognitive neuroscience.

The appeal I have just been making to the notion of a control variable is intended to replace this invocation of rationality. The question is not whether the subject is rational; the question is whether propositional attitudes figure as control variables in the subject's mental life. That is, the question is whether the propositional attitudes of the subject meet the conditions I have just indicated, of being locally manipulable and systematically mapped onto specific psychological outcomes. If the propositional attitudes function as control variables in this sense, then we do have a causally functioning mental life, whether or not the subject is rational. Of course, it is true that in the mental life of a broadly rational subject, propositional attitudes function as control variables. But it is the fact that we have control variables, not the fact that we have rationality, which means that we are 'at the right level' to talk of beliefs and desires.

We have to acknowledge, as I began by acknowledging, that when we find psychological causation without rationality, we 'look for a mechanism', since we usually think of rational connections as psychological mechanisms. When we find psychological causation with no semblance of rationality, we have a kind of 'action-at-a-distance' across psychological states that we would like to have explained in terms of some kind of mechanism, even if we are not sure exactly what kind of 'mechanism' we are looking for. One recent proposal is that there is early in development a key pathology of the prefrontal cortex.

> Disruption of prefrontal control would lead to a pathological increase in emotional responsivity of the subject, which in turn could be mediated via the amygdala's influence over the hypothalamic-pituitary-adrenal (HPA) axis. . . .
>
> (Broome *et al.*, 2005, p. 30)

This model:

> proposes that transition into psychosis is a consequence of primary prefrontal dysfunction leading to secondary enhanced subcortical stress response and dopamine transmission. . . .
>
> (Broome *et al.*, 2005, p. 30)

Dopamine dysregulation in turn may be implicated in difficulties of rational engagement with the world. Centrally, it may affect the regulation of attention and the perception of salience, so that there are problems in integrating information, registering the correct significance of events, and finding whether there are meaningful connections between distinct episodes.

> ... theories implicating impaired contextual integration and abnormal appraisal on the one hand and dopamine dysregulation on the other may be attempts at explaining the same processes at the different levels of information processing and neurochemistry, respectively.
>
> (Broome *et al.*, 2005, p. 30)

What I have been proposing is that we can think of this kind of account as explaining how it comes about that the rationality of the subject can be undermined. In this reading, the role of cognitive neuroscience is not to displace the appeal to propositional attitudes, conceived as governed by an *a priori* constraint of rationality. Nor is it to supplement the appeal to propositional attitudes, conceived as causally related to one another only by rational mechanisms. The role of cognitive neuroscience is, rather, to describe the mechanisms that make it possible for there to be causal connections between the propositional attitudes in the absence of rationality.

Acknowledgements

Thanks to Ken Kendler for many many hours discussing these topics. Thanks also to Lisa Bortolotti and Matthew Broome for their comments on an earlier draft.

References

Bayne, T. and Pacherie, E. (2005). In defence of the doxastic conception of delusions. *Mind and Language, 20*, 163–188.

Bortolotti, L. (2005a). Intentionality without rationality. *Proceedings of the Aristotelian Society,* CV, 385–392.

Bortolotti, L. (2005b). Delusions and the background of rationality. *Mind and Language, 20*, 189–208.

Broome M. R., Woolley, J. C., Tabraham, P., *et al.*, (2005). What causes the onset of psychosis? *Schizophrenia Research, 79*, 23–34.

Browning, S. M. and Jones, S. (1988). Ichthyosis and delusions of lizard invasion. *Acta Psychiatrica Scandanavica, 78*, 766–767.

Campbell, J. (2007). An interventionist approach to causation in psychology. In *Causal Learning: Psychology, Philosophy and Computation* (eds. A. Gopnik, and L. Schulz), pp. 58–66. Oxford, Oxford University Press.

Churchland, P. (2002). Eliminative materialism and the propositional attitudes. In *Philosophy of Mind: Classical and Contemporary Readings* (ed. D. Chalmers). Oxford, Oxford University Press.

Costello, E. J., Compton, S. N., Keeler, G., and Angold, A. (2003). Relationships between poverty and psychopathology: a natural experiment. *Journal of the American Medical Association, 290*(15), 2023–2029.

Currie, G. (2000). Imagination, delusion and hallucinations. In *Pathologies of Belief* (eds. M. Coltheart, and M. Davies), pp. 167–182. Oxford, Blackwell.

Davidson, D. (2001). Mental events. In *Essays on Actions and Events* (ed. D. Davidson). Oxford, Oxford University Press.

Davidson, D. (2004). Representation and interpretation. In *Problems of Rationality* (ed. D. Davidson), pp. 87–99. Oxford, Oxford University Press.

Davies, M. and Coltheart, M. (2000). Introduction: pathologies of belief. In *Pathologies of Belief* (eds. M. Coltheart, and M. Davies). Oxford, Blackwell.

de Clérambault, G. G. (1924/2002). Psychoses with base of automatism (Part 1). In *Mental Automatisms: A Conceptual Journey into Psychosis Commentaries and Translation of the Work of Gaëtan Gatian de Clerambault* (ed. P. Hriso, (2002)). Bayonne, NJ, Hermes Whispers Press.

Dennett, D. (1987). True believers. In *The Intentional Stance* (ed. D. Dennett). Cambridge, MA, MIT Press.

Maher, B. (1974). Delusional thinking and perceptual disorder. *Journal of Individual Psychology*, **30**, 98–113.

Snow, J. (1855). *On the Mode of Communicaton of Cholera*. London, John Churchill.

Spitzer, R. L., First, M. B., Kendler, K. S., and Stein, D. J. (1993). The reliability of three definitions of bizarre delusions. *American Journal of Psychiatry*, **150**, 880–884.

Startup, M. and Startup, S. (2005). On two kinds of delusion of reference. *Psychiatry Research*, **137**, 87–92.

Woodward, J. (2003). *Making Things Happen: A Theory of Causal Explanation*. Oxford, Oxford University Press.

Woodward, J. and Hitchcock, C. (2003). Explanatory generalizations, part 1: counterfactual account. *Nous*, **37**, 1–24.

Woodward, J. (In press). Cause and explanation in psychiatry: an interventionist perspective. In *Philosophical Issues in Psychiatry* (eds. K. Kendler, and J. Parnas). Baltimore, MD, Johns Hopkins University Press.

Young, A. (2000). Wondrous strange: the neuropsychology of abnormal beliefs. In *Pathologies of Belief* (eds. M. Coltheart, and M. Davies). Oxford, Blackwell.

Chapter 8

Mad scientists or unreliable autobiographers? Dopamine dysregulation and delusion

Philip Gerrans

Abstract

Delusions are currently characterized as false beliefs produced by incorrect inference about external reality (DSM-IV, 1994). This inferential account has proved hard to link to explanations pitched at the level of neurobiology and neuroanatomy. In particular, the crucial role of neurotransmitters in psychosis seems to elude theoretical capture within the inferential framework. One result is the unhappy oscillation between biological psychiatry and psychiatric approaches whose target is the phenomenology of irrational belief. This chapter provides the link between biology and phenomenology. The link is a neurocomputational theory, based on evolutionary considerations of the cognitive role of the prefrontal cortex (PFC). I develop the account by considering how it fits with with Shitij Kapur's influential attempt to link dopamine dysregulation to the phenomenology of schizophrenia.

8.1 Introduction

Recent work in computational neuroscience suggests that the role of dopamine (DA) is to make representations *salient* for a cognitive system. That is to ensure that cognitive resources are preferentially allocated to relevant information. (Barto, 1995; Schultz *et al.*, 1997; Sutton and Barto, 1998; Berridge and Robinson 1998, 2003, Berridge, 1999; Braver, 1999; O'Reilly and Munakata, 2000; Waelti *et al.*, 2001; Clure *et al.*, 2003; Kapur 2003; Gurney *et al.*, 2004; Fiorillo and Schultz, 2005; and Smith *et. al.*, 2006).

This 'DA salience' hypothesis is particularly helpful in explaining delusion, partly because DA antagonists are effective, which suggests a causal role for DA but also because the psychology of delusions is characterized by intractable and obsessive focus on delusional thoughts. Rather than allow a delusional thought, or the experience which prompts it, to recede into the cognitive background, the delusional subject allocates more and more cognitive resources to it until it produces embedded patterns of dysfunctional thought and behaviour. It does seem as if the thoughts involved in delusion are excessively salient (Kapur, 2003, 2004).

The aim of this chapter is to explore the nature and effects of this dysfunctional resource allocation and to suggest that a standard conception of delusion, the 'inferential conception' mischaracterizes it. The inferential conception of delusion treats the delusional subject as a scientist in the grip of an intractable confirmation bias. She recalls and attends selectively to evidence consistent with her biased hypothesis with the result that the delusions become ever more firmly woven into her Quinean web of beliefs (Maher, 1988, 1999; Stone and Young, 1997). I propose instead that processes of selective attention and recall exert their effects, not on a process of hypothesis confirmation but of autobiographical narrative. Someone with a delusion is not a mad scientist but an unreliable narrator. The integrated suite of processes underlying this narrative has been recently baptized mental time travel (MTT) and therefore my aim will be to show that in delusions, mechanisms of salience influence the cognitive processes which underpin MTT. The first part of the chapter is devoted to explaining what MTT is and how mechanisms of salience can influence it. This involves a slight detour to establish a computational framework which provides the necessary link between neurobiology and phenomenology and psychology. The second part defends the idea that MTT rather than hypothetical confirmation is the main culprit in delusion. In particular, I discuss cases of successful cognitive therapy for delusion which are often cited in defence of the idea that delusions are instances of faulty assignment of credence to theoretical hypotheses. I argue that where cognitive behavioural therapy (CBT) succeeds is because it actually reconfigures a subject's MTT, making her a more reliable narrator. A case study of recovery from delusion following CBT is the focus here. The view I defend here is quite consistent with the idea that pharmacological interventions are required to reduce psychosis to a manageable level while CBT helps the subject reconfigure dysfunctional thought patterns entrenched as responses to anomalous experience.

8.2 **Salience**

Essentially the mind operates in two modes: online and offline. In the online mode, the mind responds moment by moment to environmental contingencies. The cognitive systems which enable this fluent interaction are perceptual and motor systems regulated by neurochemical blockade from brainstem neurotransmitter systems (Panskepp, 1998). The brainstem systems also help coordinate limbic activation which motivates an organism towards or away from a represented stimulus or behavioural outcome (Davidson and Irwin, 1999; Davidson, et al., 2002). Normally, neural activation in online systems lasts only long enough to control the necessary behaviour and then subsides until required again. However, when the world does not cooperate and the online systems misrepresent their targets or encounter an unforeseen contingency, activation does not decay (Jeannerod, 1988; Gallagher, 2000; Pacherie, 2001; Spence, 2001). This sustained activation alerts the system to the presence of a contingency which requires additional cognitive resources. The first resource to be attracted is attention in which activation is sustained in the assembly responsible for the experience while activation in others is reduced (Fuster, 1971). The sustained activation carries information about the contingency, and under certain conditions (i.e. when that information is structured for computational purposes) may *represent* that contingency to the organism. A representation which becomes the focus of attention in this way is a *salient experience*. Moment-to-moment activation in neural assemblies generates a stream of these salient experiences. Unlike other mammals, which have only a limited cognitive and behavioural repertoire with which to respond to salient experiences, humans can plan, reflect, communicate, and deliberate to generate an appropriate response. These are all instances of offline cognition in which representations are held in working memory, meta-represented, and manipulated in novel combinations. These cognitively sophisticated responses depend on circuitry distributed between the prefrontal cortex (PFC) and posterior and limbic online systems with which it is densely interconnected (Fuster, 1997; Masterman and Cummings, 1997). The PFC evolved in mammals, first, to inhibit some automatic responses to a stimulus, while maintaining activation in assemblies responsible for a salient experience and, second, to enable the computation of appropriate responses to that experience (Knight, 1999; Wood and Grafman, 2003). Offline cognition in simple cases of mammalian cognition might consist in maintaining neural activation in systems which produce salient experience long enough to enable operant conditioning, or try out an alternative behavioural response. Humans can construct buildings and cities, narratives and theories, using the PFC to regulate the storage, retrieval, and manipulation of represented information relevant to the task. It is not just the size of the PFC but its dense interconnectivity with posterior, limbic, and brainstem areas which underwrites these abilities. These connections are both afferent and efferent which enable bi-directional signalling between PFC and posterior areas. Furthermore, while most connections from posterior networks to PFC are excitatory, the PFC has extensive inhibitory connections (via GABA interneurons) with posterior areas. This interconnectivity enables construction of transient recurrent networks distributed across the PFC and posterior networks, whose purpose is to maintain an experiential representation against interference from competing patterns of activity in other networks (Friston, 2002). This maintenance depends on selective enhancement of posterior representations which attract PFC resources and inhibition of activation levels in other posterior networks which might otherwise monopolize offline cognition (Knight, 1999). Moment-to-moment experience is a product of competition between more or less transient coalitions of active neurons, distributed across PFC-posterior network, to attract prefrontal processing resources sufficient to prevent their activation decaying. Normal experience is a constant dynamic interaction between offline and online cognition as different experiences capture prefrontal resources: a train of reflective thought is interrupted by a voice or movement, attention shifts, directing frontal resources to the new stimulus, which then recedes from attention as we habituate to it, or sustains attention as we mobilize more frontal resources to determine how to respond. Thus we can see that if the PFC is unable to selectively activate and inhibit representations appropriately, offline cognition will be abnormal. If representations cannot be inhibited or are inappropriately enhanced, they become *hypersalient*. Intrusive or recurring thoughts are a mild example, phobias and obsessions more extreme. The opposite effect would be the failure of a representation to become salient or maintain appropriate salience. Distraction is a mild example, attention deficit hyperactivity disorder (ADHD) and thought disorder are extreme cases (although the cognitive structure of each disorder is different, mechanisms of salience seem to be implicated. In ADHD, low levels of tonic DA, required to sustain patterns of thought, in the PFC make the patient vulnerable to distraction. In thought disorder, the psychosis is so hypersalient that it restructures cognition moment to moment). There is of course no single mechanism which determines the salience of a particular experience, since activation in a neural assembly is a function of numerous inhibitory and excitatory influences. Before we try and relate these essentially neurobiological facts about offline cognition to delusion, it is helpful to have a conceptual framework which enables us to talk, not just in terms of activation and inhibition of neural assemblies, but of the way in which selective activation and inhibition enables computational processes which implement psychological states such as belief.

8.3 A computational framework for understanding salience

Computationally, we can treat the neural systems which manage online cognition as interconnected neural networks whose automatic input–output relationships are determined by inflexible weights in their hidden layers (Quartz and Sejnowski, 1997; Arbib, 2003). A weight is the propensity, described as a probability, of a unit in a neural network to become active when another to which it is connected becomes active. Automaticity of processes implemented in neural networks is enabled by fixing weights. This inflexibility is an advantage when processing stereotypical stimuli (a visual system which produced different representations of the same stimulus would not be fitness enhancing, nor would a sensori-motor loop which sometimes produced aversive and sometimes exploratory behaviour towards a predator). Perceptual experience, and most representational phenomenology, is awareness of activation in output layers of these systems, which captures sustained attention. Thus a salient perceptual or sensory experience can be thought of as sustained activation in output layers of an online system which enables it to become the focus of offline cognition. In the simplest cases, offline cognition might simply consist of maintaining simultaneous perceptual representations of conditioned and unconditioned stimuli long enough for reinforcement mechanisms to bias weights in networks whose representations control conditioned behaviour (Clark and Squire L. R., 1998). Humans, as we mentioned earlier, have a larger cognitive repertoire than simple conditioning or behavioural trial and error. We can respond to experience by trawling our autobiographical memories, imagining the outcomes of alternative behavioural responses, using semantic knowledge, and *sometimes* testing conclusions using rules of inference. In the most complex cases, people write novels, solve crimes, prove theorems, or design buildings. These executive functions require the ability to detach from present experience, access stored representations, construct new representations, and manipulate them in patterns which are not determined by stereotypical associations and behavioural routines. In offline cognition, the outputs of different weight-based systems are reconstructed by memory or imagination, simultaneously held in working memory, meta-represented, compared, and manipulated into novel combinations. Hence, it can be described as *activation-based* processing because it selectively maintains activation in neural assemblies which would otherwise decay as online cognition continues its Sisyphean struggle to manoeuvre the organism through the world. Thus, an account of the delusional response to experience is an account of activation-based processing set in train by salient experiences. The difference between delusional and normal subjects lies in the way some experiences (such as the auditory hallucinations of schizophrenia) become salient and how those experiences are dealt with by offline cognition. This may not yet seem much of an advance, but putting things within this computational framework allows us to integrate the neurochemistry and neuroanatomy of offline cognition with the phenomenology and psychology. In particular, it allows us to see how dopaminergic dysregulation can cause experiences or thoughts to become hypersalient.

8.4 **Mechanisms of salience**

In the rest of this chapter, we focus on the DA system which projects from origins in the ventral tegmentum area (VTA) and basal ganglia (BG) throughout PFC, posterior, and limbic areas. The delivery of DA to neural assemblies is by no means the only mechanism which contributes to the salience of experiences, and in fact it produces its effects by interactions with other neurochemicals delivered to the PFC by reticular activating systems; but it is a very useful case study because it has recently been the focus of renewed efforts to link its molecular effects to its psychological and phenomenological effects. Neural network models which preserve biochemical parameters of the VTA-PFC and BG-PFC networks (Braver, 1999) involved in activation-based processing can be used to test the effects of dopaminergic innervation on offline cognition and provide a deeper theoretical basis for understanding the correlations between DA dysregulation and characteristic psychology and phenomenology. These models show that DA enhances the signal to noise ratio (SNR) between communicating neural assemblies. It does so via the interaction of at least two types of DA action. Phasic DA, delivered in short bursts, binds to D2 receptors on the postsynaptic membrane (Werner, 1996). It is rapidly removed by reuptake from the synaptic cleft and acts quickly. Tonic DA, which acts over longer time scales, accumulates in the synaptic cleft and binds to presynaptic DA autoreceptors triggering reuptake. Phasic and tonic DA are thus antagonists and have different effects on the assemblies they afferent. Phasic DA, acting on PFC assemblies produces a gating effect. It allows new activation patterns in the PFC-regulated networks to be formed, producing salient representations of new stimuli. Tonic DA maintains an occurrent activation pattern allowing a representation to be sustained against interference or competition. The hypothesis follows, and is confirmed by neural network models, that the balance of tonic and phasic DA is responsible for the rate of turnover of representations in the PFC-posterior networks (Grace, 1991):

> Tonic DA effects may increase the stability of maintained representations through an increase in the SNR of background versus evoked activity patterns. In contrast, phasic DA effects may serve as a gating signal indicating when new inputs should be encoded and maintained.
>
> (Braver, 1999, p. 317)

Together, phasic and tonic DA provide a mechanism for updating and maintaining representations in working memory by selectively activating target neural assemblies (Arnsten, 1998). Learning effects are longer-term consequences of DA produced by Hebbian modification of synaptic connections: when a representation is repeatedly sustained, the relevant synaptic pathways are strengthened via a cascade of chemical changes which ultimately change the receptive properties of target neurons (Braver, 1999; Kandel, 1999). Computationally, we can say that gating effects influence activation patterns and learning effects change the weights in a neural network. To summarize, offline cognition requires the construction and manipulation of representations which are transient patterns of activation across a distributed network of PFC-posterior neurons. Computational modelling captures this role for the DA system in what are called adaptive critic architectures. The adaptive critic is a cognitive system which learns through feedback which contingencies are rewarding and modulates the activity of another system which needs to choose between instrumental behaviours or cognitive activities (such as maintaining or discarding an item in working memory). In other words, it *predicts rewards for a system* (Montague, 2006). In these models, reward processing is not an accessory to central reasoning processes, but is as an essential feature of the efficient computational functioning of adaptive systems.

The human mind has evolved a similar solution, separating systems which *predict rewards and therefore motivate*, from those which *provide the reward*. DA systems confer *salience* by enhancing activation in neural systems that represent a potentially rewarding contingency (Schultz *et al.*, 1997; Berridge and Robinson, 1998, 2003; Braver, 1999; Clure *et al.*, 2003; Kapur, 2003; Smith *et al.*, 2004, 2006; Fiorillo and Schulz, 2005). The temporal structure of instrumental cognition modulated by dopaminergic activity is isomorphic to that produced by adaptive critic architectures, leading to the idea that DA is the mind's adaptive critic (Barto, 1995; Sutton and Barto, 1998; O'Reilly and Munakata, 2000; Gurney *et. al.*, 2004; Waelti *et al.*, 2004).

Keeping thoughts on track requires a subtle balance of inhibition and excitation in neural assemblies which implement the relevant representations. Whether a representation survives or not depends on DA-modulated gating and maintenance effects which modulate activation in the network. Pathological versions of these effects can lead either to offline-cognition computing over inappropriately maintained representations, as in cases of intrusive thoughts and perseverative thought patterns, or to the inability to maintain a representation as in cases of distractability or various executive disorders.

8.5 **Mental time travel and the structure of offline cognition**

> We are the only animals that can peer deeply into our futures—the only animal that can *travel mentally through time*, preview a variety of futures, and choose the one that will bring us the greatest pleasure and/or the least pain. This is a remarkable adaptation—which, incidentally, is directly tied to the evolution of the frontal lobes.
>
> (Gilbert, 2004)

Gilbert here invokes the notion of MTT to capture the idea that humans control their behaviour by imaginatively projecting themselves into future scenarios and simulating the emotional consequences.

Gilbert's work participates in a reconceptualization of episodic memory and imagination as part of a unified capacity for offline control which supports personal decision making. Recent research into episodic memory suggests that, in fact, episodic memory should not be conceived of as the ability to retrieve previous experiences but as an ability to construct experiences by activating perceptual and affective circuitry in the absence of a stimulus. The human PFC, in combination with hippocampal structures, allows us to use information about the world gathered in past encounters in order to remember *and imagine* possible futures, and recombine different aspects of experience to produce hypothetical scenarios relevant to a decision. Thus memory and imagination turn out to be aspects of the same constructive process which assembles and reassembles experiences. This is why damage to episodic memory also destroys deliberation and planning (Klein, 2002; Buckner and Carroll, 2007). As Schacter *et al.*, put it in a recent review: 'the medial temporal lobe system which has long been considered to be crucial for remembering the past might actually gain adaptive value through its ability to provide details that serve as building blocks of future event simulations' (Schacter *et al.*, 2007, p. 659). Endel Tulving baptized this ability to create experiences, through memory and imagination, in the absence of a stimulus, as MTT (Schacter *et al.*, 1997; Suddendorf, 1997; Wheeler *et al.*, 1997; Tulving, 2002; Bayley *et al.*, 2006; D'Argembeau *et al.*, 2006; Corballis and Suddendorf, 2007). As Gilbert notes, the name emphasizes the fact that offline cognition releases an organism from the stimulus-bound present, allowing us to use information from the recalled past or imagined future to guide our behaviour.

A crucial aspect of MTT is that the representations it manipulates in activation-based processing are outputs of weight-based processing. Consequently, it automatically inherits the affective associations of those weight-based online processes. This is essential, since unless those affective traces were present, the experiences summoned up in MTT could not play their essential role in deliberation. When you remember or imagine skydiving or walking down the aisle, the emotional tone of the experience helps you decide to repeat or attempt it. When you recreate the experience, you must also recreate enough of its online phenomenology to guide deliberation, while inhibiting the rest of its typical online effects such as behaviour. When you daydream about punching the boss while enduring a seminar about 'proactive management initiatives', you must not allow those thoughts to issue in behaviour. Indeed, imagining the consequences of acting on that thought may help you to sit on your hands for the rest of the meeting. It is for this reason that Gilbert regards MTT as the cognitive process essential to what he calls affective forecasting – the ability to control action by simulating the emotional consequences of an alternative course of action in the present.

Note that MTT is *not the same thing as hypothetical inference.* If I arrive at a deserted beach and see a seal colony under the cliffs where the waves are breaking, I can decide whether or not to go surfing in different ways. I can imagine myself paddling out, then the shocking impact, the rending of flesh and bone, and my screams echoing against the cliffs before I disappear beneath the surface in a welter of bloodied foam. I can recall the waves I caught last time at this beach and the relief I felt when the shadow in the water underneath my board proved to be a dolphin. Or, I can do the math about the probability of shark attack. This example shows the strengths and weaknesses of relying on autobiographical experiences alone in deliberation. Inevitably, the autobiographical representations retain their affective traces. This indexicality is good when it gives the subject information about the relevance of representations. However, MTT can also be a poor source of information where the subject's biography provides incomplete or distorted information with inappropriate affective associations. There are times when we need to be able to escape our autobiography and use information which is not based on our own experience. A very simple example would be using a map to plan a journey as opposed to imagining or recalling previous travels. Another might be consulting a book or getting the advice of a third party. In each of these cases, we use information whose representation does not essentially implicate our own experience. These types of information can also be stored and recalled in ways which do not essentially involve us – *semantic memory*, or memory for facts and propositions as it is known. However, in order to do this we have to 'switch off' or inhibit episodic MTT. It is very difficult to 'do the math' when deciding to skydive or get married. Finally, in evaluating the information we acquire through this combination of episodic and semantic sources of information, we can make use of the rules of hypothetical inference. This requires us to treat information as propositions expressing probabilities or utilities subject to rules of inference. This requires even further levels of inhibition, because the propositions stand for events which have autobiographical associations for us and which tend to produce their associated imagery automatically. When I think about the infinitesimal likelihood of shark attack, the words 'shark attack' have a far more experiential salience for me than the word 'infinitesimal' or 'P. A/B = 0.00126'. This suggests an interesting structure within offline cognition. A salient experience commands attention and requires us to deal with it. The first step is episodic MTT, in which we inhibit automatic responses to the stimulus and search our minds for alternative responses, imaging and remembering possible scenarios. Perhaps, however, our autobiographical representations do not contain enough relevant information, or continually lead to dysfunctional behaviour or patterns of thinking. In such cases, it might be best to deal with a salient experience using representations from semantic memory and other sources. Without endorsing the natural language of thought hypothesis, which has it that we think in our native language (see e.g. Carruthers, 2002 for a discussion), we can note that symbols are the obvious candidate and that much of our mental life consists in internal speech. Finally, when manipulating the information one acquires in this manner, in order to get at the truth, one can use rules of hypothetical inference to find out the likely truth of the proposition which encodes the conclusion we are interested in testing. Each stage requires progressively more inhibition as the cognitive processes involved become more abstract and distant from the salient experience which prompts the transition to offline cognition. Theorists typically note the role of the PFC in this kind of 'controlled and effortful' cognition, emphasizing that the source of the effort is the necessity of inhibiting competing cognitive routines, which are relatively automatic, in order to keep a train of reflective thought on track (Fine, 2006). When these inhibitory processes are absent, we see cases like thought disorder in which trains of semi-random thoughts jump from topic to topic. The progression between these stages is not a simple switching on and off of different cognitive systems. Fluent offline cognition is best thought of as the manipulation of different types of representation under prefrontal control as we combine autobiographical with other sources of information in order to guide action. Having calculated which superannuation plan offers the best returns, we can then imagine the experience of dying in a series of progressively bleaker and more squalid hospitals when we decide how to allocate the meagre return on a lifetime's work. In fact, it is almost impossible not to link any abstract reasoning process to an autobiographical representation. This is why abstract cognition divorced from any autobiographical or episodic context seems very difficult for most people when the problem has a real-life interpretation. The ability of the PFC to perform its inhibitory role depends almost completely on brainstem neurotransmitter delivery systems. The serotoninergic, norepinephrinergic, and dopaminergic systems, for example, project to prefrontal areas, modulating their interactions with posterior areas. The effect of these neurotransmitter systems is to change the computational properties of distributed neural networks comprised of prefrontal and posterior areas. Essentially, they lower or raise thresholds of activation required for particular distributed representations to remain the focus of cognition. We can treat the salience of a particular thought, e.g. 'I have cancer', as a resultant vector of different forces. Limbic circuitry provides an affective and motivational context for a thought made salient by dopaminergic activation while prefrontal systems can inhibit that thought while enabling the search through autobiographical space for information relevant to a response. If, however, the dopaminergic systems are malfunctioning either as a result of processes intrinsic to the mesolimbic, delivery systems or feedback between the mesolimbic systems and prefrontal and limbic systems, such a thought can become excessively salient (Broome et al., 2005).

Thus anatomical or neurochemical differences between people (or within the same person at different times) ensure different responses to experience in virtue of the differences they introduce into offline processing. The best example of how this might be the case is Shitij Kapur's account of the role DA plays in schizophrenia (Kapur, 2003).

8.6 **Delusions, dopamine, and hypersalience**

Kapur's starting point is the 'DA hypothesis' of psychosis, the foundation of biological approaches. Evidence for the role of DA in psychosis comes from two sources. The first is the fact that antipsychotic drugs are DA antagonists, whose effects are achieved by targeting DA receptors. The second is the role of DA in triggering or mimicking psychosis, evidenced by hallucinogenic drugs and heightened DA synthesis during psychosis (Crow, 1980; Jones and Pilowsky, 2002). Kapur's account builds on recent theories, of the role of DA, which treat dopamine delivery systems in the mesolimbic systems as:

> a critical component in the 'attribution of salience,' a process whereby events and thoughts come to grab attention, drive action and influence goal directed behaviour because of their association with reward of punishment . . . it provides an interface whereby the hedonic subjective pleasure, the ability to predict reward and the learning mechanisms allow the organism to focus on what it deems valuable and allows a seamless conversion of motivation into action.

> (Kapur, 2003, p. 14)

The computational models we examined earlier confirm that these effects are achieved because dopaminergic (or other neurotransmitter) modulation of target neural systems in the PFC produces both gating and learning effects. Gating effects ensure that representations, implemented in transient neural assemblies, become the focus of cognition. Learning effects, produced by Hebbian conditioning, ensure that the properties of neural assemblies change, entrenching patterns of cognitive and behavioural response to particular experiences. A clear example of this type of learning effect is seen in mood disorders such as depression. In depression, a cascade of changes, consequent on norepinephrinergic dysregulation, modifies amydala–hippocampus circuitry which associates experiences with affective tone (Ressler and Nemeroff, 1999; Davidson *et al.*, 2002). When the depressive person thinks about her past, or imagines future experiences, the representations she retrieves or constructs are saturated with negative affect. The effect is to limit her MTT to regions of the past and future in which she experiences only failure and distress. As the activation of circuitry involved in producing negative experience is repeatedly sustained, she becomes wired for despair. Kapur's theory integrates several features of schizophrenia, including the characteristic phenomenology of the prodromal period in which subjects feel that events or objects are extremely significant and/or that their senses are hypersensitive. As Kapur points out, transient episodes of this nature are not abnormal but in delusional subjects, DA dysregulation ensures that their hypersalience gives representations of objects or scenes a halo of significance and ensures that they dominate offline cognition. Kapur initially phrases his characterization of delusional response to experience neutrally as a 'top down cognitive phenomenon that the individual imposes on these experiences of aberrant salience in order to make sense of them' (Kapur, 2003, p. 15). Kapur then follows the standard inferential approach in treating the delusional response to hypersalient experiences as the adoption and maintenance of an explanatory hypothesis. Once adopted, the delusional hypothesis 'serves as a cognitive scheme for further thoughts and actions. It drives the patients to find further confirmatory evidence – in the glances of strangers, the headlines of newspapers and the tiepins of newsreaders' (Kapur, 2003, p. 16). The delusional subject is modelled as a scientist constructing and testing a hypothesis in order to explain novel or recalcitrant evidence. The effect of hypersalience is to give the delusional belief a probability approaching 100% with the result that other beliefs are revised to accommodate the delusional belief rather than the delusional belief being revised or rejected in the face of the web of background beliefs (Huq *et al.*, 1988). The experience constrains the initial abductive hypothesis, but does not determine it. Someone preoccupied by the experiences of alienation might attribute them to the occult ministrations of a shaman or to the CIA depending on their background: 'the same neurochemical dysregulation leads to different phenomeno-logical expression' (Kapur, 2003, p. 15). A similar proposal has been made by Mujica-Parodi and collaborators who explain delusion in terms of 'the failure to ade-quately restrict one's mental models' (Mujica-Parodi *et al.*, 2000). A mental model is a hypothesis which potentially explains experience and model restriction is the process by which evidence is selectively brought to bear to evaluate and revise the model. Any model is restricted by both empirical evidence and contextual hypotheses which provide the framework for reasoning. For example, that the future resembles the past is a contextual hypothesis but so are widely believed culturally based cosmological or religious beliefs. Delusional subjects both fail to seek and recognize empirical and contextual counterexamples and hence their models are not adequately restricted. Mujica-Parodi and others have demonstrated that in normal subjects, model restriction is strongly influenced by the affective valence of premises and proposed that similar processes are at work in the model restriction of delusional subjects. The model restriction hypothesis is an elegant way to conceptualize the influence of the mechanism of salience-biased thought processes (Goel *et al.*, 2004). It has the advantages of allowing that delusions need not necessarily be false or based on faulty inference (they might be valid inferences within a badly restricted model) and helping to systematize interpretations like that of Kapur. It also allows for a principled incorporation of the controversial definitional clause in the DSM concerning the 'widely held beliefs of others in the subject's culture' which can look *ad hoc* or relativist. These beliefs become contextual constraints on model restriction. The idea that delusions are the product of a confirmation bias in a system of hypothesis testing also figures very strongly in attributional-bias accounts of delusion. The essence of these attributional accounts is the interaction between attention to particular types of experience and the explana-tions of that experience. 'The preferential encoding and recall of delusion-sensitive material can be assumed to continually reinforce and propagate the delusional belief' (Gilleen and David, 2004). Subjects with paranoid delusions focus on threat-related information and tend to attribute negative experiences to external factors rather than themselves (Garety and Freeman, 1999; Bentall, 2004). The opposite tendency has been observed in people with depression-related psychoses (Leafhead *et al.*, 1996; Dudley *et al.*, 1997; Stone and Young, 1997). One theory of depression is that depres-sive subjects focus on themselves rather than the external world and tend to attribute their distressing experiences to factors about themselves (Beck, 1989; Gerrans, 2000).

Note however, that this description does not require that a cognitive model of this process of preferential encoding and recall should be derived from formal accounts of hypothesis confirmation in science. These formal accounts describe the ideal reasoning, over the long term, of a scientific community interested in theory confirmation, rather than the immediate response of an individual to experience or construction by an individual of an autobiographical narrative which integrates it with previous episodes.

8.7 Cognitive therapy: science or history?

Richard Bentall once observed that 'the unusual beliefs and experiences of psychiatric patients all seem to reflect preoccupations about the position of the self in the social universe.' Bentall is surely right that delusions are subjective responses to experience. That is, the subject is using her own cognitive resources to respond to her experience rather than the rules of hypothetical inference to demonstrate the truth of a theoretical hypothesis to others (Kaney and Bentall, 1992; Lyon et al., 1994; Kinderman and Bentall, 1996). This suggests immediately that MTT is the main culprit because it is both the first response to a salient experience and a mode of response in which the self is essentially implicated (Brune, 2004).

MTT also involves the selective attention to, encoding, retrieval, and manipulation of information in order to provide an autobiographical context for a current experience. However, those processes play a different role in MTT than in scientific inference.

The point to emphasize is that the same cognitive processes influence both MTT and hypothetical reasoning. In the former case, however, they select or create an experience and insert it as an episode in an autobiography. In the latter, they select evidence and evaluate it for consistency with a theory according to a prescriptive theory of confirmation. There is no essential role for recalled or imagined experience except to suggest a hypothesis for testing.

Earlier, I suggested that MTT is cognitively prior to hypothetical inference as a way of responding to salient experience. That is to say, confronted with an experience which captures attention, a person first consults her episodic database to determine a response. In the normal case, that is usually sufficient: one remembers or imagines an experience relevant to the current one and assembles a narrative which reconciles them.

Equally, the process can go the other way. Presented with a theoretical piece of information, such as a statistical relationship, most people will try and interpret that using their own experience. Charities do not present statistics for this reason. They present vivid vignettes or stories in order to prompt an empathetic response which a prospective donor can situate in an autobiographical context.

This does not show that people cannot reason abstractly or theoretically about the causes of experience using prescriptive norms. It just suggests that in general they do not. In the cases when they are not, processes of selective retrieval and evaluation influence MTT, not theory confirmation.

The DSM definition of delusion as depending on faulty inference has always troubled theorists since it suggests that what is restored when delusion resolves is a capacity for correct inference. Since the only theories of correct inference we have are prescriptive models, there is a tendency to think that delusion must result from the faulty application of prescriptive rules and that recovery from delusion depends on the return of the ability to apply them correctly.

Some accounts of recovery from delusion seem to support this interpretation. John Nash's description of his battle with schizophrenia is compelling:

> Initially I did not hear any voices. Some years went by before I heard voices and – I became first disturbed in 1959, and I didn't hear voices until the summer of 1964 I think, but then after that, I heard voices, and then I began arguing with the concept of the voices.
>
> And ultimately I began rejecting them and deciding not to listen, and, of course, my son has been hearing voices, and if he can progress to the state of rejecting them, he can maybe come out of his mental illness.
>
> The consequence of rejecting the voices is ultimately not hearing the voices. You're really talking to yourself is what the voices are, but it's also parallel to a dream. In a dream it's typical not to be rational.
>
> So in rejecting some of the political ideas, that had a relation to the voices, so I could think of a voice maybe as presenting what was *analogous to a political argument, and then I could say, I don't want to listen to that.*
>
> (John Nash in a PBS interview, my emphasis)

It is tempting to describe this case as instances of recovered rationality. However, when Nash treated his voices as a political argument it was so that he could say, 'I don't want listen to that.' In effect, not listening means redirecting attention away from the hypersalient experience allowing other experiences to occupy the attentional spotlight. It is interesting that Nash treated the voices as antagonists in a political argument rather than as participants in a logical or mathematical debate. Their initial power to monopolize his attention does not seem to be a matter of proof or evidence. He once said 'the ideas I had about supernatural beings came to me the same way my mathematical ideas did. So I took them seriously.'

It is important to understand that Nash is not saying that his ideas about supernatural beings arrived after months or years of intense proving and checking theorems, defending them against attempted refutation in seminars and arguments. Rather, they occurred in his mind with the same intensity and spontaneity as mathematical insights. In the mathematical case, those ideas survived and were strengthened by the process of proof but it is not clear that he ever tried to prove or disprove his delusions. Rather, while deluded 'he took them seriously' constructing elaborate narratives of persecution in which *he* was the focus of attention by global superpowers – the church, the CIA, and sometimes intergalactic forces. He constructed autobiographical episodes to fit the experience. And when he was eventually able to stop, the delusions disappeared.

Robert Chapmans's personal account of recovery from a classical case of schizophrenic delusion is equally interesting. When deluded he believed he was on the verge of worldwide fame as a modern DaVinci or the victim of global conspiracies to steal his ideas and deny him recognition.

He describes the origin of his delusion as involving preoccupations, racing thoughts, and a sense of grandiosity and significance followed by intense suspiciousness. He fitted these experiences into spectacular narratives of persecution in which he was the central focus of others' intentional activity. As he put it, he asked 'why' questions which demanded that his experience be made intelligible in terms of agency rather than 'how' questions which demand specification of causal mechanisms and logical consistency.

Thus his delusions originated in MTT prompted by salient experiences, and intensified as those experiences were made hypersalient by the allocation of meta-cognitive resources devoted to the construction of an autobiography which 'made sense' of them.

Ultimately, via an incredible effort of will, he was able to disbelieve his delusions. The transition, as he describes it, was a result of applying principles of CBT – challenging the delusional belief, gathering disconfirming evidence, developing alternative explanations, and finally 'replacing delusions with the objective truth.'

Rather than imagining being spied on and following the train of associated thoughts, Chapman found perceptual evidence that he was not. 'I look into walls floor radiators, ceiling ducts, and other orifices where I suspect a spying device is hidden, but I never find any.' By behaving as a scientist, Chapman created a new database of actual experiences to incorporate in his autobiography. 'Did I actually see it or just a "sign" of it? Did I really hear it or could I have misinterpreted it? Did I smell it, taste it or feel it?' Chapman asked, over and over.

The scientific attitude to experience involves the same meta-cognitive processes as MTT, but gives them a new focus: evidence gathering and testing instead of autobiographical narrative. Experiences relevant to theoretical disconfirmation become salient at the expense of those involved in the delusion.

Clearly, Chapman's hard-won scientific attitude to experience was crucial to his recovery, but it does not follow that the *cause* of his delusion was a failure to take a scientific attitude to his experience. The cause of his delusion was the warping of his autobiographical narrative by hypersalience of paranoid and grandiose thoughts.

The scientific attitude was required to unweave the threads of this narrative and to make available a new set of empirical materials from which to reweave a story. Out of these materials, Chapman reconstructed a story in which he was not a persecuted genius but an intrepid explorer on quest for knowledge, 'I will not allow myself to be misled and deceived anymore. As much as these strange beliefs seem awfully real I will continue to investigate them.' Instead of private fears and paranoid interpretations of his affective states, he concentrated on publicly available phenomena – not the fear of being observed by hidden spies but the sight of the empty broom cupboard.

Chapman's case is especially interesting because initially it seems to support the idea that the second factor in delusion is a reasoning impairment leading to a faulty explanation of experience. When he subjected his delusions to rational evaluation, they disappeared.

However, the fact that a delusion remitted in the face of hypothetical reasoning does not show that it *originated* as the result of an abnormality of hypothetical reasoning. Rather, the process of model restriction employed in the service of hypothetical reasoning had the effect of refocusing attention, memory, and imagination on a different set of experiences than those which prompted the delusion. Consequently, he had a new set of experiences to incorporate into his autobiography. Not only that, but the reallocation of cognitive resources involved, reduced the salience of the experiences which prompted the delusions. They receded into the meta-cognitive background as he focussed his cognitive efforts on collecting mundane veridical experiences of the external world.

When Chapman became a robust empiricist, he also became a more reliable narrator because the raw material of his narrative changed from subjective intentional interpretations of experience to perceptual experiences of publicly available information. His story about his experiences now overlapped with that of others.

8.8 **Conclusion**

I have tried to show how conceiving of delusions as faulty inferences has costs and benefits. A benefit is that it leads to a focus on biased patterns of thought and ultimately on the neural mechanisms which produce that bias. It seems very likely that those mechanisms will involve the DA regulation systems since there is convergent evidence that its cognitive role is to make representations salient, and potentially hypersalient. However, a defect of the inferential conception is that it can lead to the modelling of delusion as theory construction and revision, to conceptualizing the role of the PFC in delusion as defective hypothesis testing, and to therapeutic approaches which emphasize the restoration of a capacity for rational belief fixation. In fact, however, DA dysregulation seems more likely to be affecting the processes involved in constructing an autobiographical narrative response to experience than processes involved in a hypothetical explanation of experience. People with delusions are not mad scientists, merely unreliable narrators.

References

Arbib, M. E. (2003). *The Handbook of Brain Theory and Neural Networks*. London, Cambridge, MA, MIT Press.

Arnsten, A. F. T. (1998). Catecholamine modulation of prefrontal cortical cognitive function. *Trends in Cogntive Sciences, 2*, 436–446.

Barto, A. G. (1995). Adaptive critics and the basal ganglia. In *Models of Information Processing in the Basal Ganglia* (eds. J. C. Houk, J. L. Davis, and D.G. Beiser), pp. 215–232. Cambridge, MA, MIT Press.

Bayley, P. J., Hopkins, R. O., and Squire, L. R. (2003). Successful recollection of remote autobiographical memories by amnesic patients with medial temporal lobe lesions. *Neuron, 38*, 135–144.

Beck, A. (1989). *Cognitive Therapy and the emotional Disorders*. Penguin, Harmondsworth.

Bentall, R. P. (2004). *Madness Explained*. London, Penguin Books.

Berridge, K. C. and Robinson, T. E. (1998). What is the role of dopamine in reward: Hedonic impact, reward learning, or incentive salience? *Brain Research Brain Research Reviews, 28*, 309.

Berridge, K. C. (1999). Pleasure, pain, desire and dread: hidden core processes of emotion. In *Well Being: The Foundations of Hedonic Psychology* (eds. D. Kahneman, E. Diener, and N. Schwarz), pp. 525–557. New York, Russel Sage Foundation.

Berridge, K. C. and Robinson, T. E. (2003). Parsing reward. *Trends in Neurosciences, 26*(9), 507–513.

Braver, T. S., Barch, D. M., and Cohen, J. D. (1999). Cognition and control in schizophrenia: a computational model of dopamine and prefrontal function. *Biological Psychiatry,* **46**, 312–328.

Broome, M., Woolley, J. B., Tabraham. P., *et al.* (2005). What causes the onset of psychosis? *Schizophrenia Research,* **79**, 23–34.

Brune, M. (2004). Schizophrenia: an evolutionary enigma? *Neuroscience and Biobehavioral Reviews,* **28**(1), 41–53.

Buckner, R. L. and Carroll, D. C. (2007). Self-projection and the brain. *Trends in Cognitive Sciences,* **11**(2), 49–57.

Carruthers, P. (2002).The cognitive functions of language. *Behavioral and Brain Sciences,* **25**(6) 657–674.

Chapman, R. (2002). Eliminating delusions. A first person account. *Schizophrenia Bulletin,* **28**, 545–553.

Clark, R. S. and Squire, L. R. (1998). Classical conditioning and brain systems: the role of awareness. *Science,* **280**, 77–81.

Crow, T. J. (1980). Molecular pathology of schizophrenia: more than one disease process? *British Medical Journal,* **280**, 66–68.

D'Argembeau, A. and van der Linden, M. (2006). Individual differences in the phenomenology of mental time travel: the effect of vivid mental imagery and emotion regulation strategies. *Consciousness and Cognition,* **15**, 342–350.

Davidson, R. J. and Irwin, W. (1999). The functional neuroanatomy of emotion and affective style. *Trends in Cognitive Science,* **3**(1), 11–21.

Davidson, R. J., Pizzagalli, D. A., Nitschke, J. B., and Putnam, K. (2002). Depression: perspectives from affective neuroscience. *Annual Review of Psychology,* **53**, 545–574.

Davies, M., Coltheart, M., Langdon, R., and Breen, N. (2001). Monothematic delusions: towards a two-factor account. *Philosophy, Psychiatry and Psychology,* **8**(2–3), 133–158.

Dennett, D. C. (1987). *The Intentional Stance.* Cambridge, MA, MIT Press.

Dennett, D. C. (1991). Real patterns. *Journal of Philosophy,* **87**, 27–51.

Dudley, R. E., John, C. H., Young, A. W., and Over, D. E. (1997). Normal and abnormal reasoning in people with delusions. *British Journal of Clinical Psychology,* **36**, 243–258.

Dudley, R. E., John, C. H., Young, A. W., and Over, D. E. (1998). Conditional reasoning in people with delusions: performance on the Wason selection task. *Cognitive Neuropsychiatry,* **3**, 241–258.

Fine, C. (2006). Is the emotional dog wagging its rational tail, or chasing it? Unleashing reason in Haidt's social intuitionist model of moral judgment. *Philosophical Explorations,* **9**, 83–98.

Fiorillo, C. D. and Schultz, W. (2005). Adaptive coding of reward value by dopamine neurons. *Science,* **307**, 1642–1645.

Fodor, J. (1975). *The Language of Thought.* Cambridge, Cambridge University Press.

Friston, K. (2002). Beyond phrenology: what can neuroimaging tell us about distributed circuitry? *Annual Review of Neuroscience,* **25**, 221–250.

Fuster, J. M. (1997). *The Prefrontal Cortex: Anatomy, Physiology and Neuropsychology of the Frontal Lobe.* New York, Raven.

Fuster, J. M. and Alexander, G. E. (1971). Neuron activity related to short term memory. *Science,* **173**, 652–654.

Gallagher, S. (2000). Self-reference and schizophrenia: a cognitive model of immunity to error through misidentification. In *Exploring the Self: Philosophical and Psychopathological*

Perspectives on Self-Experience (ed. D. Zahavi), pp. 203–242. Philadelphia PA, John Benjamins.

Garety, P. A. and Freeman, D. (1999). Cognitive approaches to delusions: a critical review of theories and evidence. *British Journal of Clinical Psychology, 38,* 113–154.

Gerrans, P. (2000). Refining the explanation of Cotard's delusion. *Mind and Language, 15*(1), 111–122.

Gerrans, P. (2001). Delusions as performance failures. *Cognitive Neuropsychiatry,* 6(3), 161–173.

Gilbert, D. (2004). Affective forecasting . . . or . . . the big wombassa: what you think you're going to get, and what you don't get, when you get what you want. Interview: The Edge, the Third Culture. (2.13.04). Available at: http://www.edge.org/3rd_culture/gilbert03/gilbert_index.html (accessed October 2008).

Gilleen, J. D., David, A. S. (2004). The cognitive neuropsychiatry of delusions: from psychopathology to neuropsychology and back again. *Psychological Medicine, 35,* 5–12.

Goel, V., Shuren, J., Sheesley, L., and Grafman, J. (2004). Logical reasoning deficits in schizophrenia. *Schizophrenia Research, 66,* 87–88.

Grace, A. (1991). Phasic versus tonci dopamine release and the modulation of dopamine responsivity: a hypothesis of the etiology of schizophrenia. *Neuroscience, 41,* 1–24.

Griffiths, P. (1995). *What Emotions Really Are. The Problem of Psychological Categories.* Chicago, IL, Chicago University Press.

Gurney, K., Prescott, T. J., Wickens, J. R., and Redgrave, P. (2004). Computational models of the basal ganglia: from robots to membranes. *Trends Neurosci, 27,* 453–459.

Huq, S. F., Garety, P.A., and Hemsley, D.R (1988). Probabilistic judgements in deluded and non-deluded subjects. *Quarterly Journal of Experimental Psychology, 40*(A), 801–813.

Jeannerod, M. (1988). *The Neural and Behavioural Organization of Goal-Directed Movements.* Oxford, Oxford University Press.

Jones, H.and Pilowsy, L. (2002). The dopamine hypothesis revisited. *British Journal of Psychiatry, 181,* 271–275.

Kandel, E. (1999). Biology and the future of psychoanalysis: a new intellectual framework for psychiatry revisited. *American Journal of Psychiatry, 156,* 505–523.

Kaney, S. and Bentall, R. P. (1992). Persecutory delusions and the self-serving bias: evidence from a contigency judgement task. *Journal of Nervous and Mental Disease, 180,* 773–780.

Kapur, J. (2003). Psychosis as a state of aberrant salience: a framework for linking biology, phenomenology and pharmacology in schizophrenia. *American Journal of Psychiatry,* 160, 13–23.

Kapur, S. (2004). How antipsychotics become anti-'psychotic' – from dopamine to salience to psychosis. *Trends in Pharmacological Sciences, 25,* 402–406.

Kinderman, P. and Bentall, R. P. (1996). Self-discrepancies and persecutory delusions: evidence for a model of paranoid ideation. *Journal of Abnormal Psychology, 105,* 106–113.

Klein, S. (2002). Memory and temporal experience: the effects of episodic memory loss on an amnesic patient's ability to remember the past and imagine the future. *Social Cognition,* 20, 353–379.

Knight, R. T. (1999). Prefrontal cortex regulates inhibition and excitation in distributed neural networks. *Acta Psychiatrica Scandinavia, 101,* 159–178.

Leafhead, K. M., Young, A. W., and Szulecka, T. K. (1996). Delusions demand attention. *Cognitive Neuropsychiatry, 1,* 5–16.

Lyon, H. M., Kaney, S., and Bentall, R. P. (1994). The defensive function of persecutory delusions: evidence from attribution tasks. *British Journal of Psychiatry,* **164**, 637–646.

Maher, B. A. (1988). Delusions as the product of normal cognitions. In *Delusional Beliefs* (eds. T. F. Oltmans, and B. A. Maher). New York, Wiley Interscience.

Maher, B. A. (1999). Anomalous experience in everyday life: its significance for psychopathology. *The Monist,* **82**(4), 547–570.

Masterman, D. L. and Cummings, J. L. (1997). Frontal-subcortical circuts: the anatomic basis of executive, social and motivated behaviors. *Journal of Psychopharmacology,* **11**, 107–114.

McClure, S. M., Daw, N. D., and Montague, P. R. (2003). A computational substrate for incentive salience. *Trends Neurosci,* **26**, 423–428.

McKinney, M. (2002). Brain evolution by stretching the global mitotic clock of development. In *Human Evolution through Developmental Change* (eds. N. Minugh-Purvis and K. McNamara). Baltimore, MD, and London, Johns Hopkins Press.

Montague. R. (2006). *Why Choose This Book? How We Make Decisions.* Harmondsworth, Penguin.

Mujica-Parodi, L. R., Malapisina, D., and Sackheim, H. A. (2000). Logical processing, affect and delusion in schizophrenia. *Harvard Review of Psychiatry,* **8**, 73–83.

O'Reilly, R. and Munakata, Y. (2000). *Computational Explorations in Cognitive Neuroscience.* Cambridge, MA, MIT Press.

Pacherie, E. (2001). Agency lost and found: a commentary on Spence. *Philosophy, Psychiatry and Psychology,* **8**(2–3), 173–176.

Panskepp, J. (1998). *Affective Neuroscience.* Oxford, Oxford University Press.

PBS (1999–2002). 'A Brilliant Madness: interview with John Nash'. Available at PBS: http://www.pbs.org/wgbh/amex/nash/sfeature/sf_nash.html (accessed October 2008).

Quartz, S. R. and Sejnowski, T. J. (1997). A neural basis of cognitive development: a neuroconstructivist manifesto. *Behavioral and Brain Sciences,* **20**, 537–556.

Ressler, K. J. and Nemeroff, C. B. (1999). Role of norepinephrine in the pathophysiology and treatment of mood disorders. *Biological Psychiatry,* **46**(9), 1219–1233.

Schacter, D., Addis, R., and Buckner, R. L. (2007). Remembering the past to imagine the future: the prospective brain. *Nature Reviews Neuroscience,* **8**, 657–660.

Schultz, W., Dayan, P., Montague, P. R. (1997). A neural substrate of prediction and reward. *Science,* **275**, 1593.

Smith, A., Li, M., Becker, S., *et al.* (2006). Dopamine, prediction error, and associative learning: a model-based account. *Network: Computation in Neural Systems,* **17**, 61–84.

Spence, S. A. (2001). Alien control: from phenomenology to cognitive neurobiology. *Philosophy, Psychiatry and Psychology,* **8**(2–3), 163–172.

Stone, M. and Young, A. W. (1997). Delusions and brain injury: the philosophy and psychology of belief. *Mind and Language,* **13**, 327–364.

Suddendorf, T. and Busby, J. (2000). Mental time travel in animals. *Trends in Cognitive Sciences,* **7**, 391–397.

Suddendorf, T. and Corballis, M. C. (1997). Mental time travel and the evolution of the human mind. *Genetic, Social, and General Psychology Monographs,* **123**, 133–167.

Suddendorf, T. and Corballis, M. C. (2007a). The evolution of foresight: what is mental time travel and is it unique to humans? *Behavioral and Brain Sciences,* **30**, 229–313.

Sutton, R. S. and Barto, A. G. (1998). *Reinforcement Learning: An Introduction* Cambridge, MA, MIT Press.

Tulving, E. (2002). Episodic memory: from mind to brain. *Annual Review of Psychology,* **53**, 1–25.

Verdoux, H. and van Os, J. (2002). Psychotic symptoms in non clinical populations and the continuum of psychosis. *Schizophrenia Research,* **54**, 59–68.

Waelti, P., Dickinson, A., and Schultz, W. (2001). Dopamine responses comply with basic assumptions of formal learning theory. *Nature,* **41**(2), 43–48.

Werner, P., Hussy, N., Buell, G., Jones, K. A., and North, R. A. (1996). D2, D3, and D4 dopamine receptors couple to G protein-regulated potassium channels in *Xenopus* oocytes. *Molecular Pharmacology,* **49**, 656–661.

Werner, P., Hussy, N., Buell, G., *et al.* (1997). Toward a theory of episodic memory: the frontal lobes and autonoetic consciousness. *Psychological Bulletin,* **121**, 331–354.

Wheeler MA, S. D. and Tulving, E. (1997). Toward a theory of episodic memory: the frontal lobes and autonoetic consciousness. *Psycholl Bull,* **121**, 331–354.

Wood, J. N. and Grafman, J. (2003). Human prefrontal cortex. *Nature Reviews Neuroscience,* **4**, 139–147.

Section 4

Psychiatry and the neurosciences

Chapter 9

When time is out of joint: Schizophrenia and functional neuroimaging

Dan Lloyd

Abstract

Schizophrenia is characterized by disparate symptoms, a broad spectrum of cognitive deficits, and an equally broad spectrum of alterations in brain function and brain anatomy. Accordingly, some recent attempts to identify the brain dysfunctions responsible for schizophrenia symptoms have abandoned the search for specific loci of dysfunction, considering instead abnormal interactions among neurocognitive modules. For example, separate proposals by Andreassen, Frith, and Friston (among others) attribute some symptoms to dysregulation of recurrent circuits involving multiple brain areas. However, recurrent network models of the illness will require rethinking the role of neuroimaging in its exploration. First, an alteration in regional activity can no longer be interpreted as a simple hypo- or hyper-expression of the normal function of the region, since dysregulated interaction entails that inputs to a region are abnormal, along with the regional function itself. The resultant interactive effects may not be easy to characterize, a difficulty enhanced by recurrent feedback, which may further compound the abnormalities in function. In response to this difficulty, we explore a method for measuring the fidelity of recurrent information in the brain, using functional magnetic resonance imaging (fMRI) during an auditory oddball task. The observed alteration in recurrent information processing also lends itself to a phenomenological interpretation: Accurate recurrent information retention is necessary for the faithful representation of temporality; its dysregulation would destabilize phenomenological reality at its most basic level. Some schizophrenia symptoms may be seen as expressions of or responses to this radical dislocation.

9.1 **Introduction**

'Schizophrenia' denotes a constellation of symptoms, an array of cognitive deficits, a map of functional and anatomical differences in the brain, and a phenomenology of living hell. In each of these domains, the disorder eludes precise characterization and stable description. If its many manifestations are considered together, schizophrenia is either a mistaken name for disparate conditions, or the symbol of a diffuse, variable, and contradictory single condition. In either case, schizophrenia resists knowing. Perhaps this is a temporary gap in science, and like other complex and multiform illnesses (cancer, for example), schizophrenia will find its paradigm and a distinct science devoted to its study and cure. But it may also be that this disorder is *essentially* indefinable, and its elusiveness to definition is part of what makes schizophrenia schizophrenia. In that case, the very puzzling quality of schizophrenia is itself an important datum. In this hypothesis, what is disordered in schizophrenia is something fundamental to the core meaning-making functions of healthy cognition. Thus, for both the ill and their observers, the disorder defeats some pervasive and tacit capacity for comprehension. A person with schizophrenia experiences a deep dysfunction of this capacity, and as a result presents a configuration of properties that cannot be captured in the descriptive and theoretical frameworks of human thought. To conceive an eight-dimensional cube, or an alien sensory system completely unrelated to human senses, or even the sound of one hand clapping, may approximate the effort to contain schizophrenia in a single conceptual and theoretical frame.

An individual with schizophrenia faces a challenge to self-understanding if understanding itself is compromised. Some years ago Julius Laffal, a clinical psychologist, transcribed his therapy sessions with a schizophrenia patient of considerable intelligence and insight (Laffal, 1979). In one session, Laffal presses the patient, 'William', on his difficulties with communication. Within the dialogue, William attempts to explain his own tendency to utter 'nonsense' (73–76):

> The remarks are in process, a sort of grasping at and not conclusive.
>
> I was seeking in such an expansive way that I lost the interest in the situation.
>
> In rein of the procedure, why sometimes one has to base one's psycho-, rather subconscious, referendum in vocabulary of certain nonsensical order, nonsensical order. . . . It's a sort of an association. Number one case, it would alleviate the stress and strain of memory. Number two, would be an endeavor to record what one has said and the meaning could be accentuated by the irrelevant coinage of words and the usage of words:
>
> I'm the one who on the one hand remembering what one is saying, on the other hand forgetting through association.
>
> I'm a walking psychosomatic in that, in the event, in that I try to remember to forget. I would like to effect that, if such be the case, it has practicality, a means of therapy for those who have a strain of hysteria, who continuously broadcast a suggestive idiom.
>
> Common sense provides me at times, in which instances I can answer questions of a most serious nature, I mean, intricate. And then that ease leaves me, and I am blank. My automation is sometimes scurrilous, it's without any control, but the control of observation

merely, the consensus of remembering. I can remember irrationally. I think it's nice to stress irrationality of thought rather than action, stressing. Don't distress. I mean, don't make a plan to do it. I feel just keep your thoughts, in other words, to yourself. That, that, that sums up and it goes over my head. I suppose it will go over anybody else's.

(Laffal, 1979, pp. 73–76)

Language and thought in schizophrenia have been studied extensively (Kerns and Berenbaum, 2002; Condray, 2005; Covington *et al.*, 2005; Cummings, 2007). Impaired association of ideas is one symptom in Bleuler's original characterization of the illness, and remains the theme of the disorganized symptoms (disorganized speech, disorganized behavior, impaired attention, and behavioral disturbance) in the three-compartment conception of the illness (Bleuler, 1913; Liddle, 1987). Indeed, association is one of William's descriptors of his own experience. Laffal's transcripts open a broad window into the mind of a single patient, with whom communication is often difficult or impossible. The excerpts above, in contrast, represent William at his most lucid and insightful. Nonetheless, they display some of the properties that they also describe. Between the beginnings and the ends of his utterances something happens. William describes this sometimes as a deliberate choice of an 'expansive way' to accentuate meaning, using associations and coinage for 'broadcasting a suggestive idiom'. This can be practical as 'therapy' for a 'strain of hysteria'. But the straying thoughts can occur involuntarily as well – an 'automation' 'without any control'.

We might characterize William's difficulties as a failure to fulfill speech intentions. The thought with which he begins a sentence evaporates into a web of 'associations'. His difficulty, then, is one oriented to the immediate future, to sentences and longer units of discourse as the product of executing plans. However, William repeatedly links his deviant communication to defects in memory. According to his expressive self-report, he can 'remember irrationally'. What could this mean? He links the 'stress and strain of memory' to 'association', 'a subconscious referendum in vocabulary of certain nonsensical order'. He seems not to doubt the reliability of specific memories, but their order is nonsensical. The effort to retain a thought derails as memory presents irrelevant items for use; he cannot ignore them, being unable to 'remember to forget'.

This brief attempt to view William's self-description within a coherent frame is doubtful in many respects. His reports are obscure in large part because they are constructed within the constraints of his experiences of the processes he describes: association, irrational memory, and the like. The resulting suggestive idiom of irrelevant coinage dislocates his thought process. At the level of word choice, but also in sentence construction and the ability to sustain coherent discourse, his thoughts constantly turn awry. This is apparent to differing degrees in all his speech. The passages above have been selected for their meaning and relevance to the topic of this chapter, but even this strict filter cannot completely straighten the twists in his thought process.

Following the clues in the passage, we might summarize William's problem (from his own point of view) as one involving memory and anticipation over short time spans. The problem affects all his discourse, but may be accentuated in the self-description of the problem itself. This chapter will explore a reconceptualization of William's experience, borrowing concepts and terms from philosophical phenomenology.

Specifically, in the time span of seconds to minutes, the perception of reality rests on the ability to retain and anticipate events in the immediate past and near future. Among philosophers, Edmund Husserl developed the most detailed account of temporality, which he regarded as the essential structure of consciousness (Husserl, 1966, 1991). His phenomenology of perception will occupy the next section. The sections following will explore the features of the brain that support and embody temporal perception, and the plausibility of disruption of temporal capacities in schizophrenia. Temporality could emerge from information processing in recurrent neural networks, and even subtle distortions of normal function would lead to ramifying effects. How might this kind of dysfunction be detected? This chapter concludes with an example drawn from fMRI.

9.2 **Living in a temporal world**

Philosophical phenomenology is an ongoing attempt to characterize the structure of actual (and possible) human experience at its most basic levels (Ihde, 1977). Phenomenologists reflect on perception and action as such, and on the fundamental constitution of the world as realized by human consciousness. Being basic, many aspects of conscious experience escape notice in everyday life, and ordinary language often lacks the resources to capture them. As a result, phenomenology is often most obscure when its targets are most commonplace, and writers in the tradition have not generally under-stood their audience to extend beyond their colleagues in philosophy. Thus, where there should be an interchange between phenomenology and science, there is a gulf.

The understanding of perception is one area of difference. Perceptual psychologists have mainly understood perception to be the recovery of information about the sensible world as it appears to us here and now. David Marr, for example, directed his classic book *Vision* to the problem of constructing the three-dimensional perceptual world from the information available in the flat retinal image (Marr, 1982). Perceptual experience so conceived tracks objects in space in real time, based on occurrent, real-time information.

Phenomenology, in contrast, grounds human experience not in space, but in time. On this view, objects are not merely instantaneous constructions from sensory inputs. Instead, the immediate sensory manifold is the tip of an iceberg of nonsensory information that essentially constitutes perceptual objects. Edmund Husserl remains the most thorough expositor of temporality in perception. In Husserl's view, every moment of consciousness comprises three aspects (Husserl, 1966, 1991). We experi-ence the information flowing in via the senses, just as considered in perceptual psy-chology. Husserl denoted this sensory aspect of experience the 'primal impression'. But that information is inflected by a 'retention' of the immediate past and a 'protention' or anticipation of the immediate future. For example, a moving pendu-lum at the bottom of its swing, glimpsed in the instantaneous present, will be indiscernible from a stationary pendulum. Only in the context of what has just happened and what is expected can we distinguish moving and stationary objects. The difference is not a separate judgement, but simply the way the pendulum appears, in occurrent perception. That is, perception is always a compound of retention, primal impression, and protention. In every moment of consciousness, sensory impressions are inflected by nonsensory temporal contexts. As time passes, objects continuously slide from protention towards retention. This continual temporal flow and the tripartite temporal constitution of objects apply to every aspect of experience. Objects in the world are temporal, but so are psychological states and processes, including our awareness of temporality itself.

The temporality of all perception is phenomenologically distinct from the processes we usually call recollection and anticipation, which we experience intermittently. Husserl provides a separate account of these. In contrast, temporality is an essential feature of perception. It is always present, necessarily. The fundamental distinction between change and stasis cannot be conceived without temporality, and according to Husserl (using arguments similar to Kant's) we cannot conceive of consciousness itself without temporality. In other words, what we call reality (the real in our experience) is in every case temporally extended, and perceived as such. Accordingly, explicit temporal judgements of duration and sequence are just one expression of temporality, which implicitly operates in all perception.

Thus, in several ways, temporality is largely invisible to ordinary consciousness. Being ubiquitous, it is beneath comment, an infrastructure behind the ever-changing contents of conscious experience, whatever these may be. It cannot be turned on or off, and hence cannot be manipulated experimentally. Only technical terms can conceptualize it. In ordinary life, temporality mixes the obscure and the invisible.

That temporality can hide in plain sight also suggests that in ordinary experience, it is a stable, coherent, and reliable background. For example, if we are surprised by a change in the perceptual world, we ascribe the surprise to the world, not to our temporal construction of it. Similarly, we understand mistakes in perception as based in misconstrued sensory experience rather than a failure in retention/protention. The mistake induced by an optical illusion, for example, is not attributed to a failure of temporality. Only infrequently does misperception suggest a defect in temporality. *Déjà vu*, for example, is not experienced as a mistake in visual perception of the scene before us. Rather, the nonsensory 'feeling' of familiarity creates an illusion of anticipation, a brief dysfunction of protention.

What would it be like, then, if this sturdy backdrop to all experience destabilized over a longer period of time? Inspired by both phenomenology and proposals by Frith (1992), Gallagher suggests that aspects of the experience of schizophrenia can be cast as chronic defects in temporal perception (Gallagher, 2004). Specifically, he suggests that defects in Husserlian protention characterize alienation in schizophrenia. Intentions to act (including deliberate framing of reflective thought) give rise to specific protentions which underlie the awareness of agency and ownership. If those protentions fail, action and thought will appear 'from nowhere'.

We can generalize from this suggestion to consider possible experiences during disruptions of the ordinary scaffolding of time. Retention is the basis for the perception of duration; in its absence, the perception of change and movement, as well as the rate of change and motion, will be misperceived. As a result, fundamental perception will fail to match the mechanical regularities of physics (and the rule-following interactions of the social world). Such experiences would be deeply disturbing, and confusing as well, in that, the given appearances of things, their primal impressions, can remain approximately normal. The misperception is not exactly sensory and not captured fully by describing 'how things look'. But, as discussed, we do not have an intuitive conceptual language for temporality. Moreover, temporality is the foundation of experienced reality as such, and to suppose its failure is to doubt one's contact with the real world. This terrifying possibility is the last hypothesis one would entertain. Instead, there might be a strong desire to explain all the anomalies as individual episodes (initially), and from there develop general explanatory theories of the anomalous world. But the anomalies are random, and therefore any explanations would necessarily ramify to handle exceptions (Lloyd, 2007).

For example, the swinging pendulum will appear to accelerate oddly if retention is disrupted. The anomaly will be disturbing, conspicuous, and needing an explanation. If that explanation is not sought in temporal disturbance, then the erratic pendulum must be subject to special invisible forces causing its acceleration. In other words, one would struggle to save the appearances (of a physical object in motion), by appealing to special interventions outside of the usual causal order. From outside, to believe in occult forces is delusional. But such delusions might be the best or only way to maintain any hold on reality. Moreover, it will be inevitable to refer these occult forces to oneself (as author or victim), since the temporal misperceptions are idiosyncratic.

Disruptions in temporality would also undermine the ability to complete any complex action. Language production, in particular, depends on the accurate retention and protention of context in order to move forward. When sentential temporality is disrupted, speech and writing will deteriorate. Syntax, word choice, prosody, pragmatics, and reasoning all rely on an intact temporal stream.

In short, breaking the resilient spine of time plunges a person into a profoundly challenging perceptual world. Understanding is defeated at every turn by an inconceivably disordered stream of perception, compounded by disrupted and fragmented thought and communication. The hypothetical phenomenology of a chronic temporal disorder is conjectural, but suggestive. A disorder of temporal perception might plausibly present several symptoms of schizophrenia.

Phenomenology has its analogues in the cognitive science of schizophrenia. Temporality is the phenomenological expression of a specific awareness of context. Cognitive models of schizophrenia often cite failures to cognize context or successfully integrate contextual information with occurrent perception (Hemsley, 2005a, b). Victims of a temporal disorder would also be likely to display irregularities in their explicit judgements about time, a finding with a long history in schizophrenia research (Seeman, 1976; Davalos et al., 2003). Deficits in time estimation dissociate from more general problems with working memory or attention (Elvevag et al., 2003). These deficits in explicit time perception are consistent with a more general dysfunction of temporality.

9.3 Information and misinformation in recurrent neural networks

The neuroscience of schizophrenia has discovered a long list of anomalies in brain structure and function in individuals with the illness; this chapter will not review these. Individual studies often identify one or more regions of functional difference in comparisons between schizophrenia patients and healthy control subjects, when probing specific cognitive capacities.

For example, working memory in schizophrenia has been probed repeatedly. Several neuroimaging studies report a decrease in activity in the dorsolateral prefrontal cortex in schizophrenia patients (Callicott *et al.*, 1998, 2000, 2003; Carter *et al.*, 1998; Menon, 2001; Perlstein *et al.*, 2001; Barch *et al.*, 2002; Meyer-Lindenberg *et al.*, 2002; Wykes *et al.*, 2002; Jansma *et al.*, 2004; Mendrek *et al.*, 2004). 'Hypofrontality' thus seems to be a well-confirmed observation, except that at least five other studies showed either no change in prefrontal activity or an increase – hyper-rather than hypofrontality (Callicott *et al.*, 2000; Honey *et al.*, 2002; Sabri *et al.*, 2003; Walter *et al.*, 2003; Jansma *et al.*, 2004). A review of 22 schizophrenia experiments showed that the alterations of function characteristic of schizophrenia are not only ambivalent in the frontal cortex but conjoint with alterations in several other areas (Lloyd, in press). When patients were compared to control subjects in these experiments, on average three of four Brodmann areas in DLPFC were depressed, but one (Right area 9) was elevated. Moreover, seven other Brodmann areas outside of DLPFC were depressed at least as much as the DLPFC areas, and another four areas are elevated nearly as much as area 9 (Lloyd, in press). This is a narrow band of research, but it implicates cognitive functions and a conspicuous brain region often associated with schizophrenia. Although the frontal lobe plays some role in the illness, that role is uncertain in itself and part of a larger network of affected areas.

Individual studies also show multiple areas of abnormal function in schizophrenia (Liang *et al.*, 2006). These overlap with areas involved in time judgements. Time management in both interval production (e.g. finger tapping) and duration estimation involves a wide network of brain areas, including several frontal areas, parietal lobe, cerebellum, and basal ganglia (Volz *et al.*, 2001; Rubia and Smith, 2004), and more than one neurotransmitter system (Meck, 1996).

Overall, the studies support a hypothesis that schizophrenia is not the effect of a localized dysfunction. A similar conclusion follows from the current proposals about the relationship between neurotransmitter regulation and schizophrenia. One of these is the 'dopamine hypothesis'. Dopamine dysregulation has been observed many times in individuals with schizophrenia, and implicated in a cascade of effects that point to some of the brain areas mentioned in the survey above. These areas, especially prefrontal cortex and the mesolimbic system (including nucleus accumbens, ventral striatum, amygdala, hippocampus, entorhinal cortex, medial frontal cortex, and anterior cingulate), are targets for dopamine regulation. The details of this hypothesis and its evolution with ongoing research are once again a subject requiring a much longer review (Byne *et al.*, 1999; Carlsson *et al.*, 1999). Other neurotransmitters seem to be involved as well (Meck, 1996). However, a simple consequence of any neurotransmitter dysregulation is that multiple brain areas are affected. This, along with the overview of papers, suggests that localized dysfunction is an unlikely root cause of schizophrenia.

Motivated in part by the considerations above, several researchers have proposed that schizophrenia arises through alterations in the function of a network of regions.

Individually, function in these regions may be abnormal, but this is a secondary man-ifestation of alterations in the connections between regions.

Disconnection hypotheses take several forms. For example, in several papers Nancy Andreasen has proposed that some of the symptoms of schizophrenia arise through 'cognitive dysmetria', 'a defect in timing or sequencing the flow of information as required during normal 'thought' or speech,' involving thalamus, frontal cortex, and cerebellum (Andreasen *et al.*, 1999). Andreasen analogizes thought and action, observing that both require fine-grained coordination of sensory inputs and motor outputs. Accordingly, motor difficulties and cognitive deficits both express cognitive dysmetria.

Christopher Frith (1992) examines a 'supervisory attentional system', responsible for forming goals and plans, in interaction with a system for selecting which action to execute, i.e. a system for forming specific intentions to act. A disruption in the interactions between the supervisory system and the action scheduler could lead to several of the negative symptoms of schizophrenia. As in Andreason's proposed cognitive dysmetria, Frith's hypotheses involve an analogy between action and thought. An internal monitoring system compares the chosen action to the actual behaviour, represented by sensory feedback. Disruption of the corollary intention signal would result in actions or thoughts that appear unintended, a common theme among the positive symptoms of schizophrenia. Citing lesion studies, animal models, and behavioural experiments, Frith cautiously identifies the brain areas involved in these loops. The supervisory attentional system includes the anterior cingulate cortex, dorsolateral prefrontal cortex, and supplementary motor area. The action selector includes the striatum, especially the putamen, and the globus pallidus.

Karl Friston's 'disconnection hypothesis' again considers the prefrontal cortex, but in its interactions with the medial temporal lobe, including amygdala, hippocampus, and parahippocampal gyrus (Friston, 1999). Altered neuromodulation in this loop affects long-term synaptic plasticity, i.e. learning. Schizophrenia disrupts the learning of contingencies in the environment, including the social environment, and it disrupts the learning of complex action patterns. This could contribute to negative symptoms, especially those involving communication and social interaction, as well as positive symptoms, through misattribution of the relationships between one's own intentions and perceived events.

All the authors above draw on multiple strands of evidence, which the summaries above omit. Their common theme is the disruption of communication within net-works of multiple brain areas. Importantly, in all three proposals, the networks are recurrent. That is, they involve feedback loops. (The disconnection hypotheses iden-tify different circuits and physiologies. Andreasen and Frith seem to suggest that schizophrenic symptoms are the immediate effect of a disruption of connectivity among brain areas. Friston proposes that the symptoms are a longer term secondary consequence of disrupted modulation of otherwise normal processes of synaptic change.)

The proposals explain several schizophrenic symptoms and deficits as the effects of disruption of these recurrent networks. Localized dysfunction may therefore be a secondary manifestation of the illness. No single component fails in schizophrenia, they claim, but rather all wobble together as their interconnections slip. At scales ranging from milliseconds (Andreasen) to seconds (Frith) to years (Friston), disconnection leads to failures of coordination among the components of actions and thoughts. Here, however, we note a further commonality among these views: one function of recurrent feedback is to enable the retention of temporal information. Information transmission takes time; thus one way to bring information from the immediate past to bear on the present is to transmit it through a 'delay line' in which the time of transmission is slightly longer. Recurrent feedback connections supply their millisecond delays by the time taken for the feedback itself. As recurrent information feeds back into the primary feed-forward stream, it is information originating in a previous instant. In the simplest case, information at time $t1$ is simply superimposed on information at $t2$.

Temporal delay in a recurrent circuit may seem like a trivial aspect in a complex network, but neural network models reveal some surprising capabilities of recurrent networks. Elman, a pioneer of recurrent network models, constructed simulations of 'simple recurrent networks' (Elman, 1990). They are indeed simple, built as feed-forward connectionist models with the addition of a basic feedback circuit, in which the pattern of internal activity at time $t1$ is combined with the current input at $t2$. These networks were trained using a simple back-propagation learning algorithm, as if they were conventional feed-forward nets. Intuitively, it would seem that such a network could learn temporal contingencies only one step forward in processing, but surprisingly Elman and others have shown that recurrent networks can respond to temporal contingencies at much longer lags than the lag in the circuit itself. Simple recurrent networks were able to learn recursive grammars, for example, or anticipate meanings of terms based on context. Moreover, when the activity in the internal processing units was analysed, it revealed distinctions and structures that were only implicit in the inputs. (For example, the network distinguished nouns from verbs even though the input stream was unmarked grammatically.) How does this circuit retain information over time? Broadly speaking, as information from the past re-enters the loop, it need not be discarded. Information from times past can be encoded in the internal units and remain as needed (and according to the capacity of the network to form distinct representations). Thus, recurrent networks have shown the computational capacity to implement D. O. Hebb's conjectured cell assemblies, in which information is held by continuous recycling in the neural loop (Hebb, 1959). Rao and Sejnowski have modelled cortical recurrent circuits, lending biological plausibility to this idea (Rao and Sejnowski, 2000).

Simulated recurrent networks suggest a functional consequence of the brain's huge commitment to recurrent or reentrant circuitry. In recurrence, brains acquire a capacity to respond to temporal contingencies on a very short timescale, from tens of milliseconds to seconds. This form of information storage is functionally distinct from long-term memory and seems more comprehensive than what is usually ascribed to short-term memory. The disconnection hypotheses considered above are instances of disruptions of various recurrent circuits, and each may explain differing symptoms of schizophrenia. But a more general consequence of recurrent dysfunction involves the representation of time. In recurrent processing, we find a model sufficient for implementing the temporal capacities of retention and protention (Lloyd, 2004). That is, it is plausible that what it is like to be a very large recurrent network is to enjoy an awareness of time. But as the architecture of recurrence itself suggests, time does not find a separate representation as a time-keeper or clock, but rather is embedded in the perception of the world and the self. In an environment governed by lawful, predictable, spatial – temporal relationships, synaptic plasticity at myriad sites serves to continuously tune the circuits of perception and cognition to both retain and anticipate the behaviour of objects and other persons. To disrupt these recurrent circuits is to undermine temporal representation and processing. Thus, the conjectures above converge on a broad physiological characterization of cognition in schizophrenia, and this in turn conforms to the conjectured phenomenology of the disorder. For the individual with schizophrenia, as for Hamlet, 'time is out of joint'.

9.4 Imaging a temporal disorder

The usual application of functional neuroimaging explores contrasts between the brain in an experimental condition and the brain in a differing, control condition. The difference between images in the two conditions is presumed to indicate the regions especially committed to processing in the experimental condition, as compared to its control (or vice versa). Although oversimplified in many ways, this capsule summary nonetheless expresses the skeletal logic of many experiments in functional neuroimaging. Contrastive methods have been refined and extended, and their presuppositions examined and critiqued, by many researchers; these general considerations will not be repeated here (Friston, 1996; Price, 1996; Horwitz et al., 2000; Uttal, 2001; Lloyd, 2004; Friston et al., 2006). However, we note that the basic logic of the contrastive approach may be ineffective for probing the brain conditions associated with schizophrenia. There are several reasons for this.

First, the majority of imaging studies of schizophrenia ultimately involve a double contrast. Using the contrast between experimental and control conditions, task-related areas of activation are identified in healthy subjects; the same contrast is repeated for patients. These two contrasts are then contrasted, comparing extent of activity in patients with healthy controls. The validity of the second contrast, patient vs. control, depends on the consistency of the first. Both initial contrasts subtract control-condition activity from an experimental condition. Those contrasts are comparable only if the control conditions activate the brains in both groups in the same way. In a pervasive illness like schizophrenia, the baseline cannot be assumed to be well controlled. Whether the baseline is open-ended ('rest with eyes closed') or some component of the experimental task, individuals with schizophrenia cannot be assumed to match healthy subjects in brain activity in the control task, even if the performance of the two groups matches.

Second, if schizophrenia is indeed a disconnection disorder, the differences in activity that neuroimaging readily detect may be secondary effects. Activity in any brain area depends on the combination of inputs from other areas and the intrinsic function of the region itself. All schizophrenia studies report multiple differences between patients and control subjects, and explanatory accounts proposed in the previous section imply that inputs are altered by the illness. In other words, the disorder is at least partly in the connections among areas rather than wholly in the affected regions. Imaging studies often employ 'connectivity analysis' in which co-activation of areas provides a measure of functional connectivity (Penny et al., 2004; Friston, 2005). This is invaluable in understanding the flow of information among networks of brain regions, but the secondary contrast between schizophrenia subjects and controls cannot assume that the differences are entirely due to connectivity either, as opposed to some combination of regional and network alterations. A more robust form of connectivity analysis involves the reconstruction of white-matter tracts using a different technology, diffusion tensor imaging. This reveals anatomical differences, leaving open the relationship of structure and function. Nonetheless, combinations of methods will likely converge on a better understanding of the mechanisms of the illness, a topic beyond the scope of this chapter (Ardekani et al., 2005; White et al., 2007).

But even this level of sophistication encounters a third difficulty. Recurrent connections exhibit a robust capacity for learning contingencies across time, but the same recurrence amplifies even small dysfunctions, due to the repetition of its influence with each processing cycle (O'Reilly and Rudy, 2001). Very different brains can be equally competent in temporal cognition if they are consistently attuned to the regularities of the time-extended world. Conversely, very similar brains can differ greatly in their temporal competencies, if these abilities are globally determined by subtle mechanisms.

Finally, if schizophrenia is a disorder of a widely distributed circuit among brain areas, and if the expression of this circuit is equally ubiquitous in both temporal cognition and temporal experience, then in every contrast, both the experimental and control conditions will interweave with the continual flow of temporal processing. If temporal cognition is basic to neural function, then it will not appear when one set of temporalized images is subtracted from another. In both patients and healthy subjects, any contrastive approach will be systematically blind to the machinations of time.

Considered together, the 'standard' contrastive approach and some of its variants seem confounded by a disorder that arises from recurrent connections distributed widely across the brain. Even if the results of the standard approach were univocal, it would not rule out disconnection hypotheses, since contrastive methods eliminate commonalities between experimental conditions.

In light of these difficulties, one might dismiss functional neuroimaging as an instrument too blunt for schizophrenia research. However, here we note that the limits and confounds appear in the interpretive methods typical of this field, rather than in the technology itself (although that too faces limits of temporal and spatial resolution). Perhaps there are methods for considering brain imaging data that do not rest on contrasts. This section will conclude with the consideration of one such method. This interpretive strategy considers the brain globally, as a distributed recurrent information processor, and probes the accuracy of temporally extended representation.

Consider again the theme of recurrence, appearing above in its computational and phenomenological aspects. Recurrent processing takes time, and it is natural to think of it as an unfolding dynamic flow. However, if recurrent processing reliably encodes past or future events, then that encoding must be present at each moment in the occurrent dynamic state of the network. This is the computational analogue of the tripartite phenomenology of time, which requires that protention and retention co-occur with the primal impression in the present. Analogously, successful cognition in time requires data structures that represent occurrent inputs while at the same time representing non-occurrent facts, like the duration of the current condition, or changes in the past, or expected changes in the future. As a system moves through time, these representations must be continuously updated to reflect the passage of time. To fix an event in a stable past location requires a representation that is continually changing, to match the continuous recession and procession of time.

These two considerations combine in our expectations for neural processing in the brain. The brain must be able to support temporal phenomenology, and it must likewise support the continuously updated temporalized representations of events. Information processing and data representation will include a 'temporal spread' beyond the immediate present. Methodologically, we will need to reconsider brain images as representations of this temporal spread. However, in light of the considerations in the sections above, we can conjecture that the form of representation deployed for retention and protention is different from the representation of the immediate sensory environment; simple correlations would not detect this admixture of immediate and temporalized representation. Instead, we can attempt an indirect approach. If the current pattern of brain activity is temporalized, then it must contain information about past and future patterns of activity. Operationally, the functional image at time t must contain information about images at $t - 1$, $t - 2$, etc., and $t + 1$, $t + 2$, etc., out to an indefinite horizon for these short-term phenomena.

In the absence of an *a priori* theory of neural representation for protention or retention, we will need to cast the net very broadly. Here, we will use artificial neural networks (ANNs) as pattern detectors. For each image series, we will train a network using an image at time t as input, and an image at $t - 1$ ($t - 2$, ..., $t + 1$, $t + 2$, etc.) as its target output. If a network can learn to extract from every image specific prior or subsequent images, this will serve as indirect evidence that temporally extended information is present in each image. The trained network, in other words, is a complex mathematical function that maps from each image in a series to images before and after in the same series. That one function can make this mapping consistently for an entire image series is *prima facie* evidence that there is a consistent pattern of representation for temporal information. If this mapping can be found, then its accuracy can be measured and compared to the same analysis in individuals with schizophrenia. In effect, the accuracy of the past and future projections from each image is an operational measure of the accuracy of protention and retention.

This approach has the advantage of flexibility. ANNs can learn to recognize and interpret nonlinear interactions among brain regions, and can consider patterns in a global, distributed way. Relationships that could not appear to inspection, correlation, or linear regression can nonetheless be captured through this form of automatic pattern association. But at the same time, the pattern-detecting powers of ANNs can be too much of a good thing. They can make their associations based on spurious information too. In functional imaging, the main confound is the auto-correlation of the image series: each pixel in one image will be similar in intensity to itself measured both before and after, due mainly to the gradual rise and fall of the detected haemodynamic response over several seconds. This confound is controlled by constructing a surrogate image series. Here, we used a standard method for creating surrogate data (Schreiber and Schmitz, 1996, 2000). The oscillations of each image element were decomposed into their frequency components, and the phase of each component randomly shifted. The phase-shifted frequency components were then recombined into a surrogate signal. Importantly, the surrogate method creates pseudo-data in which auto-correlation is preserved. Then, the same ANN learning process is applied to the surrogate series, and its accuracy measured, and this measure compared to the accuracy of pattern association with the original image series. If the accuracy of learning in the original series exceeds that of the surrogate series, then that excess cannot be due to auto-correlation. That comparative value then becomes the measure of temporal information beyond the temporal smear of autocorrelation.[1] We will measure this value as the likelihood that the trained ANN accuracy exceeds the accuracy of learning in the surrogate data. This p value, subtracted from one, affords a positive measure of temporal information projected in time. In measuring a statistical parameter, the rationale and the method are parallel to statistical parametric mapping in the spatial domain.

This method for temporal analysis has been applied in 21 healthy subjects in four experiments (Lloyd, 2002), and detected protentional and retentional information in all subjects in a variety of experiments. Here, the analysis is applied with 17 schizophrenia patients and an equal number of healthy subjects, using data generously provided by the Olin Neuropsychiatry Research Center in Hartford, Connecticut. All subjects performed an auditory oddball task. A steady series of tones is punctuated at random intervals with a distinct target tone, requiring a button press. The soundstream is also interrupted by a variety of irregular noises. Each scanning session consisted of two runs of about 6 minutes; the present analysis is based on the first run. 248 images were collected at 1.5 seconds each. For this analysis, the first ten and last eight images of the series were discarded. For scanner and task protocols, see Garrity et al., 2007. Image series were preprocessed using independent component analysis (ICA) (McKeown et al., 1998; Calhoun et al., 2002). Informally, ICA discovers ensembles of voxels (fMRI pixels) that fluctuate in unison. ICA maximizes the statistical independence of each component. For this analysis, each image series was transformed into 20 independent components, sufficient for preserving most of the variance in the images over time. For the details of the ICA, see Garrity et al. 2007.

The oddball task may seem like an odd choice for probing temporality. However, if temporality is indeed a pervasive feature of all awareness, it should be present in

---

[1] ANN learning outcomes partly depend on initial randomized values in the weight matrix, or coefficients that determine the mapping from inputs to outputs. A single comparison might be skewed by initial conditions. Therefore, the analysis described here was repeated in 30 networks. The comparisons are aggregate results of the repeated analysis. In addition, the first 2/3 of the image series was used for network training, and the remainder for testing, with the statistical measures taken on the test images.

nontemporal tasks like the auditory oddball, which makes no demands on temporal judgement, short-term memory, or anticipation. Moreover, in its surprising unpredictability, the novel stimuli of the task recruit many brain areas as potentially relevant (Kiehl *et al.*, 2005). In a large-scale study of 100 subjects, Kiehl *et al.* identified more than 20 brain regions involved in the oddball task.

Temporal analysis was applied at a timescale of 15 seconds (ten images) before and after the current image, for each image analysed. In both healthy subjects and patients, each image contains information about images before and after. Fig. 9.1 displays the mean values of protention and retention, and their 95% confidence intervals, for both subject groups. Brain images of schizophrenia patients showed significantly less information about brain states before and after the current now point (Fig. 9.1), with the greatest deficits observed in retention. In this way, functional neuroimaging can reveal a deficit in image information over time. In the context of this chapter, this finding is consistent with the phenomenological conjectures, related cognitive models, the experimental and clinical observations, and the proposed computational scheme.

The network analysis can exploit global, distributed brain activity in some nonlinear combination in its determination of the past and future brain states. But it is equally possible that a subset of brain areas particularly determines temporal information. 'Localization' is vague in application, but nonetheless suggests a spectrum of functional organisations for the brain, from highly modular regional specialists at one extreme to fully distributed global processing on the other. Even qualitative distinctions between the poles of this spectrum could be useful here, in that temporal cognition and consciousness have been conjectured to rest on broad, distributed, and recurrent networks in the brain. The extent of localization for temporal information in the oddball data was probed using a 'leave one out' strategy, as follows. The ANN analysis (as above) was repeated on each image series with components omitted. That is, the analysis repeatedly used 19 of 20 components, recording the impact of omitting each component on the overall capacity of the image to project past and future images. After all 20 components have been tested by omission, the one that has the least effect on the information measures is removed, and the leave-one-out process repeated for the 19 remaining components, reducing them to 18, and so on. With each iteration, the component with the least effect on the temporal information found in the image series is deleted; conversely, then, the most temporally loaded components are preserved as the component set is incrementally reduced. This affords a measure of the localisation of temporal information according to the following rationale: if few brain areas are responsible for the temporal measures, then the deletion of the ineffectual components should have little effect on temporal information measures, because the few important components will be retained and thus continue to represent the temporal information detected by the ANN. On the other hand, if temporal information is broadly distributed among the components, then deletion of even the least of them will diminish the temporal information discovered by the ANN analysis. This strategy can be applied here to consider the localisation of temporal information in healthy subjects and patients independently, and relative to each other.

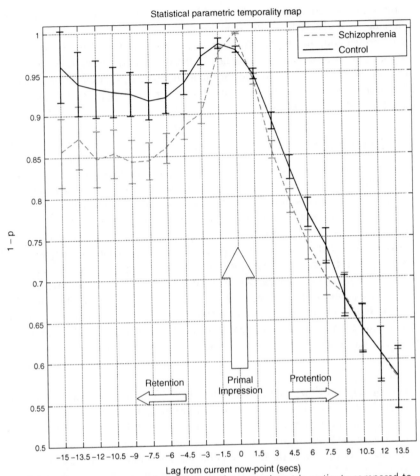

Fig. 9.1 Temporal information about the near future and past in patients compared to healthy controls.

Specifically, this analysis probed how many components were required to maintain significant protention and retention, where significance is understood as in the previous analysis, namely, the likelihood that the ANN mapping from images at differing lags was due to temporal information, and not to auto-correlation.[2] In all cases, the leave-one-out probes indicated that temporal information is highly distributed in the brains of both healthy controls and patients. Significant temporal information in healthy subjects required 16.4 out of 20 components on average (95% confidence spanned 15.4–17.4 components). In individuals with schizophrenia, significant temporal information required an average of 18.2 components (95% confidence

---

[2] Significance here is corrected for multiple comparisons using the Bonferroni method.

spanned 17–19.3 components). The healthy and patient means were significantly different, $p = 0.0228$. It should be noted that this is not an absolute measure of distributed representation in temporality, but rather one amenable to debatable thresholds and assumptions. Nonetheless, regardless of the significance threshold, large regions of the brain appear to be required for the maintenance of temporal information. Moreover, in patients, the network supporting temporal cognition is significantly more fragile than in healthy subjects.

9.5 Conclusion

Schizophrenia is such a perplexing disorder and so widely researched that it is always an act of hubris to propose a model of any aspect of the disease. Nonetheless, without models to test, both conceptually and empirically, research on schizophrenia can only continue to collect observations. This chapter has woven several strands of reasoned conjecture into a single framework, compiling educated guesses in the hope of setting a direction for further research. I proposed that schizophrenia is the expression of dysfunction or dysregulation of recurrent circuits involving many areas of the brain – so many that it makes little sense to think of the disorder as functionally localized. The chief consequence of the dysregulation is a disruption in the maintenance of an accurate representation of temporal context for occurrent mental events. The wide distribution of involved areas suggests vulnerability in action, thought, and perception. Conceiving schizophrenia as a disruption of temporality entails an experience of the illness consistent with several of its symptoms and the self-report of an articulate patient.

Functional neuroimaging provides a tool for examining temporality, following a novel strategy for analysis. The analysis measures temporal information in an image series without specifying what that information is, when it is present (or not), nor what areas of the brain might be involved. In short, it is a method appropriate for the preliminary exploration of the temporal domain. The temporal statistical parametric analysis, parallel in many ways with statistical parametric mapping of the brain, revealed a plausible distribution of temporal information with an emphasis on retention. More important, the analysis clearly distinguished individuals with schizophrenia from healthy controls. Schizophrenia patients showed diminished protention and especially diminished retention at almost every lag from the immediate present, extending at least 15 seconds into the immediate past and (on average) around 7 seconds into the future. The observed difference is large enough to suggest that temporal analysis could be a tool for diagnosis or assessment. Moreover, it was measured here in an apparently nontemporal task, suggesting that temporal analysis is an adaptable tool that could be applied retrospectively to existing datasets.

In sum, schizophrenia presents a conceptual challenge to the philosophical phenomenologist, a modelling challenge to the cognitive scientist, a diagnostic and therapeutic challenge to the clinician, and a descriptive challenge to the functional neuroimager. But of course, the greatest challenge faces individuals at the intersection of all these challenges, the sufferers of schizophrenia, for whom the other challenges are undertaken.

References

Andreasen, N. C., Nopoulos, P., O'Leary, D. S., Miller, D. D., Wassink, T., and Flaum, M. (1999). Defining the phenotype of schizophrenia: cognitive dysmetria and its neural mechanisms. *Biol Psychiatry,* **46**(7), 908–920.

Ardekani, B. A., Bappal, A., D'Angelo, D., *et al.* (2005). Brain morphometry using diffusion-weighted magnetic resonance imaging: application to schizophrenia. *Neuroreport,* **16**(13), 1455–1459.

Barch, D. M., Csernansky, J. G., Conturo, T., and Snyder, A. Z. (2002). Working and long-term memory deficits in schizophrenia: is there a common prefrontal mechanism? *J Abnorm Psychol,* **111**(3), 478–494.

Bleuler, E. (1913). Dementia praecox or the group of schizophrenias. In *The Clinical Roots of the Schizophrenia Concept* (eds. J. Cutting, and M. Shepherd). Cambridge, Cambridge University Press.

Byne, W., Kemether, E., Jones, L., Haroutunian, V., and Davis, K. (1999). Neurochemistry of schizophrenia. In *Neurobiology of Mental Illness* (eds. D. S. Charney, E. J. Nestler, and B. S. Bunney), pp. 236–257. New York, Oxford University Press.

Calhoun, V. D., Adali, T., Pearlson, G. D., van Zijl, P. C., and Pekar, J. J. (2002). Independent component analysis of fMRI data in the complex domain. *Magn Reson Med,* **48**(1), 180–192.

Callicott, J. H., Ramsey, N. F., Tallent, K., *et al.* (1998). Functional magnetic resonance imaging brain mapping in psychiatry: methodological issues illustrated in a study of working memory in schizophrenia. *Neuropsychopharmacology,* **18**(3), 186–196.

Callicott, J. H., Bertolino, A., Mattay, V. S., *et al.* (2000). Physiological dysfunction of the dorsolateral prefrontal cortex in schizophrenia revisited. *Cereb Cortex,* **10**(11), 1078–1092.

Callicott, J. H., Mattay, V. S., Verchinski, B. A., Marenco, S., Egan, M. F., and Weinberger, D. R. (2003). Complexity of prefrontal cortical dysfunction in schizophrenia: more than up or down. *Am J Psychiatry,* **160**(12), 2209–2215.

Carlsson, A., Waters, N., and Carlsson, M. L. (1999). Neurotransmitter interactions in schizophrenia–therapeutic implications. *Biol Psychiatry,* **46**(10), 1388–1395.

Carter, C. S., Perlstein, W., Ganguli, R., Brar, J., Mintun, M., and Cohen, J. D. (1998). Functional hypofrontality and working memory dysfunction in schizophrenia. *Am J Psychiatry,* **155**(9), 1285–1287.

Condray, R. (2005). Language disorder in schizophrenia as a developmental learning disorder. *Schizophr Res,* **73**(1), 5–20.

Covington, M. A., He, C., Brown, C., *et al.* (2005). Schizophrenia and the structure of language: the linguist's view. *Schizophr Res,* **77**(1), 85–98.

Cummings, L. (2007). Pragmatics and adult language disorders: past achievements and future directions. *Semin Speech Lang,* **28**(2), 96–110.

Davalos, D. B., Kisley, M. A., and Ross, R. G. (2003). Effects of interval duration on temporal processing in schizophrenia. *Brain Cogn,* **52**(3), 295–301.

Elman, J. (1990). Finding structure in time. *Cognitive Science,* **14**, 179–211.

Elvevag, B., McCormack, T., Gilbert, A., Brown, G.D., Weinberger, D.R., and Goldberg, T. E. (2003). Duration judgements in patients with schizophrenia. *Psychol Med,* **33**(7), 1249–1261.

Ford, J. M., Johnson, M. B., Whitfield, S. L., Faustman, W. D., and Mathalon, D. H. (2005). Delayed hemodynamic responses in schizophrenia. *Neuroimage,* **26**(3), 922–931.

Friston, K., Price, C., Fletcher, P., Moore, R., Frackowiak, R., and Dolan, R. (1996). The trouble with cognitive subtraction. *Neuroimage,* **4**, 97–104.

Friston, K. J. (1999). Schizophrenia and the disconnection hypothesis. *Acta Psychiatr Scand Suppl*, **395**, 68–79.

Friston, K. J. (2005). Models of brain function in neuroimaging. *Annu Rev Psychol*, **56**, 57–87.

Friston, K. J., Rotshtein, P., Geng, J. J., Sterzer, P., and Henson, R. N. (2006). A critique of functional localisers. *Neuroimage*, **30**(4), 1077–1087.

Frith, C. (1992). *Cognitive Neuropsychology of Schizophrenia*. Hove, Lawrence Erlbaum.

Gallagher, S. (2004). Neurocognitive models of schizophrenia: a neurophenomenological critique. *Psychopathology*, **37**(1), 8–19.

Garrity, A. G., Pearlson, G. D., McKiernan, K., Lloyd, D., Kiehl, K. A., and Calhoun, V. D. (2007). Aberrant 'default mode' functional connectivity in schizophrenia. *Am J Psychiatry*, **164**(3), 450–457.

Hebb, D. O. (1959). *The Organization of Behavior*. New York, John Wiley.

Hemsley, D. R. (2005a). The development of a cognitive model of schizophrenia: placing it in context. *Neurosci Biobehav Rev*, **29**(6), 977–988.

Hemsley, D. R. (2005b). The schizophrenic experience: taken out of context? *Schizophr Bull*, **31**(1), 43–53.

Honey, G. D., Bullmore, E. T., and Sharma, T. (2002). De-coupling of cognitive performance and cerebral functional response during working memory in schizophrenia. *Schizophr Res*, **53**(1–2), 45–56.

Horwitz, B., Friston, K. J., and Taylor, J. G. (2000). Neural modeling and functional brain imaging: an overview. *Neural Netw*, **13**(8–9), 829–846.

Husserl, E. (1966). *Zur Phänomenologie des inneren Zeitbewusstseins (Phenomenology of Inner Time Consciousness)* vol. 10. The Hague, Martinus Nijhoff.

Husserl, E. (1991). *On the Phenomenology of the Consciousness of Internal Time* (Tr. J. Brough). Dordrecht, Kluwer.

Ihde, D. (1977). *Experimental Phenomenology: An Introduction*. New York, Putnam.

Jansma, J. M., Ramsey, N. F., van der Wee, N. J., and Kahn R. S. (2004). Working memory capacity in schizophrenia: a parametric fMRI study. *Schizophr Res*, **68**(2–3), 159–171.

Kerns, J. G. and Berenbaum, H. (2002). Cognitive impairments associated with formal thought disorder in people with schizophrenia. *J Abnorm Psychol*, **111**(2), 211–224.

Kiehl, K. A., Stevens, M. C., Laurens, K. R., Pearlson, G., Calhoun, V. D., and Liddle, P. F. (2005). An adaptive reflexive processing model of neurocognitive function: supporting evidence from a large scale (n = 100) fMRI study of an auditory oddball task. *Neuroimage*, **25**(3), 899–915.

Laffal, J. (1979). *A Source Document in Schizophrenia*. Hope Valley, RI, Gallery Press.

Liang, M., Zhou, Y., Jiang, T., *et al.* (2006). Widespread functional disconnectivity in schizophrenia with resting-state functional magnetic resonance imaging. *Neuroreport*, **17**(2), 209–213.

Liddle, P. F. (1987). The symptoms of chronic schizophrenia. A re-examination of the positive–negative dichotomy. *Br J Psychiatry*, **151**, 145–151.

Lloyd, D. (2007). Civil schizophrenia. In *Distributed Cognition and the Will* (ed. D. Ross). Cambridge, MA, MIT Press.

Lloyd, D. (in press). Through a glass darkly: schizophrenia and functional brain imaging. *Philosophy, Psychiatry, and Psychology*.

Lloyd, D. E. (2004). *Radiant Cool: A Novel Theory of Consciousness*. Cambridge, MA, MIT Press.

Marr, D. (1982). *Vision: A Computational Investigation into the Human Representation and Processing of Visual Information.* New York, Henry Holt.

McKeown, M. J., Makeig, S., Brown, G. G., *et al.* (1998). Analysis of fMRI data by blind separation into independent spatial components. *Hum Brain Mapp,* 6(3), 160–188.

Meck, W. H. (1996). Neuropharmacology of timing and time perception. *Brain Res Cogn Brain Res,* 3(3–4), 227–242.

Mendrek, A., Laurens, K. R., Kiehl, K. A., Ngan, E. T., Stip, E., and Lidle, P. F. (2004). Changes in distributed neural circuitry function in patients with first-episode schizophrenia. *Br J Psychiatry,* 185, 205–214.

Menon, V., Anagnoson, R., Mathalon, D., Glover, G., and Pfefferbaum, A. (2001). Functional neuroanatomy of auditory working memory in schizophrenia: relation to positive and negative symptoms. *Neuroimage,* 13, 433–446.

Meyer-Lindenberg, A., Miletich, R. S., Kohn, P. D., *et al.* (2002). Reduced prefrontal activity predicts exaggerated striatal dopaminergic function in schizophrenia. *Nat Neurosci,* 5(3), 267–271.

O'Reilly, R. C. and Rudy, J. W. (2001). Conjunctive representations in learning and memory: principles of cortical and hippocampal function. *Psychol Rev,* 108(2), 311–345.

Penny, W. D., Stephan, K. E., Mechelli, A., and Friston, K. J. (2004). Comparing dynamic causal models. *Neuroimage,* 22(3), 1157–1172.

Perlstein, W. M., Carter, C. S., Noll, D. C., and Cohen, J. D. (2001). Relation of prefrontal cortex dysfunction to working memory and symptoms in schizophrenia. *Am J Psychiatry,* 158(7), 1105–1113.

Price, C. and Friston, K. (1996). Cognitive conjunction: a new approach to brain activation experiments. *Neuroimage,* 5, 261–270.

Rao, R. and Sejnowski, T. J. (2000). Predictive sequence learning in recurrent neocortical circuits. In *Advances in Neural Information Processing Systems 12* (eds. S. Solla, T. Lee, and K.-R. Muller) pp. 164–170. Cambridge, MA, MIT Press.

Rubia, K. and Smith, A. (2004). The neural correlates of cognitive time management: a review. *Acta Neurobiol Exp (Wars),* 64(3), 329–340.

Sabri, O., Owega, A., Schreckenberger, M., *et al.* (2003). A truly simultaneous combination of functional transcranial Doppler sonography and H(2)(15)O PET adds fundamental new information on differences in cognitive activation between schizophrenics and healthy control subjects. *J Nucl Med,* 44(5), 671–681.

Schreiber, T. and Schmitz, A. (1996). Improved surrogate data for nonlinearity tests. *Phys Rev Lett,* 77(4), 635–638.

Schreiber, T. and Schmitz, A. (2000). Surrogate time series. *Physica D: Nonlinear Phenomena,* 142(3–4), 346–382.

Seeman, M. V. (1976). Time and schizophrenia. *Psychiatry,* 39(2), 189–195.

Uttal, W. (2001). *The New Phrenology: The Limits of Localizing Cognitive Processes in the Brain.* Cambridge, MA, MIT Press.

Volz, H. P., Nenadic, I., Gaser, C., Rammsayer, T., Hager, G., and Sauer, H. (2001). Time estimation in schizophrenia: an fMRI study at adjusted levels of difficulty. *Neuroreport,* 12(2), 313–316.

Walter, H., Wunderlich, A. P., Blankenhorn, M., *et al.* (2003). No hypofrontality, but absence of prefrontal lateralization comparing verbal and spatial working memory in schizophrenia. *Schizophr Res,* 61(2–3), 175–184.

White, T., Kendi, A. T., Lehericy, S., *et al.* (2007). Disruption of hippocampal connectivity in children and adolescents with schizophrenia–a voxel-based diffusion tensor imaging study. *Schizophr Res*, **90**(1–3), 302–307.

Wykes, T., Brammer, M., Mellers, J., *et al.* (2002). Effects on the brain of a psychological treatment: cognitive remediation therapy: functional magnetic resonance imaging in schizophrenia. *Br J Psychiatry*, **181**, 144–152.

Chapter 10

Philosophy and cognitive-affective neurogenetics

Dan J. Stein

Abstract

Cognitive-affective neuroscience has provided a set of constructs and methods for studying psychology and psychopathology. While genetics has long been touted as potentially important in understanding mental disorders, recent work has led to specific advances in our knowledge of the role of particular gene variants in psychological phenomena. In terms of understanding the proximal mechanisms underlying mental illness, an important implication of this work is that multiple genes with relatively small effects may play a role. An understanding of functional gene polymorphisms may also shed light on the distal mechanisms contributing to mental illness; particular variants may have survival value in particular environments. The chapter considers the implications of cognitive-affective neurogenetics for some key questions in the philosophy of psychiatry. It argues that although this work may inform conceptual issues in diagnosis and treatment, a range of other considerations will continue to remain paramount in decisions about nosology and intervention.

10.1 Introduction

Behaviourism and cognitivism were key paradigms in academic psychology in the twentieth century, but cognitive-affective neuroscience is arguably a predominant paradigm at the start of the new millennium. The predominance of cognitive-affective neuroscience reflects a range of conceptual and methodological developments. At a conceptual level, the introduction of computational models of the mind, and of a multidisciplinary approach to its study, helped replace behaviourism with cognitivism during the last decades of the past century. At a methodological level, spectacular advances in brain imaging and molecular neurobiology have made it increasingly important for the cognitive sciences to include neuroscience as a key discipline. Both new theories and new data have increased awareness of the limitations of simplistic cognitive models, and have given additional impetus to the development of a more complex cognitive-affective neuroscience approach.

One of the most significant scientific achievements at the turn of the twenty first century was the sequencing of a series of genomes, both of *Homo sapiens*, and of closely related primates. Although psychologists and psychiatrists have long been interested in the heritability of individual traits and in the genetics of mental disorder, the mapping of the human genome provided the potential for integrating molecular neurobiology into the cognitive-affective neurosciences. For example, many brain-imaging studies are now addressing the extent to which particular gene variants influence neuronal activation during particular tasks. In this chapter, I address some of the conceptual questions that this work raises. I begin by considering the impact of such work on proximal and distal explanations of psychiatric disorder. I then go on to consider the extent to which such work will impact on concepts of psychiatric diagnosis, and views of psychiatric intervention.

10.2 **Proximal explanations**

Behaviourism famously explained psychiatric disorder in terms of abnormal learning. Watson, for example, demonstrated that he was able to induce fear of rabbits (conditioned response) in little Albert by making a loud noise (unconditioned stimulus) whenever the infant was playing with a toy bunny. Reversal of this process could occur by continuing to present the bunny, but in the absence of a noise (desensitization). This general approach to psychopathology and psychotherapy had a number of positive aspects, including an emphasis on the importance of rigourous empirical observation, and on the translation of basic laboratory observations into novel clinical approaches (e.g. exposure therapy for anxiety disorders). Nevertheless, behaviourism has also failed to provide adequate explanations of major psychiatric disorders (e.g. schizophrenia and bipolar disorder), and with some exceptions (Baxter *et al.*, 1992), it has failed to integrate successfully its theories and methods with the range of new brain-behaviour fields (e.g. functional imaging and molecular neurobiology).

Cognitivism, on the other hand, has favoured explanations of psychiatric disorder in terms of notions of abnormal computation or cognition. An early computational model of paranoid processes was PARRY, a computer program which incorporated several rules that effectively allowed it to simulate a paranoid conversation (Colby, 1975). Later models relied on neural networks; these often incorporate a particular 'lesion' of the network, which allows it to simulate one or other pathological phenomenon (Stein and Ludik, 1998). Cognitive therapists have developed models of a range of psychiatric disorders and their treatment; for example, depression is hypothesized to result from distorted cognitions about the self and about the world and treatment involves restructuring these cognitions. Again, a strength of the cognitive approach to psychopathology and treatment has been its rigorous empirical nature. However, although cognitive approaches have gone beyond the 'black box' behavioural approach to the mind, many cognitive therapists have remained relatively uninterested in integrating their work with biological constructs and methods.

Advances in neuropsychology and in functional brain imaging have led to a range of new information about the neuronal circuitry involved in different psychiatric disorders, and gave impetus to a cognitive-affective neuroscience approach to these conditions (Stein, 2003; Stein and Young, 1992). Here the cognitivist emphasis on the software of the mind is replaced by a focus on its wetware; particular kinds of lesions in particular circuits are thought to underpin psychiatric disorders, and these can be reversed by either pharmacotherapy (which acts in a bottom-up way to normalize these circuits) or by psychotherapy (which acts in a top-down way to normalize these circuits) (Etkin et al., 2005; Kapur, 2003; Roffman et al., 2005). Cognitive-affective neuroscience retains the rigourous empirical emphasis of behaviourism and cognitivism. However, by specifically addressing the levels of both biology and psychology, it appears to encourage a more sophisticated and integrative approach to psychopathology and its treatment than these earlier approaches.

There has long been awareness of and interest in the genetic basis of psychopathology, with early work relying primarily on family and twin studies. With advances in genetics, cognitive-affective neuroscience has increasingly begun to incorporate data from this field. Awareness of a key functional variant in the serotonin transporter (5-HTTP) gene, for example, led to brain imaging studies of differences in amygdala activation in those with different 5-HTTP variants (Hariri et al., 2002). This kind of research potentially cuts across a range of concepts and methods; certain nonhuman primates have an analogous variant in this gene allowing translation between animal and human work (Barr et al., 2003); associations of the variant with inter-individual differences can be studied in the normal population and during normal development (Arbelle et al., 2003); and the impact of this gene variant (and its interactions with the environment) on both psychopathology and treatment (Lesch, 2001) can be investigated. Thus, the inclusion of genetics data in the cognitive-affective neuroscience approach further strengthens its potential ability to integrate the biological and the psychological.

What are the conceptual implications of this move from using the explanations of behaviourism and cognitivism through to using those of cognitive-affective neuroscience and neurogenetics? One key philosophical issue for the psychological sciences is the perennial question of the mind–body relationship. For behaviourism, intimately associated with arguments in logical positivism, talk of mental states is essentially meaningless. For cognitivism, intimately associated with functionalism, mental states can be defined in computational terms. Cognitive-affective neuroscience, like behaviourism and cognitivism, holds that psychology is a science, relying on empirical observation, and rigourous explanation. However, by focussing on the particular psychobiological structures and mechanisms that emerge from new areas of scientific investigation, such as brain imaging and neurogenetics, cognitive-affective neuroscience is free to move away from logical positivism and computational functionalism towards a realist and naturalist conceptual model of the brain–mind (Bhaskar, 1978, 1979). This chapter will not attempt any defence of these different conceptual approaches in their own terms. However, I would emphasize that given the complexity of the phenomena under study, an approach that gives insight into the emergence of mental phenomena from more basic structures and mechanisms would be particularly advantageous.

Indeed, it turns out that to date, work in cognitive-affective neurogenetics, rather than reducing the psychological to the biological, has emphasized the complexity of brain–mind relations in a number of ways. First, even the most robust associations between common gene variants and inter-individual differences are relatively small (Ebstein *et al.*, 2000). Second, gene variants may have different effects at different stages of development (Schwartz *et al.*, 2003). Third, interactions between gene variants and the environment occur, adding complexity to the attempt to relate genotype to phenotype (Caspi and Moffitt, 2006). Fourth, particular gene variants are not associated in a one-to-one manner with particular psychiatric disorders, but instead may play a role in a range of normal and abnormal states, with multiple gene variants each contributing a small amount to any particular condition (Kendler, 2006). While the inability of cognitive-affective neurogenetics to account for complex psychiatric phenomena in terms of particular single gene polymorphisms may disappoint some, its success in rigorously accounting for some of the observed variance in normality and abnormality can be considered a major achievement for psychology and psychiatry. And importantly, the complexity of its findings and explanations are consistent with the complexity that would seem to be demanded of a successful brain–mind science.

10.3 Distal explanations

Medicine and psychiatry have placed particular emphasis on the proximal explanations of disease – on the specific mechanisms that underlie pathology. At the same time, since Darwin, biology as a whole has been built on a broader framework which emphasizes distal accounts – the ways in which particular mechanisms have evolved over time to enhance survival. A range of early authors noted the potential of evolutionary medicine and psychiatry; for example, early behavioural ecologists noted that some of their observations might be useful in accounting for behaviour in the clinic (Tinbergen, 1951). More recently, however, there has been significant attention to the development of evolutionary medicine and psychiatry as important fields of academic endeavour (Baron-Cohen, 1997; Nesse and Williams, 1994). Authors in these fields have put forward a range of distal explanations of psychopathology, accounting for the evolutionary basis of human susceptibility to disorders, such as psychosis, depression, and anxiety, and providing an evolutionary perspective on how interventions such as psychopharmacology work (Stein, 2006).

New knowledge in population genetics, together with advances in cognitive-affective neurogenetics, provides potential for the development of more sophisticated distal explanations of psychiatric disorder and intervention. Consider, for example, work on the brain-imaging correlations of the catechol-O-methyltransferase (COMT) gene, which has a common variant at codon 158. It turns out that subjects with methionine (Met[158]) substitutions have increased prefrontal activation during executive function tasks, while those with Val[158] alleles have an advantage in processing aversive stimuli. However, under conditions of stress, Met[158] subjects may do worse, while those with Val[158] alleles have increased prefrontal activation. Furthermore, it seems that there is an association between Val[158] alleles and disorders such as schizophrenia, while there is an association between Met[158] alleles and anxiety. Having Val[158] alleles can be considered a 'warrior' strategy, while the possession of Met[158] alleles can be considered a 'worrier' strategy; each may have greater survival value under particular environmental conditions (Stein *et al.*, 2006).

A range of conceptual questions can be asked about this kind of work. Importantly, it would seem much more difficult to confirm any particular distal explanation of a brain–behaviour phenomenon than a proximal explanation. Indeed, a criticism of much evolutionary psychology has been its reliance on 'just so' stories (Gould, 1991). This problem is redolent of some of the philosophical criticism of psychoanalytic explanations (Grunbaum, 1985). Nevertheless, creative ways have been found for testing evolutionary hypotheses, and those approaches that integrate well with other avenues of scientific discovery are particularly appealing. Indeed, while evolutionary psychology has been criticized for ignoring the brain basis of evolved modules, some evolutionary work, including research on cognitive-affective neurogenetics, has specifically explored the biological basis of adaptive psychological processes (Panksepp, 1998; Panksepp and Panksepp, 2000).

Thus, for example, basic research on the impact of particular gene variants on behaviour and survival in animals provides a way both of testing evolutionary hypotheses, and of integrating proximal and distal explanations. Consider once again the variants in the 5-HTTP gene discussed earlier. Elegant work has demonstrated that just as humans with the short allele of the 5-HTTP gene are more prone to respond to conditions of adversity with aggression, so too, nonhuman primates with the analogous allele can behave in a more impulsive way (Higley *et al.*, 1996). Thus they appear to adopt a 'live hard – die young' strategy – a strategy that arguably is associated with greater survival value under adverse environmental circumstances (Gerard and Higley, 2002). Once again, the complexity of findings and explanations in this area are consistent with the complexity that would seem to be demanded of a successful evolutionary brain–mind science.

10.4 Implications for diagnosis and intervention

What are the implications of advances in the proximal and distal explanations of cognitive-affective neurogenetics for key conceptual questions in the philosophy of psychiatry? In this section, I briefly consider three questions: (1) what is the nature of mental disorder? (2) what should a psychiatric explanation look like? and (3) should we treat psychiatric disorders?

Ontological issues around physical disorder and mental disorder lie at the heart of the philosophy of medicine and of psychiatry. Elsewhere, I have contrasted a classical and a critical approach to this issue (Stein, 1991, 2008); a classical approach to this question attempts to provide necessary and sufficient criteria for disorder, while a critical approach argues that our constructs of disorder vary from place to place and time to time and are therefore relativistic. An integrative position can perhaps be put forward; this argues that the cognitive-affective neuroscience of categorization shows that human constructs can rarely be defined in necessary and sufficient terms (Lakoff, 1987; Lakoff and Johnson, 1999), so that some exemplars of disorder are more typical and others more atypical. This does not however entail an entirely relativistic approach, in that we can provide rational arguments for including/excluding particular constructs from our nosology (for example, after considered discussion, homosexuality was excluded from the DSM system).

One attempt to use evolutionary theory in this debate has argued that mental disorder reflects evolutionary dysfunction. An immediate objection is that not all dysfunctions are harmful; Wakefield has therefore argued that disorders are harmful dysfunctions (Wakefield, 1992). While typical disorders certainly seem to be harmful dysfunctions (for example, bipolar disorder appears to involve a dysfunction in mood regulation), there are a range of more atypical conditions where this definition breaks down (e.g. social phobia, alcoholism). Social phobia may be a relatively atypical disorder insofar as some degree of social anxiety is universal (and is therefore perhaps not clearly a dysfunction); but it seems reasonable to regard this condition as a disorder insofar as high levels of social anxiety are associated with significant distress and impairment, are characterized by specific cognitive-affective neuroscience characteristics, and are potentially responsive to treatment. Alcoholism is a relatively atypical disorder insofar as it begins with a voluntary decision to consume alcohol (a decision which may not represent an evolutionary dysfunction); but it seems to be a disorder insofar as once a pattern of drinking is established, dependence is a nonvoluntary phenomenon, with particular cognitive-affective neuroscience characteristics, and potentially responsive to treatment. Thus, although Wakefield argues that social anxiety and alcoholism do not entail dysfunctions and so cannot be disorders (Wakefield *et al.*, 2005), there seem to be reasonable counterarguments. So, while evolutionary arguments may provide one set of inputs into what we define as a disorder, it turns out that there are a range of other considerations which may be paramount.

Epistemological debates in psychiatry can again be considered using a framework that contrasts classical versus critical positions(Stein, 2008). A classical approach has emphasized that science involves the discovery of covering laws, and has suggested that behaviourism is a scientific psychology insofar as it too provides new laws relating stimuli and responses. In contrast, a critical approach has argued that psychiatry is best understood in non-scientific terms; for example, psychopathology can be approached much as one approaches a narrative text, attempting to understand the patient as an agent who is responding to their context in a meaningful way. An integrative position might argue that natural science involves the discovery of real structures and mechanisms, and that although human science necessarily involves an understanding of agents, it can nevertheless similarly succeed in putting forward powerful explanations (Bhaskar, 1978, 1979).

Cognitive-affective neuroscience arguably exemplifies this kind of integrative approach to psychology and psychiatry. As noted earlier in our discussion of mind–body relations, cognitive-affective neuroscience (arguably, in contrast to earlier behaviourist and cognitivist approaches) is appropriately focussed on discovering the real psychobiological structures and mechanisms (wetware) which produce psychological and psychopathological phenomena. At the same time, cognitive-affective neuroscience does not attempt simply to reduce humans to objects; it requires an approach that understands human subjectivity and experience, and which sees humans as meaning-making agents. As pointed out earlier, neurogenetic data have increasingly been incorporated into both proximal and distal explanations in cognitive-affective neuroscience. However, as also alluded to, these data do not allow a neat reduction of human phenomena to particular genes; given the complexity of such phenomena, it is not surprising that a full understanding of any particular gene variant requires an understanding of the expression of that gene in relation to other genes, to developmental trajectories, and to environmental contexts.

Moral debates in philosophy of psychiatric can perhaps again be considered using the classical versus critical contrast (Stein, 2008). A classical approach may emphasize the importance of finding particular moral laws or ethical principles which might govern one's decision in a particular case. In contrast, a critical approach argues that such an attempt is in vain; moral decisions reflect the concerns and values of a particular place and time. An integrative position can again be attempted, perhaps by emphasizing the similarities between moral judgements and other kinds of cognitive-affective processes, and so arguing that even if such judgements necessarily depend on metaphors from a particular place and time, they often involve universal principles, and can be reasonably debated.

Some of the current interest in genetics lies in the potential it provides to a way forwards for personalized medicine – ultimately providing each person with individualized advice about treatment based on the person's unique genetic information. The examples above have indicated that this is nevertheless going to be a complex task. In clear-cut cases (e.g. typical severe psychiatric disorder, with safe psychiatric medication), there will perhaps be close to ethical convergence – agreement that treatment should be initiated. However, in more atypical cases (e.g. atypical or less severe psychiatric disorder, with unclear information about whether psychiatric medication is effective or safe), and given expectations of what might be termed 'neurodiversity' (Glannon, 2006), there will be more room for argument and for valid disagreement. While a priori principles may well have some use, in many cases, and certainly for the immediate future, only a trial of psychiatric treatment will allow the pros and cons of such intervention to be evaluated fully.

10.5 Conclusion

In this chapter I have indicated that cognitive-affective neuroscience is increasingly incorporating neurogenetic constructs and methods into its proximal and distal explanations. I argued that such an approach has many strengths, including its rigorous empirical nature, the way in which multiple scientific disciplines are brought together, and strengthening the way in which biology and psychology are interrelated. At the same time, I emphasized the complexity of neurogenetic data, arguing that complex psychobiological phenomena (such as psychopathology) cannot simply be reduced to a particular gene variant, but rather that genes need to be understood against a complex background of other factors. I then considered the implications of cognitive-affective neurogenetics for some fundamental ontological, epistemiological, and ethical questions in the philosophy of psychiatry. I argued that although genetics data may be useful in shedding light on some questions about psychiatric diagnosis and intervention, valid answers about when to diagnose and when to treat will require inclusion of a whole range of other considerations.

References

Arbelle, S., Benjamin, J., Golin, M., Kremer, I., Belmakers, R. H., and Ebstein, R. P. (2003). Relation of shyness in grade school children to the genotype for the long form of the serotonin transporter promoter region polymorphism. *American Journal of Psychiatry*, **160**, 671–676.

Baron-Cohen, S. (1997). *The Maladapted Mind: Classic Readings in Evolutonary Psychopathology*. Hove, East Sussex, Psychology Press.

Barr, C. S., Newman, T. K., Becker, M. L., *et al.* (2003). The utility of the non-human primate; model for studying gene by environment interactions in behavioral research. *Genes, Brain, and Behavior*, **2**(6), 336–340.

Baxter, L. R., Schwartz, J. M., Bergman, K. S., *et al.* (1992). Caudate glucose metabolic rate changes with both drug and behavior therapy for OCD. *Archives of General Psychiatry*, **49**, 681–689.

Bhaskar, R. (1978). *A Realist Theory of Science*, 2nd edn. Sussex, Harvester Press.

Bhaskar, R. (1979). *The Possibility of Naturalism*. Sussex, Harvester Press.

Caspi, A. and Moffitt, T. E. (2006). Gene-environment interactions in psychiatry: joining forces with neuroscience. *Nature Reviews Neuroscience*, **7**, 583–590.

Colby, K. M. (1975). *Artificial Paranoia: A Computer Simulation of Paranoid Processes*. New York, Pergammon.

Ebstein, R. P., Benjamin, J., and Belmaker, R. H. (2000). Personality and polymorphisms of genes involved in aminergic neurotransmission. *European Journal of Pharmacology*, **410**(2–3), 205–214.

Etkin, A., Pittenger, C., Polan, H. J., and Kandel, E. R. (2005). Toward a neurobiology of psychotherapy: basic science and clinical applications. *Journal of Neuropsychiatry and Clinical Neurosciences*, **17**(2).

Gerard, M. S. and Higley, J. D. (2002). Evolutionary underpinnings of excessive alcohol consumption. *Addiction*, **97**, 415–425.

Glannon, W. (2006). *Bioethics and the Brain*. Oxford, Oxford University Press.

Gould, S. J. (1991). Exaptation: a crucial tool for evolutionary psychology. *Journal of Social Issues*, **47**, 43–65.

Grunbaum, A. (1985). *The Foundations of Psychoanalysis: A Philosophical Critique*. Berkeley, CA, University of California Press.

Hariri, A. R., Mattay, V. S., Tessitore, A., (2002). Serotonin transporter genetic variation and the response of the human amygdala. *Science*, **297**, 400–403.

Higley, J. D., Mehlman, P. T., Taub, D. M., *et al.* (1996). Excessive mortality in young free-ranging male non-human primates with low cerebrospinal fluid 5-hydroxyindolacetic acid concentrations. *Archives of General Psychiatry*, **55**, 537–543.

Kapur, S. (2003). Psychosis as a state of aberrant salience: a framework linking biology, phenomenology, and pharmacology in schizophrenia. *American Journal of Psychiatry*, **160**(1), 13–23.

Kendler, K. S. (2006). Reflections on the relationship between psychiatric genetics and psychiatric nosology. *American Journal of Psychiatry*, **163**(7), 1138–1146.

Lakoff, G. (1987). *Women, Fire, and Dangerous Things: What Categories Reveal about the Mind.* Chicago, IL, University of Chicago Press.

Lakoff, G. and Johnson, M. (1999). *Philosophy in the Flesh: The Embodied Mind and Its Challenge to Western Thought.* New York, Basic Books.

Lesch, K. P. (2001). Serotonergic gene expression and depression: implications for developing novel antidepressants. *J Affective Disord,* **62,** 57–76.

Nesse, R. M. and Williams, G. C. (1994). *Why We Get Sick: The New Science of Darwinian Medicine.* New York, Vintage Books.

Panksepp, J. (1998). *Affective Neuroscience: The Foundations of Human and Animal Emotions.* Oxford, Oxford University Press.

Panksepp, J. and Panksepp, J. B. (2000). The seven sins of evolutionary psychology. *Evolution and Cognition,* **6,** 108–131.

Roffman, J. L., Marci, D., Glick, D. M., Dougherty, D. D., and Rauch, S. L. (2005). Neuroimaging and the functional neuroanatomy of psychotherapy. *Psychological Medicine,* **35,** 1385–1398.

Schwartz, C. E., Wright, C., I, Shin, L. M., Kagan, J., and Rauch, S. L. (2003). Inhibited and uninhibited infants "grown up": adult amygdalar response to novelty. *Science,* **5627,** 1952–1953.

Stein, D. J. (1991). Philosophy and the DSM-III. *Comprehensive Psychiatry,* **32,** 404–415.

Stein, D. J. (2003). *Cognitive-affective Neuroscience of Mood and Anxiety Disorders.* London, Martin Dunitz.

Stein, D. J. (2006). Evolutionary theory, psychiatry, and psychopharmacology. *Progress In Neuro-Psychopharmacology & Biological Psychiatry,* **30,** 766–773.

Stein, D. J. (2008). *Smart Pills, Happy Pills, Pepp Pills: The Philosophy of Psychopharmacology.* Cambridge, Cambridge University Press.

Stein, D. J. and Ludik, J. (1998). *Neural Networks and Psychopathology.* Cambridge, Cambridge University Press.

Stein, D. J., Newman, T. K., Savitz, J., and Ramesar, R. (2006). Warriors vs worriers: the role of COMT gene variants. *CNS Spectrums,* **11,** 745–748.

Stein, D. J. and Young, J. E. (1992). *Cognitive Science and Clinical Disorders.* San Diego, CA, Academic Press.

Tinbergen, N. (1951). *The Study of Instinct.* London, Oxford University Press.

Wakefield, J. C. (1992). The concept of mental disorder: on the boundary between biological facts and social values. *American Psychologist,* **47,** 373–388.

Wakefield, J. C., Horwitz, A. V., and Schmitz, M. F. (2005). Are we overpathologizing the socially anxious? Social phobia from a harmful dysfunction perspective. *Canadian Journal of Psychiatry. Revue Canadienne De Psychiatrie,* **50**(6), 317–319.

Chapter 11

An addictive lesson: A case study in psychiatry as cognitive neuroscience

G. Lynn Stephens and George Graham

Abstract

The proposition that addiction is a species of compulsion is popular in addiction theory and psychiatric research. This chapter examines an influential account of the cognitive neuroscience of compulsive drug seeking to learn if cognitive neuroscience can warrant the attribution of pathology to addiction. We argue that without invoking norms of autonomous agency and self-control, prudential or evaluative norms which themselves are not proper parts of brain science, no attribution of pathology to compulsive or addictive behaviour is warranted.

11.1 Introduction

It is widely assumed that the description and explanation within psychiatry and psychiatric medicine of mental disorder is and will continue to be supported and facilitated by cognitive neuroscience. Just what this facilitation should mean, however, or what might happen as a result of that support merits analysis and caution (see Murphy, 2006). It merits analysis because the forms and limits of cognitive neuroscience resist precise definition (see Kosslyn and Anderson, 1992).[1] It merits caution because it is not clear just what cognitive neuroscience can tell us about a mental disorder.

---

[1] Cognitive neuroscience is not cognitive science in the broad generic sense, but cognitive science specifically with 'a downwards direction of inquiry . . . into the brain' (Bechtel *et al.*, 1998, pp. 95, 96). Cognitive neuroscience combines results from behavioural research in cognitive psychology, neuroimaging techniques, experimentation with nonhuman animals, cognitive deficits in neuropsychological patients, as well as various related sources in order to explain how the mind works. The field has achieved remarkable results in the study of vision and a variety of other cognitive processes (Bechtel, 2001).

Consider drug addiction. In an issue of *Science* devoted to the proposition that addiction is a brain disease or neural disorder, Alan Leshner writes that the essence of addiction is 'compulsive drug seeking and use, even in the face of negative health and social consequences' (Leshner 1997, p. 46). A publication of the Institute of Medicine claims that drug addiction consists of 'drug seeking behavior involving compulsion [and] resulting in substantial impairments of health and social functioning' (Institute of Medicine 1996, p. 19).

The proposition that drug addiction is a species of compulsion is popular in the theory of addiction and clinical research. Often, it is used to identify the syndromal distress or psychological disability that makes addiction a disorder. Addiction is a source of distress and disability because it is a species of compulsion, so the assumption goes. But just what can be done with this assumption in cognitive neuroscience? If addiction truly is a type of compulsion and if its compulsive nature qualifies it as a disorder, then if cognitive neuroscience can describe just what is compulsive about addiction, cognitive neuroscience will have identified the 'pathology' of addiction. It will have explained what makes addiction a disorder. That would be an impressive result. It would help to quiet critics of cognitive neuroscience who charge that cognitive neuroscience can describe brain function but it cannot warrant or ground the normative attributions of pathology or disorder.

Terry E. Robinson and Kent C. Berridge, two biopsychologists at the University of Michigan, in an evolving series of fascinating papers spanning a period of several years, endorse the proposition that drug addiction is compulsive (see, for two primary papers, Berridge and Robinson, 1995; Robinson and Berridge, 2003). They also deploy the resources of cognitive neuroscience, broadly understood, to try to describe what makes addictive behaviour compulsive. Their last major and summary treatment of addiction is a paper entitled simply 'Addiction', which appeared in the *Annual Review of Psychology* in 2003. (Hereafter, our discussion of Robinson and Berridge (hereafter 'R/B' for short) on addiction will focus on this paper as well as on their paper of 1995. Page numbers of citations will occur in accompanying parentheses.) In the 2003 paper they write:

> Addiction is more than mere drug use. It is . . . a compulsive pattern of drug-seeking and drug-taking. [. . .] The key questions in addiction, therefore, are why do some susceptible individuals undergo a transition from casual drug use to compulsive patterns of drug use, and why do addicts find it so difficult to stop using drugs.
>
> (Berridge and Robinson, 2003, p. 26)

In 1995 and 2003 (and elsewhere) R/B propose an account of the cognitive neuroscientific basis of compulsive drug seeking. In this chapter, we propose to use their account to explore several specific interlocking questions about the ability of cognitive neuroscience to contribute to the understanding of addiction in psychiatric science and medicine. These questions are: What sort of notion of compulsion is appropriate for distinguishing casual from addictive drug seeking? How is cognitive neuroscientific evidence relevant to establishing that a pattern of behaviour is compulsive? Does the evidence support the conclusion that compulsivity is the distinguishing feature of addictive behaviour? Finally, if neuroscientific or cognitive neuroscientific evidence fails to establish that an addictive pattern of behaviour is compulsive, but if compulsion is the clinically significant feature of addiction that constitutes its pathology, what sort of conclusion follows about whether the psychiatry of addiction can rely on cognitive neuroscience to identify addiction's clinically significant distress or pathology?

Here is an overview or anticipation of our argument. As R/B understand it, compulsive behaviour is the product of excessive (their term) or over-powerful motivation. In connection with R/B's discussion of aberrant learning (their label) theories (ALT) of addiction, we point out that, as classically conceived, compulsion is not a motivational phenomenon. Indeed, the notion that a behaviour is compulsive and the notion that it is motivated are not compatible with either the classical concept of compulsion or aberrant learning theory. Nevertheless, R/B claim that any understanding of compulsion likely to be useful to distinguish casual from addictive drug use must allow behaviour to be both compulsive and motivated. With that claim we agree and we explain why we agree.

We then turn to R/B's detailed proposal concerning the psychological and neuroscientific basis of addictive drug seeking. Here we argue that the evidence that R/B cite concerning the motivational dynamics of addictive drug seeking is not relevant to establishing that addictive drug seeking is compulsive. We also argue that their construal of compulsion as excessive or over-powerful motivation needs refinement or emendation before it can support a serious discussion of whether addictive drug seeking is compulsive and of whether this fact or alleged fact, viz., that it is compulsive, captures what makes addiction a disorder.

So, we then offer a refined notion of compulsion in line with R/B's general approach. It seems doubtful, however, whether addictive drug seeking is compulsive in this refined sense. We then consider a less stringent test for compulsivity. We conclude that this less stringent notion of compulsion also is unlikely to be of much use in helping to distinguish casual from addictive and pathological drug seeking. If we are right, the prospects for a neuropsychologically inspired description of addiction that is committed to a picture of addiction as a species of compulsion look dim. Dim, too, perhaps is the related prospect of identifying the pathology of addiction in strictly neuropsychological terms.

11.2 Addictive learning

Let us start with a theory of addiction that fails to explain the 'compulsive nature' of addiction, at least in R/B's view (2003, p. 32). According to so-called ALT, 'the transition to addiction involves a transition from behavior originally controlled by explicit and cognitively guided expectations about A–O [act–outcome] relationships (i.e. the memory of drug pleasure) to more automatic behavior consisting primarily of S–R habits'(2003, p. 33) Addictive drug seeking represents an automatic, conditioned response to drug cues. So-called drug cues are stimuli that the agent has learned to associate with the rewards of drug consumption. The transition from casual to addictive drug use is a transition from deliberate to habitual behaviour.

Let us flesh this out a bit. The casual drug user seeks a drug because he expects a pleasurable high and, in his current circumstances, prefers being high to not using (being clean and sober). He consciously knows or recognizes that he has such expectations and preferences, and that they motivate him to seek drugs. However, in the course of repeated casual drug use, he learns to associate certain stimuli, such as the sight of a crack pipe, or the sound of cellophane being torn from the pack of cigarettes, with drug-seeking behaviours and their rewards. This learning is mostly implicit: he learns to associate drug cues with drug rewards but without being able to be conscious of what he has learnt or being aware that he has learnt anything. Once learnt, these associations provide the basis for 'habits'. Drug cues will trigger drug-seeking behaviour 'automatically', i.e. independent of the agent's cognitive or motivational states. Drug seeking therein ceases to be a motivated, cognitively guided action and becomes a habitual response to drug-related stimuli. Some researchers hypothesize that the pharmacological effects of drugs on the brain systems that subserve reward learning facilitate the formation of such habits, causing 'pathologically strong implicit learning' (2003, p. 33). Hence the name, 'aberrant learning theory'.

According to R/B proponents of ALT, 'suggest that over-learned habits become so automatic that they essentially become compulsive' (2003, p. 33). R/B see in this suggestion a fundamental confusion concerning the nature of compulsion viz. that 'habit learning theories mistake automatic performance for motivational compulsion' (2003, p. 33). Automaticity is a matter of whether a performance can be 'executed without need of cognitive attention' (2003, p. 33), whereas compulsivity, they say, is a matter of 'overwhelming motivational urgency' (2003, p. 34). The former (automaticity) in no way entails or presupposes the latter (motivational urgency). 'No matter how strong implicit S–R associations, no matter how over-learned or pharmacologically boosted, there is no reason to believe that automatic S–R associations per se can confer compulsive qualities' (2003, p. 34).

R/B, in both defining addiction as compulsive drug seeking and assuming that 'compulsion' is a motivational notion, suppose that ALT explanations of addictive behaviour must 'mistake automatic performance for . . . compulsion.' Certainly ALT represents the transition from casual to addictive drug seeking as a transition from behaviour controlled by the agent's motivational states to behaviour directly triggered by drug cues. Though the agent's motivational dynamics help to explain how 'automatic' connections between drug-related stimuli and drug-seeking behaviour get established, once they are in place, drug cues elicit drug-seeking behaviour without any need for motivational support. In casual drug use, drug stimuli connect up with drug-seeking behaviour via the agent's motivational states. S–R habits represent a shortcut leading directly from stimulus to behaviour (see figure 3, 2003, p. 35). But, does this nonmotivational account of drug-seeking behaviour show that ALT cannot explain the compulsive nature of addiction?

The *locus classicus* for philosophical discussions of compulsion occurs in Aristotle's *Nichomachean Ethics*. (The quotes that follow are taken from *The Nicomachean Ethics of Aristotle*, translated by Sir David Ross, and published by Oxford University Press in 1925, reprinted in 1971. See Book III, Section 1, pp. 48–52.) Aristotle claims:

> Those things, then, are thought involuntary which take place under compulsion or owing to ignorance: and that is compulsory of which the moving principle is outside, being a principle in which nothing is contributed by the person who is acting . . . [for example] if he were carried somewhere by a wind or by men who had him in their power. (p. 48)

What sorts of acts, then, should be called compulsory? We answer that, without qualification actions are so when the cause is in the external circumstances and the agent contributes nothing (pp. 48–49).

For Aristotle, an agent's behaviour is compelled only when its causes are 'external' to him and those causes dominate the agent's internal state i.e. suffice to produce the behaviour regardless of the agent's internal state. A paradigm example envisions a sailor whose boat is caught by a powerful wind and driven onto the shore of an island. From the moment the wind catches the boat, the sailor contributes nothing to determining the boat's course. What he might want or believe becomes irrelevant to the explanation of what happens to him. The outcome is entirely determined by external forces.

Although Aristotle emphasizes the externality of the causes of compulsive behaviour, internal forces (internal to an agent's body) may also dominate the agent's desires and expectations. Suppose, for instance, that a cerebrovascular accident in my left hemisphere renders me mute. My failure to respond to a request to say my own name is entirely due to the brain damage I have suffered. I might know my name and want very much to pronounce it as requested, but it matters not what I desire. My stroke has made my motivation irrelevant. I am, we might say, compelled to remain mute. What matters for compulsion (in the extended spirit if not letter of Aristotle) is not that it puts my behaviour under the control of external forces or forces outside my body, but that it removes it from the control of my own motivational states.

ALT makes addictive drug-seeking behaviour compulsive in this extended classical sense of the term. There is a motivational story to tell about how I came to be addicted – about why I initiated and persisted in the casual drug use that prepared the way for my habitual drug use. But, once I complete the transition to addiction, my current motivational states no longer figure in the explanation of my drug-seeking behaviour. Through S–R conditioning, my drug seeking has come under the control of drug-related stimuli. These drug cues have acquired the power to elicit drug-seeking behaviour regardless of my motivation for engaging in or refraining from such behaviour.

So, ALT can make sense of the claim that addictive drug seeking is compulsive. So too, R/B are not justified in charging that the theory 'mistakes' automaticity for motivation. Indeed, the relevant notion of compulsion makes for a clean conceptual distinction between compulsive and noncompulsive drug seeking and makes it easy to explain why addiction should be considered a disorder or pathology. This is because it disables the agent's normal motivational control over his behaviour.

Whatever its conceptual virtues, though, R/B have good reason to doubt that any nonmotivational account of compulsion will be of much help in distinguishing addictive from nonaddictive behaviour. The problem is that addictive behaviour is not compulsive in the classical sense of that term. The addict's behaviour cannot be explained without reference to his motivational states. So, any notion of compulsion that can serve to distinguish casual from addictive drug use must acknowledge that addiction is a motivational phenomenon.

The justification of the above position emerges from another of R/B's objections to the ALT of addiction. They write:

Many aspects of addictive drug pursuit are flexible and not habitual. Human addicts face a situation different from rats that merely lever-press for drugs. [. . .] An addict who

> steals, another who scams, another who has money and simply must negotiate a drug
> purchase – all face new and unique challenges with each new victim or negotiation.
> Instrumental ingenuity and variation are central to addictive drug pursuit in real life.
> [. . .] The formation of S-R habits may explain the rituals addicts display in consuming
> drugs, but they do not account for the flexible and deliberate behaviors involved in obtain-
> ing drugs. We believe that the flexible and compulsive nature of drug-seeking behavior in
> the addict requires an additional motivational explanation, separate from habit learning.
>
> (R/B, 2003, p. 34)

In the lab, where experimental design restricts the behavioural options for obtaining
drugs, it may seem plausible to explain addictive drug seeking in terms of direct
connections between stimuli and stereotyped responses. What constitutes drug-seeking
behaviour among human addicts in the wild is seldom so straightforward. Addicts
engage in a wide variety of drug-seeking behaviours and the sort of behaviour they
exhibit on any specific occasion shows an exquisite sensitivity to context. To explain
such flexible, creative drug seeking we need more than the hypothesis that the addict
has some stereotyped behavioural routine waiting to be triggered by an appropriate
cue. What we need, according to R/B, is the idea that the addict is motivated to attain
some objective and has the cognitive capacities to devise strategies for achieving that
end appropriate to the challenges presented by changing circumstances. If drug pursuit
is compulsive, then it must be a compulsion that works through the addict's
motivational dynamics. Compulsion classically understood, in which the causal
explanation of compulsive behaviour bypasses the agent's motivational dynamics
rather than engaging them, is not the problem in addiction.

11.2.1 Compulsion and motivation: R/B's incentive sensitization theory

Despite the criticisms of ALT, R/B agree that the transition to addiction is a transition
to a condition in which the agent's drug-seeking behaviour comes under the control
of drug cues. In their view, however, drug cues control drug seeking, not through
conditioned association linking stimuli to specific behavioural routines, but by activating or enhancing the agent's motivation to consume drugs. Drug clues trigger a
'learned motivational response' (p. 44). That motivational response, given the agent's
assessment of available ways and means for obtaining drugs, elicits a specific form of
drug-seeking behaviour appropriate to the agent's circumstances. R/B's distinctive contribution to the study of addiction lies in their account of the motivational dynamics of
this process. Here is a relevant quotation:

> The problem is not in learning *per se* but in the motivational impact of drug-associated cues,
> that is, in their ability to engage brain motivational systems . . . What is aberrant in addic-
> tion is the response of brain motivational systems to Pavlovian-conditioned drug cues.
>
> (R/B, 2003, p. 35)

R/B call their account of addiction the 'incentive-sensitization theory' (hereafter
IST). They explain the basic idea as follows:

> The incentive-sensitization theory of addiction focuses on how drug cues can trigger
> excessive incentive motivation for drugs, leading to compulsive drug seeking . . .

The central idea is that addictive drugs enduringly alter NAcc-related brain systems that mediate a basic incentive-motivational function, the attribution of incentive salience. As a consequence, these neural circuits may become enduringly hypersensitive (or 'sensitized') to specific drugs effects and to drug-associated stimuli . . . The drug induced brain change is called neural sensitization. We propose that this leads psychologically to excessive attribution of incentive salience to drug-related representations, causing pathological 'wanting' to take drugs. [NAcc' refers to the nucleus accumbens.]

(R/B, 2003, p. 36)

To begin unpacking this account of addiction, we need to explain the quotation marks around the word 'wanting'. Standard explanations of why people take drugs emphasize the hedonic effects of drug consumption.

Most expert explanations of addiction parallel the explanations likely given by the lay public: Addicts take drugs for the pleasure they produce, and to avoid the unpleasant consequences of withdrawal.

(R/B, 1995, p. 71)

But, this hedonic explanation cannot be the full story about the character of the motivation for addictive drug seeking.

The truth is that addicts continue to seek drugs even when no pleasure can be obtained, and even when no withdrawal exists. For instance, addicts seek drugs when they know those available will be insufficient for pleasure. Further, addicts crave drugs again even before withdrawal begins. [. . .] And addicts continue to crave drugs long after withdrawal is finished.

(R/B, 1995, p. 71)

R/B do not insist that 'pleasure and withdrawal play no role in the use of drugs' (*ibid.*). They do insist, however, that 'after one has accounted for all instances of drug use by addicts motivated by pleasure or withdrawal, a vast amount of compulsive drug use remains to be explained' (*ibid.*).

One might also be motivated to take drugs by more or less explicit cost-benefit reasoning. One might believe, for example, that drug use enhances one's artistic creativity or one's attractiveness to the opposite sex. One might calculate that such benefits outweigh any harm one is likely to suffer as a consequence of using drugs. Of course, such motives rarely figure in explanations of *compulsive* drug use. (Researchers who think that 'rational choice' plays a central role in so-called addictive drug use generally do not regard such drug use as compulsive. (See West 2006, pp. 29–73)). In any case, addicts frequently admit that their drug taking is not rationally justified and make rationally or prudentially motivated attempts to quit, even while continuing to use drugs. So, presumably, cost–benefit calculations do not supply the motivation for the 'vast amount of compulsive drug use' unexplained by hedonic facts.

R/B conclude, then, that there must be some other form or 'system' of motivation at work in addiction. This must be a system that is distinct from both hedonic motivation (what R/B call 'liking') and from what we will call 'rational' motivation. This other sort of motivation is (what they call) 'wanting'). What is wanting? We, following R/B, will approach the answer to this question indirectly.

First off, wanting is a motivational system but it is not the same as liking and it is not rational choice or the product of cost–benefit deliberations. Second, it is not a system whose sole or primary function is to make people (or rats, in animal models) addicted to drugs. It is a natural system that evolved 'to endow stimuli beneficial for survival, such as nutrients, water, sexual partners, and safety, with psychological reward properties' (2003, p. 26). As R/B put it, wanting 'normally establishes the motivational value of ordinary incentives' (1995, p. 72). Third, the 'psychological reward properties' with which wanting endows its objects is (something R/B call) 'incentive salience'. Indeed, R/B explicitly introduce the term wanting 'as a shorthand to refer to activation of incentive-salience processes' (R/B 2003, p. 36).

Unfortunately, it is not easy to produce an informative common sense or folk psychological paraphrase of the very idea of incentive salience. Roughly, the incentive salience of a given stimulus just is a matter of how effective it is in motivating pursuit of some goal or objective.

Things are clearer at the neurological or neurobehavioural level and this is where the resources of cognitive neuroscience are germane for R/B. In the comparison of wanting with rational choice, different brain systems appear to mediate cognitive versus incentive salience forms of motivation. 'Prefrontal and other cortical areas primarily mediate cognitive forms of desire and act-outcome representations, whereas NAcc-related circuitry (especially dopamine-related systems) play a more important role in Pavlovian-guided attributions of incentive salience' (R/B 2003, p. 42). Then, in the comparison of wanting with liking: at the (relatively) gross neuroanatomical level there seems to be considerable overlap between the brain circuitry that subserves wanting and that which subserves liking. (See R/B 1995, pp. 72–73.) But the experimental manipulation of 'NAcc-related circuitry' or of the 'mesotelencephalic dopamine system' by, for example, microinjection of amphetamine, shows that motivation for a reward as measured by various behavioural tests, can be altered without any corresponding change in the hedonic value of reward (liking) as measured behaviourally. (See R/B 1995, pp. 72–73; 2003, p. 43.) For instance, intra-accubens amphetamine injection increased the amount of work a rat would do to obtain a sucrose reward, but did not alter the liking for the rewards, as measured 'based on affective facial reactions to the taste of sugar that are homologous to the affective facial expressions that sweet tastes elicit from human infants' (R/B 2003, p. 43). So, wanting and liking turn out to be functionally distinguishable at the neurological level and are, presumably, subserved by distinct neurophysiological mechanisms.

R/B write:

> The sensitized neural systems responsible for . . . incentive salience can be dissociated from the neural systems that mediate the hedonic effects of drugs, how much they are 'liked'. In other words, 'wanting' is not 'liking'. Hedonic 'liking' is a different psychological process that has its own neural substrates (e.g. NAcc opiod transmission).
>
> (R/B, 2003, p. 36)

Finally, associative learning plays an important role in the motivational dynamics of wanting. When an agent attributes incentive salience to a reward, he will also attribute incentive salience to stimuli that 'predict' or are associatively linked to the reward. That is, the relevant stimuli or cues themselves become wanted. Further, attribution of incentive salience to cues enhances motivation for the original reward.

They write:

> [I]n addicts, the associative pairing of particular acts and drug stimuli . . . cause excessive wanting to become focused specifically on drug cues.
>
> (R/B, 1995, p. 72)

And again:

> Our hypothesis is quite specific regarding the nature of the psychological process that is sensitized to addiction. We hypothesize that it is specifically sensitization of incentive salience attribution to representations of drug cues and drug taking that causes compulsive pursuit of drugs. [. . .] Incentive salience attribution is hypothesized to transform the neural representations of otherwise neutral stimuli into salient incentives, able to 'grab' attention, and makes them attractive and 'wanted'. Individuals are guided to incentive stimuli by the influence of Pavlovian stimulus-stimulus (S-S) associations on motivational systems, which is psychologically separable from the symbolic cognitive systems that mediate conscious desire, declarative expectancies of reward, and act-outcome representations.
>
> (R/B, 2003, p. 42)

Or again:

> [T]he only plausible explanation for why a Pavlovian-conditioned cue would suddenly intensify pursuit of a reward is that incentive salience is attributed to the Pavlovian cue and its associated reward causing cue-triggered 'wanting'.
>
> (R/B, 2003, p. 43)

How does the hypothesis that addicts want (in R/B's special sense) drugs help to explain the fact that addiction is compulsive in nature? Certainly it is not because it shows that addicts are motivated to use drugs. Casual drug users are also motivated to use drugs. Nor is it because wanting is intrinsically compulsive, i.e. because all behaviour motivated by wanting is compulsive. For surely it is not. Rather, in addiction wanting becomes 'pathological' or compulsive due to drug-induced changes in the neural circuitry that subserves wanting. These changes are what R/B refer to as 'sensitization'. In their view, 'drug-induced sensitization of brain systems that mediate [attribution of incentive salience] causes drugs to become compulsively and enduringly 'wanted' independent of drug pleasure, withdrawal, habits or memories' (2003, p. 27).

So, what is sensitization? Here's what R/B say:

> Pharmacologists use the term ['sensitization'] to refer to an increase in a drug effect with repeated drug administration. In other words, the change in drug effect is in the opposite direction as seen with the development of tolerance (a decrease in a drug effect with repeated administration.
>
> (R/B, 2003, p. 37)

We refer the reader to R/B 2003, pp. 38–41, for details of the brain changes involved in sensitization to addictive drugs. What is relevant in the present context is the psychological effect of sensitization. Sensitization specifically increases the incentive salience attributed to drug cues so that drug cues 'elicit exaggerated wanting' for drugs. Thus, sensitization boosts the motivational impact of drug cues such that exposure to drug cues causes 'exaggerated' or 'excessive' wanting for drugs. Such excessive motivation compels the agent to engage in drug-seeking behaviour. As R/B write:

> Sensitization enhances the ability of drug-associated cues to trigger irrational bursts of 'wanting' for their reward, and in human addicts, who may have many years of drug experience with all the attendant opportunities for sensitization and learning, this may lead to the compulsive pursuit of drugs.[2]
>
> (R/B, 2003, p. 44)

The fact that sensitization persists once it has been established also helps to explain the phenomenon of relapse. Relapse is an important feature of addictive behaviour. It is a process 'by which a single lapse back into an old pattern of behavior leads to full resumption of that behavior' (West 2006, p. 82).[3]

> Sensitized rats attributed excessive cue-elicited incentive salience to their reward at a time when they had received no drug at all for many days . . . This situation seems to model that of the drug-abstinent and 'recovered' addict who suddenly relapses again after encounter with drug cues . . . Relapse in human addicts must also be caused by persisting sensitization in brain systems that mediate incentive salience. Upon encounter with drug cues, the addict might suddenly 'want' to take drugs again – to an excessive and compulsive degree – regardless of cognitive expectancies about 'liking', declarative goals, absence of withdrawal, etc.
>
> (R/B, 2003, p. 44)

Summarizing their view, R/B say:

> Addiction is a disorder of aberrant incentive motivation due to drug-induced sensitization of neural systems that attribute incentive salience to particular stimuli. It can be triggered for drug cues as a learned motivational response of the brain, but it is not a disorder of aberrant learning per se. Once it exists, sensitized 'wanting' may compel drug pursuit whether or not the addict has any withdrawal symptoms at all. And because incentive salience is distinct from pleasure or 'liking' processes, sensitization gives impulsive drug 'wanting' on enduring life of its own.
>
> (R/B, 2003, p. 44)

11.3 **IST, compulsion, and addiction**

Does IST explain the compulsive character of addictive behaviour?

There are two sorts of issues here in this one question. One concerns excessive wanting. The other concerns compulsion. So: apropos the first, does exposure to drug cues

---

[2] Mention of an *irrational* outburst is one of the few occasions in which R/B use a normative or evaluative term that is not somehow explained or cashed out in neurobehavioural or descriptive terms. We pass over discussion of their use since they leave the term in this quote without clarification.

[3] We do not explore here or in the body of the chapter whether there is more to relapse in the human case (as opposed to, say, that of rats in an experimental chamber) than the full resumption of old behaviour. But see footnote 4.

produce, in sensitized agents, excessive or exaggerated (i.e. for R/B, compulsive) motivation to pursue drugs. In discussing this first issue or question, we shall accept R/B's understanding of compulsion as excessive motivation. Then, apropos the second, granting that drug cues do in fact trigger excessive motivation (exaggerated wanting) in sensitized agents, should we regard the behaviour elicited by such wanting as compulsive? In discussing this second question, we shall consider whether compulsion is best understood as excessive or exaggerated wanting.

(1) *The first issue.* Do drug cues trigger excessive motivation in sensitized agents? Well, excessive relative to what? R/B cite a variety of experimental studies regarding the motivational consequences of sensitization. Using behavioural measures of motivation, these studies found that sensitizing rats 'increases their motivation to obtain' a drug reward (2003, p. 41). In fact, the studies found that sensitization (when induced by drugs) 'can also increase the incentive value of other rewards, such as sugar, food, a sexually receptive female (for male rats) and conditioned stimuli for such rewards' (2003, p. 41). For example, sensitized rats will learn more quickly to self-administer drugs, run faster in pursuit of a drug reward, and generally 'work harder than normal to gain drug rewards' (2003, p. 41). Or more exactly: they will learn faster and work harder *than unsensitized rats* will work for the same reward under the same conditions. Thus, the motivation to pursue drugs or other rewards, in sensitized rats, is excessive or exaggerated only in the sense that it is in excess of the motivation engendered in unsensitized rats in comparable circumstances. Nothing in these studies indicates that sensitized rats were irresistibly or overwhelmingly motivated or experienced motivation of any absolute degree.

R/B acknowledge that the sorts of studies alluded to above do not provide conclusive evidence for IST because they fail to rule out the possibility that factors other than wanting account for the relative increase in motivation. We need to test 'whether sensitization can specifically enhance incentive salience or "wanting" triggered by reward cues' (2003, p. 42). To this end they cite experimental work designed to carefully exclude alternative explanations of the behavioural consequences of sensitization, such as 'liking or hedonic impact of the pleasant reward, cognitive predictive expectancies about it . . . automatic stimulus-response habits' and so on (2003, p. 42). They describe an experimental design such that: 'Under these restricted conditions, the only plausible explanation for why a Pavlovian-conditioned cue would suddenly intensify pursuit of a reward is that incentive salience is attributed to the Pavlovian cue and its associated reward, causing cue-triggered wanting' (2003, p. 43). Under such excluding conditions, sensitization increased the rate of instrumental responding elicited by a reward cue. For instance: 'intra-accumbens amphetamine [injection] increased the ability of a sucrose cue to spur performance for a sucrose reward' (2003, p. 43). R/B then conclude that intra-accumbens amphetamine increased instrumental responding because it increased wanting (and as measured by observing rat facial expressions, it did nothing to increase liking). This work, claim R/B, establishes that wanting can elicit behaviour without help from any other form of motivation: wanting is independent of other motivational systems. And it establishes that sensitization can enhance cue triggered wanting vis-a-vis the effects of cue on wanting in unsensitized rats.

Finally, in an experiment which R/B regard as 'most important to our incentive-sensitization hypothesis of addiction', rats were first sensitized by several amphetamine injections (R/B 2003, p. 43). Injections were discontinued for a period of several weeks. Rats were then tested under the same conditions as the studies described earlier. Even after 2 weeks of being drug-free, in rats who have been sensitized, i.e. receive amphetamine, 'the Pavlovian-conditioned sugar cue produced a greater wanting for sugar than in non-sensitized rats' (2003, p. 44). So R/B conclude that, for the lessons of this research for understanding relapse:

> Sensitized rats attributed excessive cue-elicited incentive salience to their reward at a time when they had received no drug at all for many days. [. . .] This situation seems to model that of the drug-abstinent and 'recovered' addict who suddenly relapses again after encountering drug cues. [. . .] Relapse in human addicts might also be caused by persisting sensitization in brain systems that moderate incentive salience. Upon encountering drug cues, the addict might suddenly 'want' to take drugs again – to an excessive and compulsive degree – regardless of cognitive expectancies about 'liking', declarative goals, absence of withdrawal, and so on. [4]
>
> (R/B, 2003, p. 44)

Once again, however, these results show that drug cues trigger motivation (this time, wanting specifically) in sensitized agents which is excessive only in the sense that it is greater than the amount of wanting that the same cues trigger in unsensitized agents. This does not entail that the sensitized drug user 'wants' to take drugs to a 'compulsive degree' while the unsensitized drug user does not.

The norm or standard for what constitutes excessive wanting, or by which we should assess the motivational power of sensitized cue triggered wanting, that is relevant to the question of compulsion would be more like this: (1) is the motivation generated by drug cues in sensitized agents stronger than the motivation that supports distinctively casual drug use? For instance, is such motivation stronger than the motivation produced in casual drug users by the expectation of and desire for drug-pleasure? (2) Does cue-triggered wanting produce motivation for pursuing drugs stronger than the motivation that an addict typically has for refraining from drug pursuit. To paraphrase R/B's question (see below) concerning ALT: Would you sacrifice your home, your job, your friends, and all that is dear to you to give into your cue-triggered 'want' for drugs?

The tests that would establish the compulsive character of sensitized wanting are not comparisons of the motivation strength of sensitized as over and against unsensitized

---

[4] This may be a useful place in which to briefly clarify the suggestion made in the previous note (footnote 3) that relapse in the human case and in the case of a nonhuman animal are not entirely the same sort of phenomenon. Many human drug addicts show every sign of desiring to stop for good and yet still resume the activity. Clinics for alcohol addicts, heroin addicts, and so on, are 'largely populated by people who are in the process of making a serious attempt to stop their behavior' (West 2006, p. 128). Rats, of course, lack the capacities for negative self-appraisal and cost-benefit analysis that often motivate the human addict to try to refrain. Relapse after a deliberate effort to abstain helps to explain why relapse in a human case can appear to be normatively irrational or imprudent even in the eyes of an addict himself. Not so that of a nonhuman animal. (See also Graham, forthcoming).

wanting. They would be tests that compare wanting against other forms of motivation. Would a rat work harder when motivated by sensitized wanting than when motivated by pleasure? Suppose I am motivated by cue-triggered sensitized wanting to smoke a cigarette in the lavatory on a trans-oceanic flight. Would fear of being fined, of being publicly chastised by a flight attendant, or arrested on arrival suffice to keep me from lighting up?

R/B do not present any evidence relevant to answering such questions. One cannot conclude that since the addict is a compulsive drug user and IST explains addiction, then drug use motivated by sensitized attributions of incentive salience must be compulsive. For, unless R/B have *independent* reason to suppose that drug use motivated by sensitized wanting is compulsive, they cannot assume that IST really does explain addiction. R/B do raise the possibility, however, that sensitization might boost the motivational force of cue-triggered wanting to a level where it would count as compulsive (see their reference earlier to an irrational outburst). The very idea of a motivational boost, suitably explicated, might be an idea worth pursuing if IST is to account for the compulsive character of addictive drug use. (We shall explore that prospect a bit later in the chapter in discussing motivational dominance.) But without successfully pursuing that particular idea, they have not made the case that IST does account for addiction as compulsive.

(2) *The second issue.* Now we turn to the second issue, which, it will be recalled, is: Is compulsion really a matter of motivational strength or intensity? Of its being excessive? Would that mean that there must be some absolute scale of motivational intensity such that motivation above a certain point in the scale is compulsive and motivation below that point is noncompulsive? On the other hand, if motivational strength is always relative, a matter of one sort of motivation being stronger than another, what does this have to do with compulsion? If one form of motivation was stronger than all other forms, would that make it compulsive? Why should my doing what I am most strongly motivated to do constitute a compulsive motivation? A pathology? A clinically significant disturbance or disability? These are precisely the sorts of problems avoided by the classical account of compulsion. If you say that I am compelled only when I am moved by forces which are external to my agency (my motivational dynamics) and which dominate my motivations (i.e. move me regardless of my motivation), then you don't have to decide when one motive prevailing over another constitutes compulsion.

One might be tempted here to embrace the idea that what makes a form of motivation compulsive is that it moves us to do things that are bad for us. So sensitized wanting would be compulsive because it causes us to do self-destructive things like spending the rent money to buy methamphetamine. But in that case, it would be clear that what makes wanting compulsive or pathological is not its neurobiology or psychodynamics but simply its negative goal. The same neuropsychological process directed towards a worthy or good goal would not be compulsive. The distinction between compulsive and noncompulsive motivation would simply be a normative or evaluative distinction of a special sort. And there would be no reason to look to neuroscience or neuropsychology for an explanation of the compulsive character or, for that matter, pragmatic disability of addiction. But, of course, that is not how compulsion, as such, is or should be understood. Riding a motorcycle without protective headgear and other dangerous activities may be bad for us, but this fact, assuming it is fact, does not make engaging in such behaviour compulsive (or pathological).

11.4 **A model of motivational compulsion: the motivational dominance model**

In a discussion of the 'disease model' of addiction, Robert West offers a suggestive characterization of the compulsive quality of addictive behaviour. Addiction is a 'motivational state . . . that overwhelms the individual in totality, dominating the thoughts, feelings, and actions of the individual to the exclusion of all else.' 'It sweeps all other considerations before it in a myopic and single-minded search for the object of the desire.' For an addict, so understood, writes West, 'there is no real choice, there is compulsion' (West 2006, p. 77).

West's characterization suggests that the essential feature of compulsive motivation, as exhibited in addiction, is dominance over all competing forms of motivation: compelling motives render all other motives irrelevant to the explanation of behaviour. This notion of motivational dominance might be a proper explication of the very idea of a motivational boost that we suggested might help IST in its characterization of addiction as compulsive. Incentive salience may boost motives to dominance and such dominance may qualify a motive as compulsive. Let us see how this might work by briefly emending IST to include it. The picture of dominance might look like this.

In an agent who is sensitized, exposure to drug cues determines that the agent will engage in drug-seeking behaviour. Assuming that the agent is able to act on this motive or is not prevented from acting on it by nonmotivational prohibiting causes (e.g. is not tied down), then there is no contrary motive that can prevent the cue from eliciting drug-seeking behaviour. The agent will engage in drug-seeking behaviour, regardless of his likes, rational preferences, or other nonwanting motivational states. In addiction, so the dominance story goes, the incentive salience (wanting) system dominates all other systems of motivation. Nonwanting motivation will, at most, play a part in determining the exact form that drug-seeking behaviour takes on a particular occasion. But whether the addict will engage in some form of drug-seeking behaviour following exposure to a drug cue depends entirely upon what the addict wants. Once a drug cue triggers wanting for drugs, the addict's other motivational states are irrelevant – drug-seeking behaviour will occur, regardless.

The dominance picture is not meant to suggest that addicts will engage in drug-seeking behaviour only in response to cue-triggered wanting. Perhaps even addicts sometimes use drugs just because they like drugs or think that drugs are good for them. Rather, it supposes that once sensitized wanting for drugs has been elicited by a drug cue, no other motivational factors are relevant for determining whether the addict engages in drug-seeking behaviour.

We offer this dominance-IST model as a candidate account of what it means to say that sensitized wanting provides compulsive motivation for engaging in drug-seeking behaviour. But what is to be said for it? R/B have not shown or intended to show that sensitized wanting is compulsive in the dominance-sense. Whether or not R/B have offered empirical evidence sufficient to confirm the hypothesis that sensitized wanting is compulsive in the sense of contributing to motivational dominance (hereafter 'MD'), this hypothesis is subject to experimental testing. The most relevant tests, if feasible, would pit sensitized wanting for drugs against other sorts of factors motivating the agent to refrain from drug-seeking behaviour, for example, aversion to electrical shock. But supposing that addictive drug use is compulsive, on the MD model, why should addiction be considered a pathology or disorder? What normal function or capacity is disrupted or disabled in addiction?

Two possibilities suggest themselves: (1) wanting dominates the other motivational systems. Perhaps, wanting is particularly liable to support harmful or self-injurious behaviour. Other motivational systems must be able to overrule wanting. Such systems are 'disabled' by wanting. Or (2) normal (healthy) motivational dynamics involve 'checks and balances'. Domination of any motivational system over others is a problem or practical disability. The possibility of any motivational system being overruled by another system needs to be preserved. For example: if an essential nutrient is available only in an unpalatable form, then wanting should overrule liking. Or if drug pleasure decreases as tolerance develops, then liking should overrule wanting (so that the agent will no longer take the drug). Or, if a subject must behave a certain way (e.g. refrain from taking drugs in order to secure a high-paying job), then rational preference or reasoned cost-benefit analysis should overrule wanting. Or, if an agent is unaware that an 'expensive' nutrient is essential, wanting should overrule rational preference.

But note that such possibilities aside the MD model imposes quite stringent conditions on compulsivity. For, even if an agent expects that pursuing a drug will exact high personal costs, given sensitization of wanting circuitry, such expectations cannot prevent wanting from eliciting drug-seeking behaviour. True, addicts sometimes do maintain drug-seeking behaviour despite very high costs. R/B themselves speak of sacrificing 'your home, your job, your friends, and all that is dear in life' (2004, p. 34). And they speak of drugs inducing neuronal changes in the frontocortical areas subserving rational choice. These changes may cancel the inhibitory effect of rational considerations on incentive-salience-driven behaviour in addicts.

Despite the cancellation of inhibitions that does occur in addiction, there is considerable evidence that addicts sometimes do exercise motivational or inhibitory control over their drug seeking, in least on occasion or in the short term. For example, in one experimental setting, alcoholics were given access to a fifth of liquor, but told that they would lose certain hospital privileges if they drank more than five ounces. Most managed to stay within the limit (Cohen et al., 1971, pp. 434–444; see also Cohen et al., 1971; Schuckit, 1984).

Of course, long-term control is more of a problem, as witness the emphasis on relapse in R/B's discussion. However, in order to 'relapse' into drug use, a person has to first quit or abstain for a while. R/B invoke *persisting* sensitization in order to explain relapse, so they themselves presume that even sensitized agents may refrain from drug-seeking behaviour on occasion. But if so, then how is this so? It is implausible to suppose that all pre-relapse abstinence is explained by nonmotivational factors (such as the unavailability of drug cues or physical restraint) or by lack of exposure to drug cues. It would seem then that sensitized agents are not mired in motivational dominance. One can be sensitized and yet motivationally abstain.

Actually, R/B leave themselves a number of options to explain why drug cues might fail to elicit drug-seeking behaviour even in a sensitized agent. One hypothesis is that after sensitization is established, whether the sensitized behaviour is 'expressed . . . at any given place or time' depends on a variety of contextual factors (2003, p. 40). So, for example, rats sensitized by drug treatment in one environment may fail to exhibit drug-seeking behaviour when placed in another environment.

Given environmental shifts, this might make it seem appealing to develop a case-by-case model of compulsion. Instead of seeing the addict as being in a persisting state in which wanting dominates other forms of motivation, we would suppose that the addict is susceptible to occasional episodes in which wanting dominates other motivational systems. Perhaps, other motivational systems often are able to prevent the expression of cue-triggered wanting in drug-seeking behaviour, but on some occasions, sensitized wanting makes drug-seeking behaviour motivationally irresistible.

However, any such case-by-case or circumstance-by-circumstance account of the compulsive nature of addiction threatens to remove the distinction between casual and addictive drug-seeking behaviour. The fact that wanting may sometimes prevail over competing forms of motivation does not show that wanting provides compulsive motivation. It is likely true of any form of motivation that sometimes (under certain circumstances etc.) it prevails over competing motives.

Of course, in order to retain the MD theory of compulsion, one might argue that the mark of motivational compulsion is not that some form of motivation did prevail in a particular instance, but that, in that instance, it would have prevailed regardless of any incentive to refrain provided by other forms of motivation. That is, on this occasion, once I was exposed to that drug cue, I could not have refrained from lighting up even if you had offered me a million dollars or threatened to shoot my dog. But how could we ever know that something like that is true?

In our view, one has to establish something pretty stringent about addictive drug use in order to justify calling it compulsive (see section 11.5, Conclusions). Establishing merely that it is 'strongly' motivated and sometimes occurs despite the agent's cost–benefit judgement or in the absence of hedonic pay offs is just not enough to show that addictive drug-seeking behaviour is compulsive. All that is just as true of nonaddictive behaviour.

11.5 **Conclusions**

As we see things, IST does not explain what makes addiction compulsive (assuming it is compulsive) for it fails to distinguish between casual and addictive drug use. Likewise, IST does not show that addictive behaviour is a clinically significant disability or disorder insofar as it is compulsive. No doubt the drugs to which people are addicted can have long-term effects on the brain and these effects can be harmful. But many habitual behaviours are harmful (risk loss of family etc.) though we do not pathologize them.

Perhaps the main or overarching problem with IST is that it tries to offer an account of both compulsion and addiction in terms of effects on behaviour of the neurological substrates of drug consumption, whereas the difference between casual and compulsive or addictive drug consumption cannot be described, we would argue, without also invoking the sorts of norms that persons use in assessing the rationality, prudence, or desirability of behaviour. A normatively neutral or purely descriptive cognitively neuroscientific account of either addiction or compulsion just does not have the conceptual tools or resources necessary to explain what makes addiction 'addiction' or compulsion 'compulsion'.

To briefly explain, one of the powers or abilities that we all value or want for ourselves as intelligent human beings is the power or ability to understand our impulses or motives and reflectively evaluate them, and to act in terms of motives that we judge to be best or in conformity with our values or ideals. Agents who lack such a power or ability (such as the severely retarded or severe cases of Alzheimer's disease) are frequently described as disabled in autonomy or incapacitated in reflective self-control. It is significant that addicts (especially after relapse) often complain or feel ashamed or lowered in self-esteem over their inability to control themselves i.e. to act in conformity with their values or ideals (see e.g. Knapp, 1998). Philosophers like Harry Frankfurt, Gary Watson, and others argue that no behaviour is compulsive or addictive (subject to some conceptual provisos that we do not mention here) unless it contravenes an agent's reflective self-evaluation and desire for self-control (see Kane, 2005 for references and discussion). If this sort of argument is sound, that is a pretty stringent norm if a behavioural pattern is to qualify as compulsive or addictive. It means that a motive or want does not qualify as compulsive or addictive in character or purport unless it contravenes or violates a contrary motive or want which the agent holds self-reflectively dear.[5] Destructive effects on a person's life may be relevant to other sorts of disorders (like delusions, for example) independent of an agent's evaluation of consequences, but what seizes attention in the behaviour of people who are addicted or compelled is the personally negative appraisal of their own behaviour. One may somehow try to revise the cognitive neuroscience of addiction to somehow reflect the normative role or presence of such negative self-appraisals, but as things stand, the lesson of IST is that if psychiatry is to be conducted as a cognitive neuroscience, then normatively neutral descriptions of brain activity cannot warrant the attribution of pathology in cases of addiction. Some sorts of prudential, self-appraisal or rationality norms (at least in the mind of the addict) must be violated by the behaviour.[6] Whether this

[5] The notion that a pattern of behaviour counts as compulsive only if it contravenes a contrary want or motive that the agent holds self-reflectively dear is loosely continuous conceptually with the Aristotelian picture of compulsion. Compulsive behaviour, so understood, is moved not literally by a physical externality like the wind, but by the 'wind' of motives external to an agent's self endorsement or positive appraisal.

[6] In closing the chapter, we bypass (with no room to discuss in this context) the entire issue of how the addict's self-reflective evaluation or valuational activities may itself presuppose rationality or prudential norms.

lesson about addiction or similar lessons may hold true of other sorts of disorders cannot be discussed here. But if some such lessons do hold, then, as noted at the beginning of the chapter, just what support cognitive neuroscience may be able to give psychiatric medicine merits both caution and analysis. Psychiatry has a lot to learn from cognitive neuroscience but the clinically significant pathology of a disorder may not be among its addictive lessons.

Acknowledgements

We would like to thank our two co-editors, Matthew Broome and Lisa Bortolotti, for the invitation to contribute to this volume and for helpful editorial comments on the penultimate draft. Neil Levy also offered useful comments.

References

Bechtel, W. (2001). Decomposing and localizing vision: an exemplar for cognitive neuroscience. In *Philosophy and the Neurosciences: A Reader* (eds. W. Bechtel, P. Mandik, J. Mundale, and R. Stufflebeam), pp. 225–249. Malden, MA, Blackwell.

Bechtel, W., Abrahamsen, A., and Graham, G. (1998). The life of cognitive science. In *A Companion to Cognitive Science* (eds. W. Bechtel and G. Graham), pp. 1–104. Malden, MA, Blackwell.

Berridge, K. and Robinson, T. (1995). The mind of the addicted brain: Neural sensitization of wanting versus liking. *Current Directions in Psychological Science,* **4,** 71–76.

Cohen, M., Liebson, I., Fallace, L., and Allen, R. (1971). Moderate drinking by chronic alcoholics: a schedule-dependent phenomenon. *Journal of Nervous and Mental Disease,* **153,** 434–444.

Cohen, M., Leibson, I., Fallace, L., and Speer, W. (1971). Alcoholism: controlled drinking and incentives for abstinence. *Psychological Reports,* **28,** 575–580.

Graham, G. (forthcoming). *The Disordered Mind.* Routledge.

Institute of Medicine (1996). *Pathways to Addiction: Opportunities in Drug Abuse Research.* Washington DC, National Academy Press.

Kane, R. (2005). *A Contemporary Introduction to Free Will.* New York, Oxford University Press.

Knapp, C. (1998). My descent into alcoholism. In *Abnormal Psychology in Context* (eds. D. Sattler, V. Shabatay, and K. Kramer), pp. 167–170. Boston, MA, Houghton Mifflin.

Kosslyn, S. and Anderson, R. (eds.) (1992). *Frontiers in Cognitive Neuroscience.* Cambridge MA, MIT Press.

Leshner, A. (1992). Addiction is a brain disease. *Science,* **278,** 45–47.

Murphy, D. (2006). *Psychiatry in the Scientific Image.* Cambridge, MA, MIT Press.

Robinson, T. and Berridge, K. (2003). Addiction. *Annual Review of Psychology,* **54,** 25–53.

Schuckit, M. (1984). *Drug and Alcohol Abuse.* New York, Plenum.

West, R. (2006). *A Theory of Addiction.* Oxford, Blackwell.

Phenomenology and scientific explanation

Chapter 12

Understanding existential changes in psychiatric illness: The indispensability of phenomenology

Matthew Ratcliffe

Abstract

This chapter argues that phenomenological reflection is indispensable when it comes to interpreting at least some psychiatric conditions. I distinguish 'phenomenological' from 'psychological' and 'personal' understanding. For the phenomenologist, a background sense of reality that is presupposed by both psychological and personal understanding is itself an object of enquiry. As many of the experiential changes reported in psychiatric illness involve alterations in the sense of reality, a 'phenomenological stance' is required in order to understand them. To illustrate this point, I discuss some of the *existential changes* (by which I mean alterations in the sense of reality and belonging) that can occur in depression. The remainder of the chapter addresses the relationship between phenomenology and neuroscience, and shows how interaction between these disciplines can be mutually illuminating.

12.1 **Introduction**

This chapter makes a case for the view that phenomenological reflection is indispensable when it comes to interpreting at least some psychiatric conditions. It then goes on to show how phenomenological and neurobiological perspectives can be mutually informative. I begin by distinguishing 'phenomenological' from 'psychological' and 'personal' understanding. For the phenomenologist, a background sense of reality that is presupposed by both psychological and personal understanding is itself an object of enquiry. Given that many of the experiential changes reported in psychiatric illness involve alterations in the sense of reality, a 'phenomenological stance' is required in order to understand them. To illustrate this point, I sketch some of the *existential changes* (by which I mean alterations in the sense of reality and belonging) that can occur in depressive illness. In addition to arguing for the utility of a phenomenological stance, I suggest that some of the phenomenological analyses that are offered by Husserl, Merleau-Ponty, and others can aid us in interpreting these changes.

Following this, I turn to the relationship between phenomenology and neuroscience. Any attempt to explore the neural correlates of a kind of *experience* will presuppose at least some appreciation of what the relevant experience involves, and misleading conceptions of experience can obfuscate scientific studies in a number of ways. I suggest that phenomenology can inform scientific enquiry by offering detailed accounts of the structure of experience that avoid certain commonplace confusions. I go on to argue that scientific work can also play a valuable role in clarifying and refining phenomenological claims. Amongst other things, scientific studies can generate conceptual distinctions that have the potential to inform phenomenological reflection. I conclude that, although interaction between these disciplines is mutually illuminating, the goal of 'naturalizing' phenomenology through neurobiology is an untenable one. Neurobiology presupposes the experientially constituted sense of reality that phenomenology seeks to describe. So the fruits of phenomenological research cannot all be integrated into an objective, scientific account of neurobiological processes.

12.2 **Phenomenological understanding**

What is it that neurobiological accounts of psychiatric illness fail to include? One concern is that they sideline the *psychological*. For example, Garner and Hardcastle (2004, p. 368) refer to a division between 'psyche' and 'soma', upon which most neurobiological studies are premised. This, they say, is accompanied by a tendency to prioritize an understanding of the 'material world', with the result that 'mind and the mental become marginalized, perhaps even erased entirely' (p. 368).[1] The complaint that neurobiology excludes the *personal* is quite different; it relates to the objective, impersonal *standpoint* adopted by empirical science, rather than to the *subject matter* of empirical science. One can adopt an impersonal attitude towards psyche just as well as to soma, and treat it as a poorly understood part of the objective, scientifically described world. However, responding to someone as a person requires the adoption of a different kind of stance or attitude towards her. A personal stance is not about positing minds in certain moving objects that one observes. It is a way of experiencing and understanding others as *persons*, which depends upon adopting (usually without thought or effort) a perspective very different from that which a scientist might on occasion adopt. R. D. Laing (1960) compares the shift between impersonal and personal perspectives to a gestalt switch; in adopting a personal perspective towards another individual, one perceives that individual very differently. He also suggests that there

---

[1] Such complaints need not presuppose a specific metaphysical account of the relationship between mind and matter. Indeed, Garner and Hardcastle suggest that imposition of a distinction between psyche and soma upon the world is misleading. Their concern is that those features of human beings which we label as 'psychological' get neglected, regardless of what the 'psychological' might ultimately be found to consist of.

are no grounds for regarding the impersonal stance as epistemically privileged over the personal or as the only stance that is legitimately adopted in the context of scientific enquiry:

> The science of persons is the study of human beings that begins from a relationship with the other as a person and proceeds to an account of the other still as a person.
>
> (Laing, 1960, p. 20)

Laing is not alone in claiming that the impersonal perspective misses out something important. For example, Binswanger (1975, p. 210) similarly observes that 'as soon as I objectify my fellow man, as soon as I objectify his subjectivity, he is no longer my fellow man'. The difference between impersonal and personal stances is also stressed by phenomenologists such as Edmund Husserl (1989) and Alfred Schutz (1967).[2]

The understanding of experience sought by phenomenological enquiry differs from both psychological and personal understanding. When one experiences or thinks about another human being in a personal or an impersonal way, one does so in the context of a world that is shared by interpreter and interpreted. The background sense of belonging to the same world as one's object of study is itself a constituent of experience, rather than a judgement based on experience, to the effect that (1) some entity, the 'world', exists and (2) we are both located within it. Hence any study of experience that restricts itself to how we experience specific people, objects, events, and situations within the world will be incomplete. In everyday life, we tend to obliviously take for granted the fact that we find ourselves in a world. As Husserl notes, 'more than anything else the being of the world is obvious. It is so very obvious that no one would think of asserting it expressly in a proposition' (1960, p. 17). This background acceptance of the world, overlooked by both personal and psychological understanding, is something that the phenomenologist seeks to describe.

In order to study the structure of world experience, Husserl advocates a methodological shift that he calls the epoché. This, he says, is a suspension of the 'natural attitude' of believing in the existence of the world, a 'universal depriving of acceptance, [an] "inhibiting" or "putting out of play" of all positions taken towards the already-given Objective world and, in the first place, all existential positions' (1960, p. 20). Performing the epoché is not a matter of *doubting* that the world exists. Instead, one *abstains* from any judgements concerning what is and is not. In so doing, one ceases to immerse oneself in the usual habitual, unthinking acceptance of the world's existence and instead makes that acceptance a focus of study. Rather than enquiring as to what the world contains or how we know what it contains, and taking the world's existence for granted in the process, we study the structure of our experience of the world as 'existing'.

Although Husserl refers to a sense of the world's existence as a kind of 'believing', it is quite different from any of the 'beliefs' we might have about the world's contents.

---

2 For more recent defences of the view that understanding others involves experiencing them as persons through a distinctive kind of stance, and for discussion of what a receptivity towards others as persons consists of, see Hobson (2002) and Ratcliffe (2007, chapter 6).

In fact, it is a condition of possibility for any such belief. Consider walking into a room and seeing a cat on a chair. One believes that there is a cat on the chair but what form does this 'belief' take? It is not, first and foremost, an affirmation that the sentence 'there is a cat on the chair' is true. One takes it to be the case that there is a cat on the chair before taking the sentence 'there is a cat on the chair' to be true. Taking something to be the case in this way does not consist of a judgement that is made after experiencing what looks like a cat sitting on a chair. Rather, one *experiences* the cat as 'really there'. A sense of there being a cat present is integral to the experience; there is a 'believing inherent in perceiving' (Husserl, 2001, p. 66). When we experience something, our experience usually incorporates a sense of the perceived object as *really there*. On other occasions, we might have a sense of doubt; we might encounter it as 'possibly not what it seems' or 'possibly not really there'. However, only some experiences involve uncertainty. In most cases, the reality of what we experience is not in question. Our experience also incorporates a range of other distinctions, such as that between 'really there', 'imagined', and 'remembered'. An experiential *sense of reality* is not a matter of judgements that are made about the reality of entities, but of the ability to distinguish 'really there' from other possibilities, to experience some things and not others as 'real'. In the absence of this ability, it is not the case that everything would simply be experienced as unreal or 'not there'. Without a contrast between 'really there' and other possibilities, one could not experience things in either way; the *sense of reality*, of what it is for something to be real, would itself be gone.

The *world*, for Husserl, is not an entity that we take to be real but a nonconceptual background of belonging that is constitutive of the sense of reality:

> It belongs to what is taken for granted, prior to all scientific thought and all philosophical questioning, that the world is – always is in advance – and that every correction of an opinion, whether an experiential or other opinion, presupposes the already existing world . . .
>
> (Husserl, 1970, p. 110)[3]

What is suspended and then reflected upon by means of the epoché is not a belief or even the totality of one's beliefs but the sense of reality that is presupposed by all beliefs. As all of our beliefs are dependent upon it, they are suspended in the process. Personal and psychological understanding, both take the world for granted and so are unable to access this aspect of experience. Phenomenology, in contrast, seeks to describe the structure of our ordinarily presupposed sense of belonging and reality.

There is some debate over what exactly the epoché is and whether it is something that human beings are capable of performing (e.g. Merleau-Ponty, 1962, p. xiv). If it is conceived of as a way of experiencing one's own experience, whereby the phenomenologist preserves the sense of belonging to a world wholly intact but at the same time somehow wholly detaches herself from it and studies its structure, it is not at all clear

---

[3] Heidegger's (1962) account of being-in-the-world is in many respects complementary. Like Husserl, Heidegger holds the view that our relationship with the world consists in a sense of practical belonging that is presupposed by everyday experiences and thoughts. The relationship is not, first and foremost, a matter of our attending to the world as an object of experience or thought.

that such a stance is psychologically possible. Even if the epoché is construed in methodological rather than experiential terms, as an attitude of enquiry that one adopts towards experience rather than a kind of experience, it seems unlikely that any method will be able suspend the natural attitude in its entirety; one will always end up taking something for granted. Furthermore, it is doubtful that a reflective attitude can be adopted towards an experience without altering that experience in some way.

Rather than worrying any more about the nature of the epoché and whether it is possible, I will adopt a more modest conception of phenomenological method here. A phenomenological stance is not a radical transformation of all experience, where one becomes, as Husserl puts it, 'the "non-participant onlooker" at himself' (1960, p. 37). Instead, it is a methodological shift, whereby one comes to appreciate that there are certain questions which cannot be satisfactorily addressed from the standpoint of empirical science or from any other standpoint that takes a sense of reality for granted. This stance does not demand a total *removal* of all existential commitment from one's methodological orientation. What is required is the *acknowledgement* that there is an experientially constituted sense of reality and belonging, coupled with a commitment to study and attempt to describe this and other aspects of experience, using whatever means are at our disposal.

Although a complete *removal* of the sense of reality from experience is not required for phenomenological enquiry, examining *changes* that occur in the background structure of experience can, I suggest, play an important role. Aspects of experience that we ordinarily overlook can become apparent to us when they are altered in some way.[4] Methods that continue to presuppose the world cannot be employed to interpret such alterations. They will misconstrue what we might call *existential changes* – shifts in the background sense of belonging and reality – as changes in experiences of things within the world.

Reflecting upon existential changes can also assist in orientating the enquirer towards a phenomenological stance in the first place. Descriptions of experience, which may well start off as vague and metaphorical, can help draw attention to the fact that there is a genuine realm of enquiry here, which demands a distinctive kind of methodological orientation. The relevant experiences can then be described in a clearer, more detailed way by means of phenomenology. There is thus an ongoing commerce between a phenomenological stance and its subject matter. Phenomenological description does not begin from a neutral, wholly detached perspective. It is something that proceeds gradually; interpretations are progressively refined, elaborated, and revised through engagement with one's subject. We cannot suspend all that we habitually accept in one swift move. As Merleau-Ponty (1964, p. 21) puts it, 'what is

---

[4] Heidegger (1962, p. 232) makes this point with respect to a change in the background structure of world-experience that he refers to as 'anxiety'. Heideggerian anxiety is a total eradication of all significance from the world, a loss of the practical connectedness that is constitutive of our more usual sense of belonging to a world. Anxiety plays an important role in Heidegger's phenomenological method. The way in which we ordinarily take the world for granted becomes conspicuous in its absence and thus amenable to phenomenological study. See Ratcliffe (2008, chapter 9) for the claim that a wide range of different changes in the structure of experience can similarly inform phenomenological enquiry.

given is a route, an experience which gradually clarifies itself and proceeds by dialogue with itself and with others'.

What does all this have to do with psychiatric illness? As I will illustrate in what follows, at least some patients experience quite significant changes in the sense of belonging and reality. It is not that they take the real to be unreal or vice versa. Rather, the overall structure of experience has changed and the patient no longer experiences or believes anything in quite the same way anymore. It follows that her experience cannot be adequately interpreted if it is assumed from the outset that she occupies the same background 'natural attitude' as oneself. One has to cease presupposing the usual sense of reality and recognize that her existential orientation has shifted, sometimes radically. Phenomenology therefore plays an indispensable interpretive role.

12.3 **Existential changes in depression**

Various authors have stressed the need to interpret some anomalous experiences existentially. For example, the difference between specific experience/thought contents and existential changes is recognized by Jaspers in his *General Psychopathology*, the first edition of which was published back in 1913. In his discussion of delusions, Jaspers states that 'to say simply that a delusion is a mistaken idea which is firmly held by the patient and which cannot be corrected gives only a superficial and incorrect answer to the problem' (1962, p. 93). Delusions, he says, are not just mistaken beliefs. They need to be understood as arising in the context of alterations in the sense of reality and belonging; they involve '*a transformation in our total awareness of reality*'(1962, p. 94). Complementary claims have been made by several more recent authors, especially in relation to schizophrenia. For example, Laing (1960, p.15) states that 'the mad things said and done by the schizophrenic will remain essentially a closed book if one does not understand their existential context'. Sass and Parnas (2007) similarly argue that symptoms of schizophrenia need to be interpreted in terms of alterations in the overall structure of world experience. A phenomenological approach, they maintain, allows us to 'make sense out of seemingly bizarre actions or beliefs that might otherwise seem completely incomprehensible' (2007, p. 65).

In order to illustrate the role of phenomenological understanding, I will focus upon depression, rather than schizophrenia.[5] One reason for this choice is that depression (in its less severe forms, at least) is not quite so far removed from everyday experience as schizophrenia. Hence the existential alterations involved may well be more readily

---

[5] There are many other psychiatric conditions where existential interpretations are plausible. For example, the kinds of experience referred to as 'depersonalization' seem to involve overall shifts in the structure of experience, rather than changes that are restricted to how only certain perceptual contents appear (Ratcliffe, 2008, chapter 6). Indeed, depersonalization frequently occurs in depression and some of the existential changes that occur in depression may be attributable to depersonalization. See Baker *et al.* (2007) and Simeon and Abugel (2006) for recent descriptions of depersonalization. It is also arguable that some allegedly 'monothematic' and 'circumscribed' delusions such as the Capgras and Cotard delusions are better understood in terms of existential changes than in terms of a combination of anomalous experiential contents and propositional attitudes (see Ratcliffe, 2008, chapters 5 and 6).

accessible to phenomenological reflection and thus a better case study with which to illustrate the need for a phenomenological stance. Another reason for focusing on depression is that it deserves more attention from phenomenologists (and from philosophers more generally) than it has received.[6] Although many millions of people suffer from depression, the nature of the experiential changes involved is far from clear. Depression is of course frequently discussed and written about, and there are many lengthy and detailed autobiographical accounts. One might therefore assume that the experience is in fact very well understood. But it is not. Almost all descriptions eventually lapse into metaphorical or figurative language and many authors explicitly state that some aspects of the experience of depression are indescribable (see e.g. Styron, 2001, p. 14).

In the remainder of this section, I will draw attention to some aspects of the phenomenology of depression that consistently feature in autobiographical accounts. My aim in so doing is to make clear that depression involves existential changes that cannot be understood if they are interpreted against the backdrop of a presupposed reality.[7] Hence I will focus on shifts in the overall structure of experience, rather than on more specifically directed emotions, perceptions, and thoughts. However, this is not to suggest that the latter have no role to play in depression.

The depressed person does not find herself depressed within the world; the depression is, amongst other things, an alteration of her sense of being in the world. Central to this alteration, I will suggest, are changes in her sense of what is possible. What I offer here will not add up to anything like a comprehensive account of the phenomenology of depression. Nevertheless, I hope that it will at least provide an indication of the kinds of experiential changes that such an account will need to address and of how one might draw on the work of phenomenologists in order to interpret them.

In his *Principles of Psychology*, William James describes the experience of what is now known as 'depression' in the following way:

> In certain forms of melancholic perversion of the sensibilities and reactive powers, nothing touches us intimately, rouses us, or wakens natural feeling. The consequence is the complaint so often heard from melancholic patients, that nothing is believed in by them as it used to be, and that all sense of reality is fled from life. They are sheathed in india-rubber; nothing penetrates to the quick or draws blood, as it were. [. . . .] 'I see, I hear!' such patients say, 'but the objects do not reach me, it is as if there were a wall between me and the outer world!'
>
> (William James, 1890, p. 298)[8]

---

6 There has, however, been at least some recent discussion of the phenomenology of depression (see, for example, Stanghellini, 2004; Fuchs, 2003, 2005a).

7 I appreciate that there are many different kinds of depression, that classifications of 'depression' and 'melancholia' are historically changeable, and that the proper classification of depression is a matter of ongoing debate. Hence I do not want to insist that the existential changes I discuss are common to all forms of depression, that they occur in quite the same way in all cases, or even that they occur only in depression.

8 In suggesting that what James describes in this particular case is covered by the modern term 'depression', I do not wish to imply that historical uses of the term 'melancholia' map neatly onto current use of the term 'depression'. See Radden (2003) for a discussion of how the two differ.

In this passage, James seems to appreciate the difference between an existential alteration and a change in experience or thought contents. He does not say that *everything looks unreal* or that patients have *altered beliefs* but that the *sense of reality* is itself gone. Without it, the possibility of experiencing or thinking about anything as 'real' or unreal' is gone. The passage also draws attention to another aspect of the condition that is often reported. There is a suffocating sense of estrangement from people and things, like being 'sheathed in India-rubber'. Many authors describe a similar experience of estrangement from the world, of being irrevocably cut off from everything, as if by some impenetrable substance. For example, Andrew Solomon remarks that the air seemed 'thick and resistant, as though it were full of mushed-up bread' (2001, p. 50) and later recalls that 'I felt as if my head had been encaged in Lucite, like one of those butterflies trapped forever in the thick transparency of a paperweight' (2001, p. 66).[9] The problem is not that specific things seem practically and emotionally inaccessible but that the possibility of connecting with anything in the world is gone from experience. The world no longer incorporates the opportunity for certain kinds of practical and affective connectedness.

There is more to this loss of possibilities than the *absence* of something from experience; the absence itself is *there*. It is conspicuous, a very real part of the experience; there is a painful awareness of the loss of feeling. This is at least partly because one continues to experience the possibilities as *there* but only as *there for others*. So there is an experience of irrevocable isolation from other people, of being not contingently or temporarily cut off but cut off with no possibility of return:

> I felt completely alone. Everyone else, my wife, my kids, coworkers, friends, the guy who sold me the morning coffee – seemed to be moving through their days peacefully, laughing and having fun. I resented them because they were having such an easy time of it and because I felt utterly cut off from them emotionally.
>
> (Karp, 2001, p. 143)

In addition to a loss of practical significance, there is also a loss of the appreciation that the depression itself is a contingent state, that a different way of being in the world is possible. The inconceivability of recovery, of things being otherwise, is frequently reported. No situation offers potential reprieve; all experience is structured by the depression and the possibility of having an experience that transcends the depression is gone:

> My father would assure me, smilingly, that I would be able to do it all again, soon. He could as well have told me that I would soon be able to build myself a helicopter out of cookie dough and fly it to Neptune, so clear did it seem to me that my real life, the one I had lived before, was now definitively over.
>
> (Solomon, 2001, p. 54)

> [My psychiatrist was] extremely reassuring, telling me again and again that depression is self-limiting and that I would recover. I did not believe a single word. It was inconceivable to me that I should ever recover. The idea that I might be well enough to work again was unimaginable and I cancelled commitments months ahead.
>
> (Wolpert, 1999, p. 154)

---

9 Solomon also recalls Sylvia Plath's 'bell jar' metaphor (Plath, 1966).

Loss of practical possibilities and a sense of inescapability are closely associated with alterations in the experience of time. The future is the dimension of potential activity and change. Because the world no longer offers up possibilities for action or alternatives to one's current predicament, the structure of temporal experience is different. There is no possibility of significant change, of things being different or of their ever having been different and so the phenomenological distinction between the dimensions of past, present, and future is eroded: 'You cannot remember a time when you felt better, at least not clearly; and you certainly cannot imagine a future time when you will feel better' (Solomon, 2001, p. 55). How one finds oneself in the present moment becomes an eternity from which there is no escape; the contingency and transitory nature of the present are lost (Wyllie, 2005).

Not all kinds of possibility are absent or diminished however. Things no longer appear as opportunities for action but certain other kinds of possibility can become unusually salient. The anxiety that is so often associated with depression involves all experience being structured by a sense of existential threat. Everything appears relevant only to the imminent extinction of one's own being. The threat is not only experienced as possible or likely but as looming, inevitable; 'there is something in the future which is coming. […] I am afraid that it will suck out my core and I will be completely empty and anguished' (Thompson, 1995, p. 47).

Again, it would be a mistake to interpret this experience as being restricted to an experience of specific things, even very many things, as threatening. It is an existential shape that structures all experience; what used to be a possibility only some things offered has become the constant form of world experience as a whole.

Although the changes I have outlined above all concern experience of one's relationship with the world and other people, almost all authors also describe distinctive changes in bodily feeling, including a wide range of somatic symptoms. For example, Solomon states that even in mild depression or 'dysthymia':

> Such depression takes up bodily occupancy in the eyelids and in the muscles that keep the spine erect. It hurts your heart and lungs, making the contraction of involuntary muscles harder than it needs to be.
>
> (Solomon, 2001, p. 16)

Nearly every author has his or her own story to tell about the nature of the relationship between the psychological and the somatic (see e.g. Solomon, 2001, p. 20; Styron, 2001, p. 43). Descriptions tend to distinguish them, perhaps under the assumption that a feeling of bodily states must be different from a way of experiencing things outside of the body. Yet, at the same time there is an emphasis on the inextricability of bodily symptoms and an altered sense of being in the world. It is the depression that 'takes up bodily occupancy', the same depression that manifests itself as a relationship with the world. Often, bodily complaints and existential predicament seem to be one and the same. For example, Thompson (1995, p. 246) describes her experience as follows: 'I felt myself hurtling once more into the abyss. The mental pain was physical, as if the marrow of my bones were being ground into dust'.

The language used to describe the experience of depression is consistently metaphorical or figurative, with frequent references to 'blackness', 'darkness', and 'being weighed down' complementing more elaborate descriptions such as being encased in Lucite, sheathed in india-rubber, on the outside of life looking in, and so on. It is often unclear what kind of experience an author is trying to express. Even so, it is at least plausible to maintain that existential changes of some kind contribute to depression. Almost all accounts try to convey something that is not a specific experience but a shift in the shape of all experience. Many authors describe a disconnection from the world that amounts to a diminishing of self and a loss of reality from experience. A sense of practical connectedness and significance is lost, and with it experience of the body as a locus of potential activities. When the world no longer offers up possibilities, the body is no longer experienced as something through which those possibilities can be actualized. It becomes object-like, conspicuous, strange, and inanimate.[10] And a world drained of all practical significance is a world that no longer appears as real; in offering nothing it is *not quite there*. The self does not survive this existential change intact; it is impoverished, stripped of possibilities for experience and thought that are partly constitutive of selfhood. Susanna Kaysen offers a vivid description of the predicament:

> The worst thing about depression – the thing that makes people phobic about it – is that it's a foretaste of death. It's a trip to the country of nothingness. Reality loses its substance and becomes ghostly, transparent, unbelievable. The perception of what's outside infects the perception of the self, which explains why depressed people feel they aren't 'there'.
>
> (Kaysen, 2001, p. 43)

Some authors not only say that this feels like death; they report having wondered whether they really were dead. There are frequent reports of feeling that the self has been extinguished with only the body staying on in a kind of lingering, living death. For example:

> I became, to myself, more and more like a ghost, or a shadow. What I more and more felt, as the trauma deepened, was that while my body survived, the self that I had been had lost its life.
>
> (McMurtry, 2001, p. 69)[11]

Such descriptions strongly suggest that what is involved in depression is, in part at least, a change in the background sense of belonging to a world. Hence the relevant experiences cannot be adequately interpreted without the adoption of a phenomeno-logical stance, which suspends the ordinarily presupposed sense of reality so as to explore its structure and clarify the ways in which it might be altered.

----

[10] Stanghellini (2004) and Fuchs (2005a) argue that the kind of corporealization reported in depression is different from changes in bodily experience that occur in schizophrenia. In the former case, one is trapped inside a prison-like body and, in the latter, one is detached from one's body, disembodied. However, I doubt that the two kinds of experience are quite so different and think it very likely that some of the same kinds of existential change can occur in both depression and schizophrenia (see Ratcliffe (2008, chapter 7) for a discussion).

[11] This description refers to a period of depression that followed major heart surgery. However, similar experiences are reported by people who have not undergone surgery or suffered any obvious bodily trauma.

12.4 **Bodily feeling, world-experience, and possibility**

Although I have suggested that a phenomenological stance is required in order to understand the experience of depression, I have not yet offered much by way of phenomenological analysis, other than emphasizing that changes in a sense of what is possible are central. Hence I will now draw on some claims that phenomenologists have made concerning the structure of experience.[12] Of central importance are accounts that are offered of the relationship between our bodily phenomenology and the experience of possibilities. First of all, consider the phenomenology of bodily feeling. It is commonplace in philosophy, science, and everyday life to think of feelings as experiences of bodily states – a bodily feeling is an experience that has one's own body or part of one's body as its exclusive object. It follows that bodily feelings need to be clearly distinguished from experiences of things outside of one's body. This kind of bodily experience/world experience division often features in accounts of depression. Authors stumble to express the relationship between two things that must be separate but seem to be one and the same. We can draw on phenomenology in order to argue that the division rests upon a misconception of bodily feeling. Bodily feelings do not always have the body as their primary object. In many cases, the body is that which *feels* rather than that which is *felt*. In other words, the feeling body does not operate as an object of perception but as an organ of perception, a means of perceiving other things. As Sass (2004, p. 134) puts it, bodily feeling is often 'the tacitly inhabited medium of an attitude'.

I find an analogy with touch helpful here. When we explore the world through touch, the part of our body that touches is *felt by us* in some way, as exemplified by the phenomenological difference between how one's hand usually feels and the experience of having lost feeling in it (after having slept upon one's arm, for example). However, as one runs one's hand along a surface, it is more often the surface than the hand that is the primary object of feeling. The hand is what feels rather than what is felt (Ratcliffe, 2008, chapter 3). Even when the body is a conspicuous object of experience, the feeling can contribute to perception of other things too. Consider, for example, running the sole of one's foot across a surface that tickles. The same lesson, I suggest, applies more generally. Many kinds of bodily feeling are at the same time ways of experiencing other things. Furthermore, it seems that certain bodily feelings are not just ways in which specific objects or situations are experienced. Instead, they are constitutive of how one relates to the world as a whole, of an existential background that frames all experience. Consider the following description:

> A law clerk friend invited me to a party one Saturday night, and I went. The noise and bright social talk were almost physically painful. Standing in that crowded room holding a beer, I felt like some poor creature that had been boiled and peeled.
>
> (Thompson, 1995, p. 246)

---

[12] Working towards a clear phenomenological account of depression is not merely an intellectual exercise. The unbearable isolation that patients so often complain of can be exacerbated by an inability to communicate what it is that they are going through and by others' lack of understanding. Hence such an account, in offering a better understanding of the relevant experience, has the potential for therapeutic application.

The discomfort here is bodily and at the same time a way in which the overall situation is experienced; there is no distinction to be drawn between the two.

The inextricability of bodily feeling and world experience has been emphasized by a number of phenomenologists. For example, van den Berg (1962) observes that psychiatric patients seldom complain of psychological symptoms but more often of 'physical complaints' (pp. 22–23), these complaints being seamlessly entwined with a sense of how they find themselves in the world as a whole. The world, he says, is 'our home', rather than a collection of objects that we relate to as detached spectators (pp. 29–40). It is a context of practical significance that we inhabit, and it is through our feeling bodies that we perceive significance. Hence changes in bodily feeling can at the same time be changes in world experience. Being ill, van den Berg remarks, "means first and foremost that the surroundings have changed' (p. 45).

Others indicate that our sense of belonging to the world is very much like a felt bodily 'hold' or 'balance,' as opposed to being an intellectual achievement. To quote Binswanger:

> When we are in a state of deeply felt hope or expectation and what we have hoped for proves illusory, then the world – in one stroke – becomes radically 'different'. We are completely uprooted, and we lose our footing in the world. [. . .] . . . our whole existence moves within the matrix of stumbling, sinking, and falling.
>
> (Binswanger, 1975, pp. 222–223)

He maintains that references to 'sinking' and 'falling' are not merely metaphorical. A type of existential predicament and an experience such as losing one's balance or falling have certain features in common. On those occasions when we physically lose our balance and fall down, certain kinds of possibility are salient. Some things appear as no longer offering support, others as posing a threat that we have no control over. We experience ourselves as out of control; we lose our grip, our hold or our footing. The same kinds of experienced possibility, Binswanger indicates, can come to characterize the overall structure of world experience. Rather than being contingent, concrete possibilities, they become a shape that all objects of experience take on, an existential 'matrix' through which all experiences are structured. This seems to be the case with the anxiety that so often occurs in depression. Solomon (2001, p. 50) describes it as akin to falling. It is like 'when you feel the earth rushing up at you' but instead of being temporary and offering the possibility of eventual relief, it is constant and inescapable: 'I felt that way hour after hour after hour'.

The relationship between bodily feelings, possibilities, and existential changes can be clarified by means of an analysis that is offered, in slightly different forms, by Husserl (e.g. 1989) and Merleau-Ponty (e.g. 1962). Both phenomenologists emphasize that the 'lived body', the body through which we perceive, act, and think, is not just an *object* of experience with which we are especially well acquainted but a framework that structures all experience: 'The Body [*Leib*] is, in the first place, the *medium of all perception*; it is the *organ of perception* and is *necessarily* involved in all perception' (Husserl, 1989, p. 61).

Central to the phenomenological role of the body is the part it plays in our experience of possibilities. Husserl and Merleau-Ponty both appreciate that experiencing something is not just a matter of perceiving what actually appears. We also perceive a range of salient possibilities, which partly constitute both a sense of *what* the perceived thing is and also the sense *that* it is. For example, when I look at the cup in front of me, it appears as something that I or others could see from different angles (revealing some of its hidden aspects in the process), and as something that could be touched, manipulated, and used in certain salient ways. The possibilities incorporated into object-perception are intersensory, something that is again noted by both Husserl and Merleau-Ponty: 'any object presented to one sense calls upon itself the concordant operation of all the others' (Merleau-Ponty, 1962, p. 318).[13] For instance, the cup as seen offers possibilities for tactile contact and the cup as touched offers possibilities for vision.

The possibilities that we experience can have varying degrees of determinacy ('turn me around to reveal my hidden aspects' is less specific than 'turn me around to reveal something red with a specific shape') and there are also different *kinds* of possibility. For example, things can appear as having a practical significance 'for us', 'for me and not them' or 'for them and not me'. Experienced possibilities can be variably enticing. Actions are sometimes solicited, called for, and on other occasions they appear as merely possible. And available actions may present themselves as easy, difficult, or even as impossible.

Not all the possibilities that experience includes are possibilities for action though. There are also potential happenings, which can appear as inconsequential, as having consequences 'for us', 'for them but not me', and so on. These happenings can take a range of forms, such as 'pleasurable', 'threatening', 'interesting', 'unavoidable', 'merely possible', 'likely', or 'unlikely'. And again, they appear with varying degrees of determinacy. A threat, for instance, can be vague or quite concrete. The structured systems of possibilities that surround objects are referred to by Husserl and Merleau-Ponty as 'horizons'. Horizons are not static in nature but have a temporal structure; as certain possibilities are actualized, others are revealed.[14]

Importantly, horizons are at the same time felt, bodily potentialities. It is through the feeling body that we perceive possible ways of revealing hidden features of things, of affecting them, and being affected by them. The body is the indissociable counterpart of structured horizons; it is 'constantly there, functioning as an organ of perception; and here it is also, in itself, an entire system of compatibly harmonizing organs of perception' (Husserl, 2001, pp. 50–51). The role of the body is not restricted to specific, concrete possibilities that surround particular entities. It also sets up an existential context that shapes all experience. For anything to be experienced as 'tangible', 'accessible to others', 'practically significant', and so on, the structure of experience has to incorporate possibilities such as 'tangibility', 'accessibility to others', and 'practical significance'. The sense that there are such possibilities is constituted by bodily potentialities. The feeling body is at the same time the situation in which one finds oneself,

---

[13] See also Husserl (1989, section I, chapter I).

[14] The account of possibilities and the phenomenology of the body that I provide here is only a cursory sketch of something that Husserl calls 'passive synthesis' (meaning the way in which perception is effortlessly structured so that we experience a structured world of interrelated objects). For a detailed discussion, see Husserl (2001).

the space of possibilities that one inhabits; it *is* one's existential orientation. To quote Merleau-Ponty (1962):

> To have a body is to possess a universal setting, a schema of all types of perceptual unfolding and of all those inter-sensory correspondences which lie beyond the segment of the world which we are actually perceiving.
>
> (Merleau-Ponty, 1962, p. 326)

> The natural world is the horizon of all horizons, the style of all possible styles, which guarantees for my experiences a given, not a willed, unity underlying all the disruptions of my personal and historical life. Its counterpart within me is the given, general and pre-personal existence of my sensory functions. . . .
>
> (Merleau-Ponty, 1962, p. 330)

If we acknowledge that experience has this general structure, we can begin to understand what the existential changes that occur in depression consist of. Existential changes can be analysed in terms of the *kinds* of possibility that are incorporated into the structure of experience. These possibilities are constituted by the feeling body. Hence some changes in the feeling body are at the same time changes in a possibility space that shapes all experience. Elsewhere, I refer to variants of the possibility space as 'existential feelings', as they are both bodily feelings and at the same time ways of finding ourselves in the world (Ratcliffe, 2005, 2008).[15]

All existential feelings can be described in terms of the kinds of possibility that experience incorporates. There are different kinds of existential shift, the character of each shift depending on which kinds of possibility are heightened, diminished, or absent. For example, experience as a whole might lose all sense of practical significance or, alternatively, everything might appear as significant. The world as a whole could take on the form of threat or of irrelevance. The possibility of tangibility might be removed or perhaps that of accessibility to other people. In other cases, the temporal flow of possibilities could lose its usual harmonious structure, leading to a way of experiencing that is not irrevocably lacking any *kind* of possibility but is however disordered or even chaotic (Ratcliffe, 2008, chapter 7).

The fact the experience includes possibility in addition to actuality serves to dissolve an apparent paradox concerning what Jaspers (1962) refers to as 'delusional mood' or 'delusional atmosphere'. In a delusional mood, everything looks markedly different and yet the experience is hard to convey because everything also looks exactly as it did before. If one had to point to what had changed, one would have to say 'nothing':

> . . . . perception is unaltered in itself but there is some change which envelops everything with a subtle, pervasive and strangely uncertain light. A living room which formerly was felt as neutral or friendly becomes dominated by some indefinable atmosphere.
>
> (Jasper, 1962, p. 98)

---

[15] My account of existential feeling draws on Heidegger's account of mood [*Stimmung*] in *Being and Time* (Division One, V), as well as the work of several other phenomenologists.

What Jaspers is referring to, I think, is some kind of change in the possibility space. Hence, although experience is significantly altered, the alteration in question cannot be conveyed in terms of concrete differences in how things look (Ratcliffe, 2008, chapter 5).[16] What exactly this particular change consists of is a question I leave open. Indeed, it could be that the term 'delusional mood' encompasses a range of subtly different existential predicaments. It does after all seem that many different kinds of existential change can occur in psychiatric illness. R. D. Laing employs the term 'implosion' to refer to one such change:

> . . . the full terror of the experience of the world as liable at any moment to crash in and obliterate all identity, as a gas will rush in and obliterate a vacuum. The individual feels that, like the vacuum, he is empty. But this emptiness is him.
>
> (Laing, 1960, p. 47)

In cases like this, the world no longer offers possibilities for action. It offers only the impossibility of action. All experience is shaped by existential threat, with all experienced possibilities taking a 'self-involving' and more specifically 'self-destroying' form.

Other kinds of existential change are referred to by the term 'sense/feeling of unreality'. However, it is important to recognize that a sense of unreality may well take a range of different forms. For example, an intangible world is not the same as a world that is no longer experienced as including possibilities for other people. To further complicate matters, depression can involve experience of things as strangely unreal and yet there is also a way in which the world of depression might be experienced as *more* real:

> His world is even more real than ours; for, whereas we are able to rid ourselves of the spell of a depressing landscape, the patient is unable to liberate himself from his gloomy scenery.
>
> (van den Berg, 1972, p. 20)

Because the possibility of alternative ways of experiencing the world is gone, so is the possibility of doubt. What the depression reveals is inescapable, unavoidable, immutable and indubitable. This is partly why, as Solomon (2001, p.16) observes, depression 'feels like knowledge'.

The descriptions of depression that I discussed in the last section indicate that it sometimes or always involves a range of other existential changes too, most of which are closely associated with each other or even phenomenologically inextricable. All of them can be described in terms of the loss, diminution, or heightening of kinds of possibility. For example, the practical significance of things is diminished; things no longer offer up the usual possibilities for activity. Associated with this, there might be a sense of impossibility; possibilities can appear as 'there but impossible to actualize'. There might also be a sense of estrangement, as the possibilities that are inaccessible to the self appear as 'accessible to others with little effort'. Other people continue to offer possibilities for emotional and communicative relatedness but these possibilities at the same time appear as 'impossible for me to take up'. Combined, these alterations in

---

[16] See also Fuchs (2005b) for an account of 'delusional mood' that adopts this kind of approach.

the possibility space constitute a feeling of irrevocable isolation. It is irrevocable because the experience of depression does not incorporate a sense of its own contingency but is a form that determines the scope of all experience. A feeling of estrangement from the world and a loss of practical significance constitute a diminishment and change in the usual sense of reality. Things no longer strike one as available; they seem strangely distant, not quite there anymore. The loss of possibilities also amounts to an altered sense of self. Partly cut off from a diminished world that offers no hope of communion, one is an impoverished spectator who lacks a practical connectedness that is integral to the sense of being there, of being part of things, of belonging to a world. The self that is estranged is not 'wholly intact but cut off from things'. Experience of self cannot be wholly separated from a sense of belonging to the world or from the possibility of standing in various kinds of relation to other people. So the estranged self is a diminished self. All of this is at the same time a way that the body feels, which is why the existential shift is also an unpleasant way of experiencing one's own body, often akin to a form of pain. Added to all this, it is frequently the case that certain kinds of possibility are heightened. A world that no longer offers up invitations to act can at the same time be an all-encompassing and imminent threat, before which one is passive, helpless and utterly alone.[17]

Of course, this is only a very brief sketch of the relevant phenomenology. Nevertheless, I hope it at least serves to illustrate that both a phenomenological stance and specific phenomenological analyses have considerable potential to illuminate at least some of the experiential changes that are reported in psychiatric illness, including several of those that are commonly associated with depression.[18]

12.5 **Phenomenology and neuroscience**

A phenomenological understanding of the kind I have just outlined can make a significant contribution to the neurobiological study of depression and to scientific work on depression more generally. Suppose one wanted to study the neurobiology of some phenomenon 'x'. In those cases where x can be described without explicit or implicit reference to any kind of experience, phenomenology has no contribution to make. However, at least some of the subject matter of neurobiology is phenomenological in nature. For example, there are frequent references to the neurobiological correlates of consciousness and of various types of emotion. So, let us restrict our considerations to cases where x has a phenomenological character. In these cases, we must have at least some understanding of what x is in order to study the neurobiological correlates of x. Otherwise our enquiry would have no subject matter. Assuming we do have some conception of x, that conception – at least to begin with – will not be

---

[17] As noted earlier, all of this is also inextricably bound up with alterations in the structure of temporal experience. For a good survey of how phenomenological analyses of time can contribute to the interpretation of anomalous experience in psychiatric contexts, see Wyllie (2005).

[18] For a more detailed account of horizons, feelings, and possibilities, and of how such an account might be put to work in interpreting psychiatric illness, see Ratcliffe (2008).

a *product* of neurobiological study. x is something that we have identified independently of scientific enquiry and then undertaken to study scientifically. The initial understanding we have of x need not be comprehensive or even accurate. We can acknowledge that the results of further study might lead us to revise our conception of x or even, conceivably, to abandon the view that there is such a thing as x. Nevertheless, the goal of attempting to describe x as well as we can before we start exploring its neurobiology is surely not inconsequential to the neurobiologist.

If a patient complains that nothing seems real anymore, that her body feels peculiar and that the world is drained of significance, one might well be inclined to identify three distinct phenomena here. There are the bodily feelings, which need to be distinguished from altered experiences of things, and there are also beliefs that are formed on the basis of those experiences, such as 'x believes that for all p, where p is an entity in the mind-independent world, p looks somehow different from how p used to look'. Having done this, the neurobiologist might go on to investigate the neurobiological correlates of one or more of these. However, by drawing on phenomenology, we can show that the changed bodily feeling *is* the altered experience. Furthermore, the belief 'nothing seems real' is not an attitude directed at many entities in the world but the expression of an existential change. It is a transformation in the sense of reality rather than a change in the appearance of certain things, which once looked real but now look unreal. Hence references to 'feelings', 'experiences', and 'beliefs' can all express the same unitary existential change. Phenomenological clarification, in this case, is clearly relevant to scientific study. If one undertakes to study one or more of phenomena x, y, and z, when in fact the terms x, y, and z all refer to the same thing, confusion will inevitably arise. A partial description of experience may suffice but a confused description will not. It is difficult to make scientific discoveries about experience 'x' if one has no idea or very little idea of what one is talking about when one refers to x.

The point applies to a range of anomalous experiences. For example, it is commonplace to distinguish the positive symptoms of schizophrenia from the negative symptoms or signs, where the former are additions to the patient's psychology (e.g. delusions or hallucinations) and the latter are absences of something that is more usually present (e.g. loss of affect). These different classes of symptom are often construed as being distinct from each other (e.g. Frith, 1992, p. 12). However, once it is recognized that changes in bodily feeling can at the same time be alterations in the structure of world experience, it becomes apparent that many negative signs, such as diminished affect, are identical to or at least phenomenologically inextricable from positive symptoms such as a strange experience of unfamiliarity. This claim is argued at length by Sass (2003), who suggests that all so-called 'positive symptoms' cannot be adequately interpreted unless it is appreciated that they are intelligible only in the context of an existential shift.

Hence phenomenological reflection can aid us in understanding an aspect of experience that is frequently described in a confused way due to the imposition of tidy distinctions between experience, bodily feeling, and belief, and an associated tendency to overlook the existential background of experience. By facilitating the reconceptualization of at least some experiences, phenomenology can clarify phenomena that neurobiology seeks to explore and also aid in the interpretation of results. Phenomenology also has the potential to influence experimental design, something that Gallagher (2003) refers to as 'front-loading phenomenology'. For instance, one would not set up an experiment to distinguish the contribution made by x to depression from the contribution made by y, if one appreciated from the outset that x and y were in fact the same thing. Alternatively, an experiment could conceivably be devised to *test* the phenomenological claim that x and y are identical. As this might suggest, neurobiology has the potential to inform phenomenological enquiry too. Phenomenology does not get its conceptualizations of experience from nowhere. Just as the neurobiologist might assume the presence of distinct components x, y, and z when there is just the one existential shift, it is also likely that the conceptual distinctions employed by phenomenologists serve on occasion to mislead. Amongst other things, the process of scientific enquiry can serve to generate fine-tuned or revised conceptualizations, which can then be put to work in phenomenological reflection. I will offer just one example here, that of how we should conceive of the phenomenology of motivation, pleasure, and reward.

There is a long-running debate in neurobiology concerning the role of mesolimbic dopamine in relation to perceived reward. One hypothesis is that it determines the impact of reward. However, whether or not a stimulus *appears* rewarding can be distinguished from whether it *does* generate pleasure. Hence an alternative hypothesis is that it regulates anticipation of reward. A third hypothesis is that dopamine plays a role in 'incentive salience'. One might gain a reward from something and anticipate that one will gain that reward but still not be motivated to act. The incentive salience hypothesis is that dopamine plays a role in motivation, rather than contributing to actual or anticipated reward. According to Berridge (2007), current evidence favours this third hypothesis, as dopamine does not seem to be required for 'hedonic "liking"' or for learning to anticipate outcomes (p. 391). The research he appeals to is not phenomenological in nature. Indeed, much of it involves behavioural studies on rats. A behavioural conception of motivation, anticipation, and reward needs to be distinguished from a phenomenological conception. As Berridge recognizes, 'none of these basic reward components are equivalent to their respective subjective feelings of reward' (2007, p. 408). Even so, I suggest that this distinction between motivation, anticipation, and reward, which arose as a product of empirical scientific research, has the potential to inform phenomenology. Regardless of whether or not the distinction is employed in a phenomenological way in neurobiology, we can still ask whether this is the kind of distinction we should adopt when reflecting phenomenologically. Without empirical scientific data that indicate a decoupling between anticipation of reward and motivation, one might assume that perception of something as rewarding is at the same time a motivation to acquire it. But once the distinction is available, we can ask whether it is one that our experience respects.[19]

Scientifically informed phenomenology can then feed back into scientific research. For example, our phenomenologist might propose that there are several subtly different varieties of motivation, anticipation, and reward, and that scientific research into the role of dopamine therefore needs to further fine-tune the categories it employs.

---

[19] Thanks to Henrik Walter for drawing my attention to this example.

There is thus the potential for ongoing and mutually informative interaction between these two very different fields, where phenomenology serves to clarify the subject matter of neurobiology, a subject matter that is then further clarified by ongoing interaction between phenomenologists and scientists. Each generates possibilities for the other to explore and we can strive for consistency between them. For instance, if the phenomenologist claims that x and y are inextricable and the neurobiologist claims that they can be decoupled, one view, the other, or both should be revised. Hence phenomenology and neuroscience can be mutually constraining (Varela, 1999, p. 267).

A more specific and stronger claim regarding the nature of the relationship between phenomenology and neuroscience is that the latter should seek to 'naturalize' the former, meaning roughly that we should aspire to understand all aspects of experience in empirical scientific terms.[20] Although I welcome interaction between phenomenology and neuroscience, I reject the goal of naturalization, the reason being that the phenomenological stance reveals a sense of reality that is not accessible to the standpoint of empirical science. The phenomenologist studies aspects of experience that are presupposed by all empirical, scientific investigation into what the world contains. One cannot distinguish between what is and is not the case in the world without having a sense of what it is to be the case. Hence scientific practices do not escape existential backgrounds and then confront them as objects of empirical study. Rather, scientific practices and scientific conceptions of the world arise within the space of possibilities that the phenomenologist describes. We find statements of much the same point in the writings of many phenomenologists. For example, here is how Heidegger puts it, in one of his *Zollikon Seminars*:

> One must see that science as such (i.e., all theoretical-scientific knowledge) is founded as a way of being-in-the-world – founded in the bodily having of a world.
>
> (Heidegger, 2001, p. 94)[21]

Husserl makes a similar claim in several writings. Here is how he puts it in his final work, *The Crisis of European Sciences*:

> Objective science, too, asks questions only on the ground of this world's existing in advance through prescientific life.
>
> (Husserl, 1970, p. 110)

---

[20] See Dennett (e.g. 1991) for an example of this general attitude. Dennett offers numerous compelling examples of how scientific studies can inform philosophical theorizing. However, his conception of the relationship between phenomenology and science is very different from my own. Dennett assumes from the outset that the goal should be to integrate phenomenological data (in the form of reports gathered by a 'heterophenomenologist', meaning a phenomenologist who relies on third-person reports rather than first-person experience) into a construal of the world that is dictated solely by the empirical sciences. He does not recognize anything like the phenomenological stance or the possibility that there are experiential achievements which the standpoint – or standpoints – of empirical science continue to quietly presuppose.

[21] These seminars were held at the home of the psychiatrist Medard Boss, over a 10-year period between 1959 and 1969.

> [Science] is an accomplishment which, in being practiced and carried forward, continues to presuppose this surrounding world as it is given in its particularity to the scientist.
>
> (Husserl, 1970, p. 121)

We also find versions of it in Merleau-Ponty's work, such as in his proposal that the philosopher rediscover:

> ... the world of actual experience which is prior to the objective world, since it is in it that we shall be able to grasp the theoretical basis no less than the limits of that objective world.
>
> (Merleau-Ponty, 1962, p. 57)

An objective, scientific account of what exists within the world cannot incorporate the *sense of reality* because the intelligibility of any such account will itself presuppose the phenomenological achievement under investigation. A science that did succeed in accommodating the sense of reality would look very different from any of the current empirical sciences. First of all, it would need to include the employment of a phenomenological stance, as the relevant aspects of experience are inaccessible to any stance that takes the being of the world for granted. And second, it would need to acknowledge that its own intelligibility depended upon its object of study, rather than attempting to assimilate everything into an objective, scientific conception of the world that quietly presupposes phenomenological achievements. It would thus be quite unlike the kind of naturalistic picture advocated by many philosophers.[22]

Acknowledgements

Thanks to Lisa Bortolotti, Matthew Broome, Martin Wyllie, and audiences at the University of Central Florida and the Institute of Psychiatry at the Maudsley for helpful comments on an earlier version of this chapter.

References

Baker, D., Hunter, E., Lawrence, E., and David, A. (2007). *Overcoming Depersonalization and Feelings of Unreality: A Self-Help Guide Using Cognitive Behavioral Techniques*. London, Robinson.

Berg, J. H. van den. (1972). *A Different Existence: Principles of Phenomenological Psychopathology*. Pittsburgh, PA, Duquesne University Press.

Berridge, K. C. (2007). The debate over dopamine's role in reward: the case for incentive salience. *Psychopharmacology*, **191**, 391–431.

Binswanger, L. (1975). *Being-in-the-World: Selected Papers of Ludwig Binswanger*. (Tr.J. Needleman,). London, Souvenir Books.

Dennett, D. C. (1991). *Consciousness Explained*. London, Penguin.

Frith, C. (1992). *The Cognitive Neuropsychology of Schizophrenia*. Hove, Psychology Press.

---

[22] My criticisms here are not directed at all those doctrines which go by the name of 'naturalism'. See, for example, Rouse, (2002) for a much more sophisticated and quite different conception of 'naturalism'.

Fuchs, T. (2003). The phenomenology of shame, guilt and the body in body dysmorphic disorder and depression. *Journal of Phenomenological Psychology*, **33**, 223–243.

Fuchs, T. (2005a). Corporealized and disembodied minds: a phenomenological view of the body in melancholia and schizophrenia. *Philosophy, Psychiatry and Psychology*, **12**, 95–107.

Fuchs, (2005b). Delusional mood and delusional perception – a phenomenological analysis. *Psychopathology*, **38**, 133–139.

Gallagher, S. (2003). Phenomenology and experimental design: towards a phenomenologically enlightened experimental science. *Journal of Consciousness Studies*, **10**(9–10), 85–99.

Garner, A. and Hardcastle, V. G. (2004). Neurobiological models: an unnecessary divide – neural models in psychiatry. In *The Philosophy of Psychiatry: A Companion* (ed. J. Radden). Oxford, Oxford University Press.

Heidegger, M. (1962). *Being and Time* (Tr. J. Macquarrie, and E. Robinson) Oxford, Blackwell.

Heidegger, M. (2001). *Zollikon Seminars: Protocols – Conversations – Letters*. Evanston, IL, Northwestern University Press.

Hobson, R. P. (2002). *The Cradle of Thought*. London, Macmillan.

Husserl, E. (1960). *Cartesian Meditations: An Introduction to Phenomenology* (Tr. D. Cairns). The Hague, Martinus Nijhoff.

Husserl, E. (1970). *The Crisis of European Sciences and Transcendental Phenomenology* (Tr. D. Carr) Evanston, IL, Northwestern University Press.

Husserl, E. (1989). *Ideas Pertaining to a Pure Phenomenology and to a Phenomenological Philosophy: Second Book* (Trs. R. Rojcewicz, and A. Schuwer). Dordrecht, Kluwer.

Husserl, E. (2001). *Analyses Concerning Passive and Active Synthesis: Lectures on Transcendental Logic* (Tr. A. J. Steinbock). Dordrecht, Kluwer.

James, W. (1890). *The Principles of Psychology*. vol. II. New York, Holt.

Jaspers, K. (1962). *General Psychopathology*. Manchester, Manchester University Press.

Karp, D. (2001). An unwelcome career. In *Unholy Ghost: Writers on Depression* (ed. N. Casey), pp. 138–148. New York, William Morrow.

Kaysen, S. (2001). One cheer for melancholy. In *Unholy Ghost: Writers on Depression* (ed. N. Casey), pp. 38–43. New York, William Morrow.

Laing, R. D. (1960). *The Divided Self: A Study of Sanity and Madness*. London, Tavistock Publications.

McMurtry, L. (2001). From *Walter Benjamin at the Dairy Queen*. In *Unholy Ghost: Writers on Depression* (ed. N. Casey), pp. 67–74. New York, William Morrow.

Merleau-Ponty, M. (1962). *Phenomenology of Perception* (Tr. C. Smith). London, Routledge.

Merleau-Ponty, M. (1964). *The Primacy of Perception. And Other Essays on Phenomenological Psychology, and Philosophy of Art, History and Politics*. Evanston, IL, Northwestern University Press.

Plath, S. (1966). *The Bell Jar*. London, Faber & Faber.

Radden, J. (2003). Is this Dame Melancholy? Equating today's depression and past melancholia. *Philosophy, Psychiatry & Psychology*, **10**, 37–52.

Ratcliffe, M. (2005). The feeling of being. *Journal of Consciousness Studies*, **12**(8–10), 43–60.

Ratcliffe, M. (2007). *Rethinking Commonsense Psychology: A Critique of Folk Psychology, Theory of Mind and Simulation*. Basingstoke, Palgrave Macmillan.

Ratcliffe, M. (2008). *Feelings of Being: Phenomenology, Psychiatry and the Sense of Reality*. Oxford, Oxford University Press.

Rouse, J. (2002). *How Scientific Practices Matter: Reclaiming Philosophical Naturalism*. Chicago, IL, University of Chicago Press.

Sass, L. A. (1992). *Madness and Modernism: Insanity in the Light of Modern Art, Literature and Thought*. New York, Basic Books.

Sass, L. A. (2003). Negative symptoms, schizophrenia, and the self. *International Journal of Psychology and Psychological Therapy*, **3**, 153–180.

Sass, L. A. (2004). Affectivity in schizophrenia: a phenomenological view. In *Hidden Resources: Classical Perspectives on Subjectivity* (ed. D. Zahavi), pp. 127–147. Exeter, Imprint Academic.

Sass, L. A. and Parnas, J. (2007). Explaining schizophrenia: the relevance of phenomenology. In *Reconceiving Schizophrenia* (eds. M. C. Chung, K. W. M. Fulford, and G. Graham), pp. 63–95. Oxford, Oxford University Press.

Schutz, A. (1967). *The Phenomenology of the Social World* (Trs. G. Walsh, and F. Lehnert). Evanston, IL, Northwestern University Press.

Simeon, D. and Abugel, J. (2006). *Feeling Unreal: Depersonalization Disorder and the Loss of Self*. Oxford, Oxford University Press.

Solomon, A. (2001). *The Noonday Demon*. London, Chatto and Windus.

Stanghellini, G. (2004). *Disembodied Spirits and Deanimated Bodies: The Psychopathology of Common Sense*. Oxford, Oxford University Press.

Styron, W. (2001). *Darkness Visible*. London, Vintage.

Thompson. T. (1995). *The Beast: A Reckoning with Depression*. New York, Putnam.

Varela, J. J. (1999). The specious present: a neurophenomenology of time consciousness. In *Naturalizing Phenomenology* (eds. J. Petitot, F. J. Varela, B. Pachoud, *et al.*), pp. 266–314. Stanford, CA, Stanford University Press.

Wolpert, L. (1999). *Malignant Sadness: The Anatomy of Depression*. London, Faber & Faber.

Wyllie, M. (2005). Lived time and psychopathology. *Philosophy, Psychiatry & Psychology*, **12**, 173–185.

Chapter 13

Delusional realities

Shaun Gallagher

Abstract

Recent accounts of delusions involve either top-down or bottom-up, or some hybrid version of theories that rely on internalist, brain-based, or purely belief-based approaches. My intent in this chapter is to explore an alternative explanatory framework, to raise some questions that lead in a different, externalist, and existentialist direction, and to provide a broader account that treats other factors – body, affect, social, and environmental factors – as important in the constitution of delusional realities. This account makes use of the concept of multiple realities, deriving from William James and developed by Alfred Schutz. The account does not provide a causal explanation of delusions, but aims to work out a more adequate characterization of delusions that would provide a framework for any such explanation.

13.1 Introduction

A number of recent papers have addressed the question of whether accounts of delusions should be top-down (rationalist), bottom-up (empiricist), or some hybrid of top-down-bottom-up (Campbell, 2001; Bayne and Pacherie, 2004, 2005; Gallagher, 2004, 2007; Hohwy, 2004; Hohwy and Rosenberg, 2005; Mundale and Gallagher, 2009). There is growing consensus that neither top-down accounts nor bottom-up accounts on their own are able to explain all issues concerning delusions. Nonetheless, even if one combines the top-down and bottom-up accounts, the accounting does not quite add up to a full explanation. Some aspects of delusions remain puzzling from either or both approaches.

In this chapter I first provide a brief review of bottom-up and top-down proposals and outline what they fail to explain. I note that on either kind of approach, brain processes (organic malfunctions) are viewed as playing a causal role, whether to explain delusional experiences caused by bottom-up neural dysfunction or delusional beliefs resulting from meta-cognitive or introspective problems. Various neural disruptions can account for generating aberrant experience as well as for higher-order cognitive difficulties. As a result, all of these accounts share a certain internalistic bias; they frame the explanation of delusions in terms of what is happening 'in the head' of the subject. Of course, it seems right to say that delusions are 'in the head' since they do not reflect the world as it objectively exists. We know as a matter of objective fact that the schizophrenic who claims that his actions are being controlled by someone or something else is incorrect, at least in the literal sense in which the patient claims; we know that the relatives of the Capgras patient are in fact not impostors; we know for a fact that the Cotard patient is not dead, and so on. Accordingly, such delusions simply do not match up to the way the world is; so, they seemingly must be errors in the mind–brain system that completely mis-takes the world.

My main intent here is to explore an alternative explanatory framework and to raise some questions that might lead in a different direction, in terms of both theoretical explanation and possible therapeutic practices (although I have little to say about the latter). Is it possible to take a more externalist approach that can answer some of the unanswered questions about delusions? If we take cognition to be generated in a system that includes brain, body, and environment, or if we take seriously the idea that the brain–body system puts us *in-the-world* in a certain way – in a world with specific kinds of affordances – can we get a different characterization of delusions? To be clear, my aim is not to provide a causal explanation of delusions, but to work out a more adequate characterization that would provide a framework for any such explanation.

13.2 **Top-down accounts**

The *DSM-IV* defines a *delusion* as 'a false belief based on incorrect inference about external reality that is firmly sustained despite what almost everyone else believes and despite what constitutes incontrovertible and obvious proof or evidence to the contrary. The belief is not one ordinarily accepted by other members of the person's culture or subculture.' Placing the emphasis on the concept of belief, this definition reflects a top-down view. The distinction between top-down (or rationalist) views and bottom-up (or empiricist) views is nicely summarized by John Campbell (2001, p. 89).

> On what I will call a rationalist approach to delusion, delusion is a matter of top-down disturbance in some fundamental beliefs of the subject, which may consequently affect experiences and actions. On an empiricist approach, in contrast, delusion is a rational response to highly unusual experiences that the subject has, perhaps as a result of organic damage.

Campbell defends a rationalist approach, suggesting that a delusion is a special kind of belief expressed by what Wittgenstein had called a framework proposition. Naomi Eilan (2000, pp. 108–109) also supports this view and explains it as follows.

> Our framework beliefs are those fundamental beliefs we do not question, and which globally constrain our inferences and our interpretation of our experiences . . . The suggestion is that primary paranoid beliefs, such as that the IRA is out to get one, should be treated as constraining one's reasoning and interpretation of one's experience in an analogous manner. They are resistant to counter-evidence because of their fundamental framing role . . . (But . . . this does not render their expression senseless.).[1]

---

[1] Whether this is a good interpretation of Wittgenstein is open to question. It may be possible to view Wittgenstein as proposing something closer to a pre-conceptual, habitual, experiential background, which would make his proposal consistent with the alternative view proposed below. My thanks to Matthew Ratcliffe for pointing this out.

So framework propositions in some sense act as implicit and background presuppositions with regard to our normal beliefs about the world. They remain implicit in the sense that we do not usually question them and may not be conscious of them at all. Campbell (2001, p. 96) cites the following examples from Wittgenstein: 'There are a lot of objects in the world', 'The world has existed for quite a long time', 'There are some chairs and tables in this room', and 'This is one hand and this is another'. Such framework propositions or beliefs are those against which we test our normal factual beliefs. Delusions if they function as framework propositions can remain relatively circumscribed and heterogeneous, but within their particular area of relevance, they can govern a variety of factual beliefs. So the delusional subject may hold perplexing and paradoxical beliefs with regard to some areas of his life, but be relatively rational in others (see Klee's (2004) discussion of Davidsonian fragmentation). The idea, then, is that if one (or more) of our framework propositions is delusional, it will have an effect on a number of our factual beliefs, but not necessarily all of them, and the framework proposition would not be something that we would normally test out or doubt. It would stand, as the DSM suggests of delusions, as 'firmly sustained despite what almost everyone else believes and despite what constitutes incontrovertible and obvious proof or evidence to the contrary'.

Campbell's rationalist proposal is top-down because, as he puts it, 'delusion is a matter of top-down disturbance in some fundamental beliefs of the subject' (2001, p. 89). His account does not offer much of an explanation of what causes the delusion (likely, he suggests, some organic disturbance) or why a subject might adopt the delusional belief. A different, but equally top-down account offered by Graham and Stephens (Graham and Stephens, 1994; Stephens and Graham, 2000), does try to explain this. They propose that in some way our natural 'proclivity for constructing self-referential narratives', an introspective competency that allows us to explain or rationalize our behaviour retrospectively, breaks down. For example, having a sense of agency for my action depends on whether I can explain the action in terms of a general set beliefs or desires with which I normally explain or rationalize such actions. Thus, whether something is to count for me as my action

> depends upon whether I take myself to have beliefs and desires of the sort that would rationalize its occurrence in me. If my theory of myself ascribes to me the relevant intentional states, I unproblematically regard this episode as my action. If not, then I must either revise my picture of my intentional states or refuse to acknowledge the episode as my doing.
> (Graham and Stephens, 1994, p. 102)

On this approach, non-schizophrenic, first-order experience of agency appears the way it does because of properly ordered second-order interpretations; in contrast, schizophrenic delusional experience appears the way it does because of second-order *mis-interpretation*. Delusions, then, are the result of inferential mistakes made on the basis of higher-order introspective or perceptual self-observations. '[W]hat is critical is that [in the case of the delusion of thought insertion] the subject finds her thoughts inexplicable in terms of beliefs about her intentional states' and this inability to explain the thought or the action leads to the delusional belief that someone or some thing else caused it (p. 105). In effect, the delusion is simply the result of a (mis)judgement made about the incongruence between the content of the current experience and what the subject takes to be her more general conception of her intentional states (see, Stephens and Graham, 2000, p. 170). If problems in the process of introspective judgement can account for why one might hold a delusional belief, Graham and Stephens do not offer any indications of why the process of introspective judgement goes wrong. Presumably, like Campbell, they would gesture to something going wrong in the brain that causes the introspective problems that lead to delusions.

Certain two-factor models of delusion combine aspects of top-down and bottom-up accounts and suggest a more central role for neurological problems.[2] In some two-factor models, delusions are seen as an erroneous, cognitive attempt to explain an anomalous experience generated by neurological disruptions. The first factor consists of an anomalous experience, such as an odd feeling (or lack of appropriate feeling), anomalous perception, or hallucination; the second factor consists of a cognitive or reasoning error that generates the delusion in attempting to explain the anomalous experience (see, e.g. Garety et al., 2001). Recent explanations of Capgras delusion illustrate this two-stage approach (e.g. Ellis and Young 1990; Ramachandran 1998; also see Davies et al., 2001). In such accounts, the first factor is the anomalous perceptual experience of seeing one's parents or other loved ones without simultaneously experiencing an emotional response to them. This sets the stage for the second factor, which is the attempt to rationalize this experience by regarding the loved one as an impostor. The second factor generates the delusional component, and it is either immune or very resistant to revision.

Before moving on to consider bottom-up accounts, let us take a look at what top-down and two-factor explanations fail to explain. The common complaint against these models is that they never explain why the delusions have the specific thematic contents that they do. Consider the explanation of the Capgras delusion. A person may see his wife and at the same time fail to experience the appropriate emotional response to her. But why should he come to hold the delusional belief that the person he sees is not really his wife, but an impostor; rather than, for example, that he no longer loves his wife? In schizophrenia, a person may experience a lack of agency for a particular movement she makes; but why should she come to the delusional explanation that someone else is making her do things, rather than that something is wrong with her own motor control system? There seems to be no resources in these models to answer such questions (but cf. Sass, 2004).

---

[2] I think of the two-factor model as a hybrid, although sometimes the two-factor model is categorized as bottom-up, or empiricist. It depends, however, on how one defines the two factors, i.e. first-order experience and higher-order (e.g. introspective) cognition. For example, the experience can be specified as anomalous and as motivating a higher-order reflection or rationalization that generates the delusion (see e.g. Ellis and Young, 1990; Ramachandran, 1998). Campbell (2001) calls the two-factor model empiricist since experience is a motivating factor, and Bayne and Pacherie (2004) endorse this but distinguish it as explanationist in contrast to an endorsement model. In contrast, a one-factor approach is clearly empiricist and bottom-up. In this view, experience itself is considered delusional, while higher-order cognition simply reports (endorses) the delusion (and, as things develop, perhaps enhances). The delusion is generated (by neurological problems) in the experience itself (see e.g. Maher, 1999; Gallagher, 2004, 2007; Hohwy and Rosenberg, 2005; Mundale and Gallagher, 2009).

A similar question can be raised against Campbell's proposal that delusions are akin to framework propositions, since it is not clear how the subject arrives at such delusional propositions. One example of a delusional proposition, as suggested by Campbell, is 'My wife has been replaced by an imposter.' But from whence does one derive this proposition? Campbell suggests that the subject 'assigns' a certain epistemological status to such propositions (p. 96). But, given the nature of framework propositions, they are not the sort of propositions assigned status by subjects (unless perhaps the subjects are philosophers doing epistemology). Rather, such propositions tend to remain implicit, unconscious, and they operate more as summaries of our worldly experience than as first principles of knowing the world. We can paraphrase Wittgenstein here: we do not explicitly *assign* framework propositions. We discover them subsequently 'like the axis around which a body rotates. This axis is not fixed in the sense that anything holds it fast, but the movement around it determines its immobility' (Wittgenstein, 1969, §152). As Thornton (in press) puts it: 'They are not learned before more problematic beliefs which might be justified in terms of them. So they cannot be identified as what is first held to be the case. They have instead to be identified piecemeal from "within" a mature world-view.' In other words, the delusional proposition does not impose the delusion onto the way that I understand the particular realm to which it applies; it reflects my delusional understanding of that realm. In this sense, as Bayne and Pacherie (2004, p. 7) note, delusional framework propositions are not necessarily top-down; they may in some sense be derived from my experiential understanding of things.

It also seems clear that framework propositions are usually shared, and in some cases may derive from cultural forces. The idea that 'the world has existed for quite a long time', is not something I invented on my own, and it tends to be something that I assume (even if implicitly) that most other people believe. But as Andy Young (1999) points out, a delusional patient can think it very strange if you express your agreement with his delusion (see Bayne and Pacherie (2004) for discussion).

Another problem that the top-down approach does not address is what Louis Sass calls the 'double bookkeeping' paradox connected with some schizophrenic delusions, although this may be a relatively rare phenomenon.[3]

> [M]any schizophrenics who seem to be profoundly preoccupied with their delusions, and who cannot be swayed from belief in them, nevertheless treat these same beliefs with what seems a certain distance or irony . . . A related feature of schizophrenic patients is what has been called their 'double bookkeeping' . . . A patient who claims that the doctors and nurses are trying to torture and poison her may nevertheless happily consume the food they give her; a patient who asserts that the people around him are phantoms or automatons still interacts with them as if they were real.
>
> (Sass, 1994, p. 21)

---

3 This may more frequently occur in chronic patients who are partially treated or those with comorbidity (negative symptoms, depression, neuropsychological impairment). Most delusional patients seen by psychiatrists are fully in their delusions, act on them, without irony, and in a relatively consistent manner. My thanks to Lisa Bortolotti for this point.

Likewise, in cases of Capgras and Cotard there are sometimes inconsistencies between certain beliefs about relevant persons, and between beliefs and actions. In the Cotard delusion, for example, the subject may claim that he is dead, but will continue to eat and drink and so forth. In the Capgras delusion the subject may claim a loved one is an impostor but fail to express any concern about the whereabouts of the genuine loved one (Coltheart and Davies, 2000, p. 10; Young, 2000, p. 49). The idea of Davidsonian fragmentation or the circumscribed and heterogeneous nature of delusions (understood as framework propositions) is not sufficient to address this paradox since belief and action with respect to a particular person or situation should consistently fall within the same framework even if they do not link up to beliefs or actions that fall under other framework propositions. Failure of a cohesive introspective or narrative capacity does not fare well either in respect to explaining this kind of discrepancy.

Top-down accounts, whether of the sort that Campbell proposes or of the sort that Graham and Stephens propose, have another problem. Bayne and Pacherie (2004, p. 8) put it this way: 'We are also puzzled by the question of how a top-down account of delusions could explain the damage to the autonomic system that one finds in the Capgras and Cotard delusions. Is this caused by the delusional belief? That seems unlikely.' It may be better, however, to say that the top-down accounts do not really provide a clear picture of how organic malfunction is related to the cognitive mechanisms that generate delusions. Campbell suggests that organic malfunction could be the cause of the delusional proposition, but it is not clear how precisely that would work. Likewise, if some kind of organic damage resulted in problems with introspective or narrative capabilities that result in delusions, as Graham and Stephens would have it, it is not clear why the subject's delusions are selectively about certain topics and not others – that is, why the subject is delusional in regard to some topics but not delusional in regard to everything he believes, or why some actions or thoughts are considered alien, but not others. This has been called the problem of specificity (Gallagher 2004), and, as Pacherie, Green, and Bayne (2006, p. 575) note, it remains unsolved.

13.3 **Bottom-up accounts**

Bottom-up theories deny the claim that delusions are cognitively derived, second-order processes. Gold and Hohwy (2000) have recently offered a good example of a bottom-up model, not unlike ones developed by a variety of phenomenologists (see, e.g. Sass, 1994; Parnas and Sass, 2001). They refer to 'experiential irrationality' as a way to capture the experiential nature of delusion. In their view, this new category of rationality is needed because neither the standard categories of content rationality nor procedural rationality adequately capture the irrational nature of schizophrenic delusion. As they explain:

> We claim . . . that the source of thought insertion and related delusions is the experience itself of the schizophrenic subject, and, in particular, its alien quality. The elaboration of the delusion in hypotheses and ancillary beliefs should be understood to be derivative from, or secondary to, this experience. Thus the violation of egocentricity does not merely produce strange experiences that form the basis of delusional beliefs as the result of pathological processes of thought or reasoning. Rather, it is *the experience of non-egocentric*

thought as alien that is the delusion itself. The alien quality of the delusional experience is part of its content, and it is the content of experience that is the locus of the delusion and thus of the irrationality. At least some delusions, therefore, are best explained as *disorders of experience* rather than disorders of belief, desire, or reasoning.

(Gold and Hohwy, 2000, p. 160)

Experiential irrationality suggests the non-derivative immediacy of at least some forms of delusion. In this view, the subject is not led *into* a deluded belief, his experience is itself delusional. Subjects experience certain thoughts as *intrinsically* alien. In contrast with top-down models, Gold and Hohwy insist that, 'A hallucination is an unusual form of experience, but no subsequent judgment is required on the part of the subject for the experience to become delusional' (p. 162).[4]

Similar to Gold and Hohwy, I have also argued for a bottom-up model where I distinguish between (1) first-order experience, that is, the phenomenological level of immediate, pre-reflective, lived-through experience of the world, and (2) higher-order cognition, a reflective experience which supports the ability to make attributive judgements about one's own first-order experience. Both first-order experience and second-order cognition depend on a third level of the cognitive system, (3) the non-conscious, sub-personal processes that are best described as neuronal or brain processes (Gallagher 2004; Mundale and Gallagher 2009). Schizophrenic delusions such as thought insertion, alien control, and other misattributions of agency are experienced by the subject at the first-order phenomenological level. Such experiences are immediate, non-inferential, and non-introspective. This is especially clear starting with prodromal symptoms, i.e. early symptoms that precede the characteristic manifestations of the fully developed illness (Gallagher 2000a, 2004b, 2007). While the higher-order, cognitive report of the delusional experience may be confused, it is not necessarily mistaken; the subject recounts what he or she is experiencing at the phenomenological level.

On this kind of account, the problems with self-agency that manifest themselves in the first-order phenomenology of thought insertion and delusions of control, for example, are generated on a neurological level. Farrer and Frith (2002; Farrer *et al.* 2003) have shown contrasting activation in the right inferior parietal cortex for perception of action caused by others, and in the anterior insula bilaterally when action is experienced as caused by oneself. The role of the anterior insula in providing a sense of self-agency involves the integration of three kinds of signals generated in self-movement: somatosensory signals (sensory feedback from bodily movement, e.g., proprioception), visual and auditory signals, and corollary discharge associated with motor commands that control movement. They suggest that a 'close correspondence between all these signals helps to give us a sense of agency' (p. 602). Accordingly a disruption in one or more of these signals, a disruption in their integration, or some other kind of malfunction in the anterior insula or the right inferior parietal cortex, or in the mechanism that allows for

---

4 In later work, Hohwy (2004) appears to favour a combination of bottom-up and top-down models and thinks neither is adequate by itself. But he does not appear to revoke his claim about the non-derivative nature of (at least some) forms of schizophrenic delusion.

the proper dicrimination between self and non-self (Georgieff and Jeannerod 1998), may generate a loss of the sense of self-agency, or a sense of alien control at the level of first-order experience (de Vignemont and Fourneret, 2004; Gallagher, 2004b; Pacherie *et al.*, 2006). Indeed, in schizophrenic patients, delusions of alien control during a movement task have been associated with an increased activity in the right inferior parietal lobe (Spence *et al.*, 1997). There may be a more general or basic disruption of neuronal processes that affect not just the sense of agency for motor action, but also disrupt the sense of agency for cognitive processes, resulting in symptoms of thought insertion. The sense of agency for thought may depend on the anticipatory aspect of working memory (Gallagher, 2000b, 2004b), something that may also malfunction in schizophrenic subjects with delusions of control (see Singh *et al.*, 1992; Daprati *et al.*, 1997; Vogeley *et al.*, 1999; Franck *et al.*, 2001).

Delusional experiences may of course motivate second-order introspective processes, which may take on a defensive role in an attempt to explain or justify the alien experience. In this way, higher-order processes iterate and perhaps enhance problems first manifested at the experiential level. Thus, a key point of contrast between bottom-up models and top-down models concerns the location of causal power. According to the top-down approach, the misattribution of agency to someone or something else is caused by a cognitive error. According to the bottom-up approach, the primary cause of delusional experience is to be found in the brain pathology; at best, whatever higher-order cognition does is secondary to the alien experience.[5]

Although the idea that cognitive errors are involved in delusion is at the core of top-down approaches, one could argue that there are very basic kinds of errors that, while often referred to as cognitive errors, are so deeply entrenched in perception, and so automatic, that they are an integral part of our *immediate, phenomenological experience*. Well-known examples of such errors may include salience effects, attribution errors, primacy and recency effects, contrast effects, and various other biases and distortions. Such biases may exert a bottom-up, or background influence on first-order experience. In other words, their influence can be pre-cognitive and non-inferential. This would allow for some of the appeal of the cognitive approaches to delusion, while preserving the idea that delusional experience is immediate and not derived from faulty inference (Mundale and Gallagher, 2009).

---

[5] Frith's (1992) influential model of schizophrenic delusions of control and thought insertion is sometimes regarded as a bottom-up account, but in fact it is in some regards a mixture of top-down and bottom-up explanations. Frith postulated problems with mechanisms of self-monitoring, where self-monitoring was sometimes defined as a meta-representation, i.e., a full-fledged second-order act of reflection. But the failure of meta-representational introspection is attributed to neurological dysfunctions associated with sub-personal efferent copy and comparator mechanisms (for discussion, see Gallagher, 2000, 2004b; Stephens and Graham, 2000, pp. 141ff). In later papers, however, Frith focusses more on the neurological dysfunctions in motor-control mechanisms and adopts a more bottom-up approach. Still, as Pacherie, *et al.* (2006) point out, Frith's recent model remains explanationist, and to that extent, still, in our view, top-down.

Salience effects and their role in misattribution, for example, are a prime example of the sort of effect, which in the case of schizophrenic delusion exerts important pre-cognitive, or background effects. Patients report such things as having a new awareness of their surroundings, a heightened sense of consciousness, unusually sharp sensory abilities, newfound clarity of thought, etc. This exaggerated sense of significance starts to shape a delusional experience. Kapur proposes a model that explains the experiential aspect of certain delusions in terms of such salience effects, and that the heightened significance that schizophrenics may attach to ordinary objects, sensations, events, or ideas is due to a higher than normal dopamine release in the brain. In the psychotic state, Kapur insists, it is not just that dopamine mediates salience, but that the rush of dopamine 'becomes a creator of saliences, albeit aberrant ones' (2003, p. 15). Salience effects may also help to explain the problem of specificity – for example, the fact that in the case of thought insertion, specific kinds of thought contents, but not all kinds, appear to be thought inserted (Gallagher, 2004b) – if specific events, things, or persons trigger the dopamine release. In effect, schizophrenics may experience a certain semantic or content consistency amid the inconsistency of their delusions. Although it is difficult to explain the problem of specificity in purely subpersonal terms (e.g. Frith's 1992 suggestion about the dysfunction of a sub-personal comparator), salience effects at the first-order level of experience may contribute to an explanation.

There remain, nonetheless, several problems with bottom-up accounts, especially if they are taken to be models for delusion in general. First, the suggested pathogenesis of delusions of control that might lead to attributing one's own actions to another person does not necessarily lead beyond that to the extravagant delusional narratives that one can find in schizophrenia. In effect, experiential content may not be rich enough to explain all aspects of the delusion. In the case of Capgras delusion, the experiential lack of emotion in relation to specific others does not necessarily point to anything like an impostor or substitution hypothesis. It may be possible that via an anomalous perception, the other person actually looks unreal, fake, like a fake spouse, or like a statue, or robot-like. As Matthew Ratcliffe (private correspondence) points out, there are frequent references in the literature to robots and aliens, rather than just impostors. The experiential content may actually be 'this entity is an impostor spouse' rather than 'this perceived p is not that remembered q'. It also seems possible that delusional content is added by some kind of top-down confabulation, although as I noted above, there seems no motivation to arrive at just this specific delusional idea rather than some other conclusion (*pace* Sass, 2004).

Precisely these kinds of considerations have motivated the two-factor approaches. One can take seriously the idea that experience itself may be delusional, but that top-down contributories enhance the delusion or take it to the more extravagant extremes. Kapur, for example, feels the necessity to invoke a two-stage, top-down process for completing the full-blown generation of the delusion, claiming that, '. . . once symptoms are manifest, delusions are essentially disorders of inferential logic . . .' and that delusions are 'a "top-down" cognitive explanation that the individual imposes on these experiences of aberrant salience in an effort to make sense of them' (Kapur, p. 15).

Still, this account does not succeed in explaining why the delusions have the specific thematic content that they do.

13.4 **The multiple realities hypothesis**

A standard but narrow view of the cognitive system that takes it to be composed of a brain which produces experience and higher-order cognitive events (often modelled as propositional attitudes) can be contrasted to a broader view that understands the experiencing subject as a brain–body–environment system. Both the top-down and bottom-up models are predicated on the standard view. If in all cases, dysfunctions in the brain ultimately cause delusional mental states, these accounts never go beyond experiential or propositional outcomes. They remain, as the theorists rightly put it, either empiricist or rationalistic, and narrowly so. In either case, everything of importance happens 'in the head'. In contrast, in the spirit of embodied, situated, and phenomenological views of cognition, I want to propose an alternative model.[6]

A hint of this alternative view can be found in Jaspers, who explicitly dismisses what today is the orthodox conception of delusion:

> To say simply that a delusion is a mistaken idea which is firmly held by the patient and which cannot be corrected gives only a superficial and incorrect answer to the problem . . . [A]ll experience of reality [. . .] has a root in the practice of living . . . Delusion proper [. . .] implies a transformation in our total awareness of reality.
>
> (Jaspers, 1913/1963, pp. 93–94)

The alternative model begins with the idea that the experiencing subject is *in-the-world*, in the way that phenomenologists like Heidegger and Merleau-Ponty define this. That is, the subject is not first and foremost an intellectual creature who perceives the world objectively and then formulates her beliefs about this, and accordingly acts upon those beliefs. Rather, the experiencing subject is first and foremost an embodied pragmatic agent who finds herself already physically, affectively, and socially situated in a world that is defined as a set of practical involvements. On this view, the 'world' is not the objectively defined physical place that we inhabit, but, in some respects, a set of affordances (Gibson) that we relate to.

Is it possible to define delusions from this perspective? To see our way to the concept of delusion on this phenomenological model, we need to borrow an idea that originally comes from William James (1890, II, pp. 291–306) but is developed further by the phenomenologist Alfred Schutz (1974, pp. 207–259). Schutz explains James's concept of 'sub-universes' in the following way. The experiencing subject does not live in the one unified world of meaning that is defined objectively (in a view from nowhere), but

---

[6] To the embodied/situated terminology, one could add enactivist models, i.e., the proposals of Varela *et al.* (1991), Hurley (1998), and the recent work of O'Regan and Noe (2001; Noe 2004). For our purposes here, however, nothing of great importance hinges on these terms. In general our approach is externalist in the sense that we want to emphasize the importance of embodied, affective, and environmental contexts that are both physical and social.

in *multiple realities*, sub-universes or finite provinces of meaning. There is, as both James and Schutz suggest, a 'paramount reality' – the reality of shared everyday life (and a set of everyday, relative language games) that we normally engage in. This is the world where we work, earn our salary, socialize, enjoy family life, and so forth. But there are also multiple other realities that take us away from everyday reality. If, for example, I read a novel, or go to the theatre or the cinema, or play a video game, I spend a couple of hours escaping into a different sort of reality which opens up in the pages, on the stage, or on the screen. In such realities, I may not have a role to play as myself, and I may identify with one or more of the characters presented in these different media. In dreams or even daydreams or various fantasies, I may more actively play a part as myself, or as a modified variation of myself, but not one that I usually play in my everyday reality.[7]

The various 'realities' (and their particular rules) are not necessarily commensurable, and my actions or virtual actions are of course different in these different realities. More basically, the changes are existential involving a transformation of background familiarity and of the sense of reality. Usually, however, I can make sense of my behaviour in these realities and can understand it from the perspective of everyday reality. I can say, 'I didn't really slay a dragon; I was playing a game.' There are normally clear transitions as I move from one reality to another. In everyday reality I can go to the theatre; once in the theatre, however, I enter a different reality. At some level, when I enter into a virtual world, such as Second Life, I keep account of the fact that from the perspective of everyday reality, I am playing a game. I can distance myself from the various roles that I might play or fantasize about. If I am truly engaged in one of these alternative realities, however, it is not simply that I adopt an alternative set of beliefs or values. Rather, I may enter into it *body and soul*, so to speak, or to some varying lesser degree. Indeed, the alternative reality has a certain 'presence' and salience that makes it more than an intellectual exercise (see Gallagher, 2006). I am *in-the-world* of the play, the film, the game, etc.; I can get excited and emotional, or remain cool under pressure; I may adopt a certain physical posture, I may act virtually (which itself requires physical movement of my body), and I may engage in such action explicitly or implicitly.[8] Sometimes, as I come back out of such realities, everyday reality can seem oddly unreal in relation to what I have been doing.

It seems quite possible that one can enter into a delusional reality just as one can enter into a dream reality, or a fictional reality, or a virtual reality. Like other multiple realities, some delusional realities are ones that are *more or less* cut off from one's everyday reality; ones that are incommensurable with the normal rules of reason that govern one's everyday normal lifeworld, and ones that offer a different set

---

7 Scientific reality may be one of these alternative realities that my work leads me to. That is, if as a physicist, in the lab or the realm of theory, I inhabit a world composed of quarks and sub-atomic particles, my affordances are quite different from the kind of affordances that define my everyday action.

8 Even when I imagine doing a certain action, my body does not remain neutral. The same motor areas of the brain activated when I act, are activated when I see someone else act, or even when I simply imagine doing the action (see Decety and Sommerville, 2003).

of affordances.[9] As Sass (1992, p. 109) puts it, the delusional subject 'inhabits a world radically alien to that of common sense.' Accordingly, *the multiple realities (MR) hypothesis* is this: when a subject enters into a delusional state, he or she is entering into an alternative reality. Unlike other multiple realities, however, this one may be 'firmly sustained . . . [and] is not one ordinarily accepted by other members of the person's culture or subculture' (*DSM-IV*). If it is firmly sustained, this may vary in degree. A dream is something that ends and too quickly dissipates as we wake up, although one sometimes revisits it; a drama comes to an end when the theatre lights come on. One can slip in and out of a delusional reality. Some delusions, however, may progress to the point where they are more like being in a theatre where the lights fail to come on. Thus delusional patients sometime report pervasive feelings of strangeness, where everything seems somehow unreal or unfamiliar (e.g. Stone and Young 1997, p. 337). Furthermore, and importantly, realities created in theatre, film, novels, and games are socially constructed realities, they are *for others*, and by definition are understandable to many people. Some delusions are more like dreams; they are in some regards idiosyncratic, or as Louis Sass (1994, 2004) puts it, 'quasi-solipsistic,' although they may share certain themes, such as being controlled by others, seeing others as impostors, and so forth. Thus, although delusions are not 'for others' they do not exclude others from appearing within the delusional reality.

To think of delusions in terms of multiple realities is not to rule out a slightly different way of putting it, namely, that delusion involves a radical or structural (or existential) change in the way that the subject relates to everyday reality. In Capgras delusion, for example, although rare, a subject may consider a set of tools as having been replaced by exact doubles (Ellis, 1996). One might say that the tools remain part of the person's everyday reality, but that her relation to the tools has been radically reconfigured (see, e.g. Dreyfus 1987; also Kafka, 1989). This may in some cases be a more apt description than saying that the person has entered into a delusional reality where her tools have been replaced by replicas. The difference in the way of putting this, however, reflects how comprehensive or pervasive, or 'firmly sustained' the delusion is or to what extent the subject's interactions with objects in everyday reality are close to normal. For example, the subject may still uses the tools as tools

---

[9] Both James and Schutz hint that psychopathological delusion could constitute a sub-universe or reality, but neither develops this idea. Kafka (1989) uses the term 'multiple realities' in the context of clinical psychoanalysis, but cites neither James nor Schutz. In contrast to them, he conceives of multiple realities as different organizations of everyday reality, or what he calls different 'reality organizations.' But he comes closer to the Schutzian concept when he describes schizophrenic patients who between bouts of psychotic episodes are able to live normal and relatively productive lives. Concerning the idea that delusional realities offer different affordances, consider a description offered by Renee, a schizophrenic patient cited by Sass (1992, p. 118; originally cited in *Autobiography of a Schizophrenic Girl* (Sechehaye 1968): A jug appeared to her 'not as something to hold water and milk, a chair not as something to sit in – but as having lost their names, their functions and meanings; they became "things" and began to take on life, to exist.'

rather than treat the tools as instruments with magical powers. In extreme cases, however, the delusional reality rather than everyday reality becomes paramount.

In contrast to the *DSM-IV* definition, a delusion is not 'a false belief based on incorrect inference about external reality'. To consider a delusion to be merely a belief is, as Jaspers suggested, to abstract it from something much richer – something that the delusional subject experiences and lives through. To consider a delusion to be a framework belief or the result of a dysfunctional introspection about something in everyday (external or objective) reality, is not just to remain too cognitive; it may also target the wrong world. The delusion may not be about external or everyday reality, but may be tied to an alternative reality, in the same way that events that take place in a play are tied to a fictional reality.[10] If I believe that Hamlet killed Polonius, this is not a false belief about the objective world; if you tried your best to convince me that Hamlet did not kill Polonius because neither Hamlet nor Polonius existed, I would think that you were either practising your metaphysical wit or going a bit mad. The MR hypothesis does have something to say about belief in the case of delusion, however. If I am able to maintain an objective perspective on the fact that I am in a theatre or playing a game, etc., it is because in some sense I have suspended my belief about the ontological actuality of the particular world opened up by the play or the game. The delusional subject seemingly enters into the delusional world without this suspension of belief. The delusional subject may take on a number of beliefs (or even a framework belief) about the delusional reality, beliefs that may be true of the delusional reality even as they are false with regard to everyday reality. In terms of belief, however, this is not the primary problem. The primary problem is the failure to suspend belief in the ontological actuality of the delusional reality.

---

[10] That delusions are not composed of false beliefs or propositions about the everyday world can be seen in the accounts that many schizophrenics give of their delusions. Sass (1992, pp. 113, 116) remarks on just this point, and provides some examples. 'In the famous memoir of his psychosis, for example, Daniel Paul Schreber describes what he calls his "so-called delusional system" in terms very different from those used by his psychiatrist. He does not, in fact, make claims about actual characteristics of the objective, external or consensual world– the sort of statements that could be shown to be false by reference to evidence independent of the experiences in question. Thus, when he describes a delusional belief about himself, he typically says not "I am a scoffer at God" or "I am given to voluptuous excesses", but, rather, I am "represented" [*dargestellt*] . . . as one of these things. In one passage, Schreber even talks about . . . being "subjectively certain" . . . that his body manifests female organs. Similarly, another patient described the objects he hallucinated as appearing in "their own private space peculiar to themselves"; the sight of such objects could not, he said, be blocked by real objects, nor could they appear simultaneously with real ones . . . For a patient to believe such a thing would imply a profoundly altered conception of the everyday physical world–of those laws of gravity, object constancy, or spatial organization that preclude material objects from flying about, materializing instantaneously, or existing inside one's skull. If such were the case, one would expect profound confusion or mistakenness about the physical world; whereas in fact schizophrenics are usually well-oriented and quite capable of practical activity when this is called for.'

To consider a delusion to be an alternative reality, in the sense defined by Schutz, requires that we see it, neither as a set of false beliefs about the objective or everyday world, nor as merely a set of odd beliefs about an alternative world. Rather, it is primarily something experiential. As such the MR hypothesis does not require that we give up either the component of neurological dysfunction or the component of cognitive dysfunction, since being-in such a world would involve all of this, and more.

As Heidegger defines being-in-the-world, it entails a threefold existential structure. One fold of this structure involves the idea of attunement (*Befindlichkeit*) which Heidegger cashes out as a certain kind of affectivity that manifests itself as mood.[11] We can think of attunement as a fundamental kind of emotional stance and link this idea up with some suggestions made by Eilan (2000), taking things somewhat beyond the notion of framework propositions. Commenting on the structural feature reflected in framework propositions, she remarks that it 'could indeed capture at least one sense in which one might want to say, with Jaspers that the schizophrenic's *worlds* are different' (109). She also suggests that at least in some cases, the schizophrenic's occupation of a delusional world comes along with the subject's finding herself affectively attuned in a very idiosyncratic way. Eilan recounts the reports of a schizophrenic who was delusional about bombs falling on her, but not on others around her:

> The bombs were directed at her in a way that made the rest of the world, her family and friends, wholly irrelevant. What brought home the awfulness of this fear, its otherworldliness, was her response to the question of whether her past delusions felt continuous with her current life, with her autobiographical sense of who she is. The answer was that they were completely continuous, and what was clear was that the connection with the present was through the live horror the delusions embodied.

> (Eilan, pp. 111–112)

The continuity expressed here between this delusional world and her everyday reality suggests that the delusional world was framed not by a mere proposition, but by a strong attunement at an affective (emotional) level.[12] This delusional world was more real, more salient, than the everyday world inhabited by her relatives and friends. Yet, were her friends to voice their agreement about fearing the bombs, the subject would likely find that odd, as Young (1998) suggests, because they are not part of the delusional world in that way.

---

[11] Heidegger (1968; see 2001). Medard Boss (1979), a psychiatrist who developed a Heideggerian approach to psychiatry, writes: 'The prevailing attunement is at any given time the condition of our openness for perceiving and dealing with what we encounter.... What we call moods, feelings, affects, emotions, and states are the concrete modes in which the possibilities for being open are fulfilled. They are at the same time the modes in which this perceptive openness can be narrowed, distorted, or closed off' (p. 110). In effect, various kinds of attunement open up possible ways of relating to the world, and close off others. This Heideggerian approach to psychopathology has not previously been framed in terms of multiple realities, which might also be understood as possible ways of relating to the world.

[12] See Ratcliffe (2004), and e.g. Green *et al.* (2006) and Freeman and Garety (2003) for the connection between emotion and delusion.

The level of detachment from everyday reality (or the feeling of irreality that characterizes many delusions) may vary from one form of delusion and one delusional subject to the next. On the one hand, the Capgras patient who claims that his wife is an impostor when he sees her, may, in some cases, be perfectly accepting of her when he speaks with her on the phone. On the other hand, the feeling is not restricted to perception of the person who seems to be the impostor; it colours the world more generally. Thus Capgras patients 'commonly report more pervasive feelings of strangeness, loss of affective response, and feelings that everything is somehow unreal or unfamiliar' (Stone and Young 1997, p. 337), and 'when questioned carefully, they report a more widespread feeling that things have changed in a way that makes them seem not quite right – strange, somehow unfamiliar, almost unreal' (Young 2000, p. 59). The schizophrenic who is emperor of the world and all-powerful in his delusional world, in his everyday world completely lacks power and is incapable of acting in accordance with his delusional self. The Cotard patient is dead and rotting in the delusional world, but eats and lives in everyday reality. Cotard patients may complain of 'feelings of derealisation,' and 'more general feelings of unreality' (Young and Leafhead 1996, p. 155). In some cases, the delusional world displaces everyday reality, and becomes paramount; and in others it is more or less detached from everyday reality, which remains paramount to some degree.

A second fold of being-in-the-world is what Heidegger calls understanding (*Verstehen*) and is manifested in terms of a process in which we are always and already projecting meaning onto things and events, and planning our actions. Certain kinds of attunement, however, can disrupt this kind of projective understanding – paralysing it (in the case of psychotic depression, for example), or making it more intense (as in the case of existential *Angst*), and in either case making various entities (even of the most ordinary type) within the world more salient than they necessarily are. This kind of aberrant saliency, which is more than a cognitive error and may reflect abnormal levels of dopamine (Kapur, 2003), may characterize certain features of the delusional reality.

The third fold, which Heidegger associates with expression (*Aussage*), brings us closer to the cognitive level, and indeed very close to Campbell's model, if we think of delusional framework propositions as expressive of the kind of being-in-the-world experienced by the delusional subject. The subject's everyday speech may very well be nonsensical from the perspective of the socially constituted everyday reality that most of us live in most of the time, but it is so because it is closely tied to the affective attunement and understanding that puts him in the delusional reality. The subject expresses the logic of the delusional reality from the perspective of that reality. From the perspective of our everyday, shared reality, this may very well be (more or less) non-sensible. This is not reducible to simply having inconsistent or conflicting beliefs – something that, to a certain degree, may occur in non-pathological subjects. It is more like living in a different world, which may or may not come into conflict with one's everyday world.

13.5 Solving some problems

Does the MR hypothesis give us a better understanding of delusion? Again, the aim here is not to offer the MR hypothesis as an explanation. It is certainly more descriptive than explanatory. The proposal, however, is that it can function to stage or frame the proper explanatory account.[13] The MR hypothesis is consistent with something like a hybrid account that incorporates both top-down and bottom-up explanations, since it does not rule out explanatory contributions in terms of brain dysfunction or higher-order cognition. But the MR hypothesis importantly includes other contributories – embodied, social, affective, and environmental factors. The concept of a delusional reality on this account is defined across all of these factors.

Can this hypothesis help in exploring related theoretical issues (I leave aside more practical or therapeutic issues, but see Kuipers *et al.*, 2006 for related discussion)? Does this broader view offer any theoretical purchase for developing a more adequate account of delusions? Does it solve any of the troublesome issues that bottom-up and top-down explanations seem unable to solve?

One problem that neither bottom-up nor top-down accounts are able to explain is what Sass (1994) calls the *double-bookeeping paradox* connected with schizophrenic delusions. As mentioned above, many schizophrenics are preoccupied with their delusions, but nonetheless treat these delusions with a certain distance or irony. In the MR hypothesis, the possibility of gaining distance from or taking an ironic attitude towards the delusion can be explained to the extent that the subject is able to consider the delusion from the perspective of everyday shared reality. That is, they may be unable to maintain distance as they are caught up in the delusional reality, but to the extent that they can shift back to everyday reality, they may be able to feel the strangeness of the delusion. This may also explain why a patient can view doctors and nurses as poisoners (in delusional reality) but happily eat the food they give her (in everyday reality), or why a patient who treats people as phantoms or automatons (in delusional reality) still interacts with them as if they were real (in everyday reality). What needs to be investigated here is the frequency and degree to which a patient can shift between multiple realities as they move in and out of delusional states, the nature of the transitions, whether this shifting is more frequent in prodromal cases, or in cases of partial remission, and so on.

A second problem involves the *extravagantly complex nature* of some delusional narratives. This is something that bottom-up accounts are unable to address. In effect, experiential content considered merely in terms of odd sensory-motor processes or simple feelings, even if they can explain the loss of the sense of agency, or the feeling of alterity, are not rich enough to explain all aspects of the delusion. Top-down accounts might suggest that this complexity is found fully within the subject's delusional belief system, but beliefs that are consciously explicated (as in delusion) usually need some kind of support to be sustained. Everyday reality and the things that make up our normal everyday life do not offer this kind of support but instead show up the contradictions of delusion. A delusion that starts out in a prodromal experience as a

---

[13] There may be some worry about how to cash out the MR hypothesis in scientific terms. We hope it is clear that the concept of delusional reality is not cashed out purely in neurophysiological terms; it involves intersubjective and normative dimensions that depend on physical, social, and cultural environments. Our intention in this paper, however, is not to work out all of the details of this alternative approach to the question of delusions.

simple feeling of alien forces can develop in complexity if there is a different way to be-in-the-world, a different experiential framework, an alternative reality where it can grow and find support.

The idea that certain emotional states or certain social or environmental factors might set off the delusional experience could also help to address the *problem of specificity* in schizophrenic delusions, for example. Why is a subject delusional with regard to some topics but not delusional with regard to everything he believes, or why are some actions or thoughts considered alien, but not others? Neither bottom-up nor top-down explanations on their own seem able to explain this. For example, a schizophrenic who has delusions about thought insertion will report that a particular person inserts certain thoughts, which are always about a specified topic. Such patients often feel controlled by specific others or by machines and in very specific ways (see, e.g. Bovet and Parnas, 1993). A bottom-up explanation in terms of brain dysfunction does not entirely resolve this, since brain dysfunction is not usually something that turns on or off without some other factor being involved. If the other factor is simply another sub-personal mechanism, then delusions should be randomly about anything, rather than, with a certain degree of consistency, about specific topics or things. Why, in particular cases of Capgras delusion, for example, would a patient think only her husband, but not her children or other people, to be an impostor? (Passer and Warnock, 1991). If it is a matter of disrupted connections between the face-recognition area of the brain and the limbic system (Ramachandran), why would such connections be specific for only one or a few people rather than all familiar people?[14]

In the MR hypothesis, the specificity may in fact be tied to (or motivated by) the experiential presence of social or environmental factors encountered in everyday reality, factors that transition the subject into the delusional reality. Emotional reactions to such specific worldly experiences may trigger the sub-personal dysfunction.[15] For delusional subjects, in the presence of certain significant individuals, but not others, or in certain kinds of situations but not others, or confronted with

----

[14] Capgras delusions most often occur alongside other psychotic symptoms in disorders like schizophrenia, Alzheimer's etc. The face-recognition-affect account may be relevant to an unusual, 'local' form of Capgras, and may not generalize to all cases. Lisa Bortolotti (private correspondence) indicates that the commonest form of delusional misidentification, especially in dementia, is for place, e.g. this is not a hospital but the hotel we stay in on holiday.

[15] There is growing evidence for the connection between social and physical environments, emotion, and delusion. Freeman and Garety (2003) note a link between emotional disturbance in the onset of psychosis and social and cultural factors. 'The role of social and cultural factors in the development of psychosis has recently been highlighted by the finding of higher rates of psychosis in [a variety of immigrant groups] ... [These] findings have been linked with socio-demographic variables such as living in inner-cities, unemployment, living alone, fewer social contacts, and also with the effects of racism (see review by Sharpley, Hutchinson, Murray, & McKenzie, 2001). It is plausible to speculate that these variables, reflecting social deprivation and adversity, may create emotional distress and enduring negative schemas, particularly about other people, which leave individuals especially vulnerable to developing distressing psychotic beliefs.' Also see Ellett *et al.* (2008) and Garety *et al.* (2007). In addition, Raune *et al.* (2006) stress the connection between stressful events and psychosis.

certain objects, or on the occasion of an unbidden thought, a resulting unruly emotion (anxiety or fear, for example) might trigger the brain dysfunction. The force of the emotion, if not consciously experienced, might be cashed out in terms of embodiment – in measurable autonomic processes, for example, and may show up phenomenologically as a certain way of being-in-the-world.

One other thing that needs to be explained here is not that there are specific differences from one person's delusions to the next – such differences are to be expected – but rather the fact that there are shared types of delusions. Many schizophrenics complain about alien control; all Cotard patients claim that they are dead; all Capgras patients fall upon the impostor or substitution explanation. Each group shares type but not token realities. Bottom-up approaches suggest possible areas of brain damage that can open the door to a delusional reality of that sort for the subject, and can, at the same time, for the scientist, make sense out of some typical aspects of schizophrenic delusions of control (lack of a sense of agency, feeling of alterity). Neural explanations of Cotard and Capgras delusions are less clear. The MR hypothesis suggests that we examine certain shared features of our cultural environments (our other multiple realities) that may lead to the particular types found in delusion. Why there are typical kinds of delusions may call for the same kind of answer that we would give to the question of why there are typical scenarios developed in pretend games and imaginary play in childhood, or 'universal' literary themes found in novels, plays, and other media.

13.6 Conclusion

The MR hypothesis suggests that delusions are more than false beliefs, or even very complex belief systems; they are more than disorders of inferential logic; they are more than what can be explained by a problematic framework proposition. Although one can say that delusions involve delusional experiences, the concept of delusional experience seems inadequate to account for many of the more complex and extravagant aspects of delusion. The MR hypothesis is an attempt to provide an explanatory framework (although not a explanation) that can integrate both the top-down and bottom-up aspects of delusion into a broader account that treats other factors – body, affect, social, and environmental factors – as important in the constitution of delusional realities. As a personal-level or existential description, the MR hypothesis would surely have implications for both cognitive neuroscientific attempts to explain delusions and for psychiatric practice. At the very least, it suggests the involvement of both top-down and bottom-up processes, and that we have to think of delusions at a level that is more global than that offered by doxastic accounts.

Acknowledgements

My thanks to Jennifer Mundale, Matthew Ratcliffe, and Louis Sass for reading earlier versions of this chapter and making helpful comments. I have also benefitted from the helpful comments of the editors of this volume.

References

American Psychiatric Association (2000). *Diagnostic and Statistical Manual of Mental Disorders, Text Revision. Fourth Edition. (DSM-IV)*. Washington DC, American Psychiatric Association.

Bayne, T. and Pacherie, E. (2004). Bottom-up or top-down: Campbell's rationalist account of monothematic delusions. *Philosophy, Psychiatry and Psychology,* **11**(1), 1–11.

Bayne, T. and Pacherie, E. (2005). In defense of the doxastic conception of delusions. *Mind and Language,* **20**(2), 163–188.

Boss, M. (1979). *Existential Foundations of Medicine and Psychology* (Trs. S. Conway and A. Cleaves). New York, Jason Aronson.

Bovet, P. and Parnas, J. (1993). Schizophrenic delusions: a phenomenological approach. *Schizophrenia Bulletin,* **19**, 579–597.

Campbell, J. (2001). Rationality, meaning, and the analysis of delusion. *Philosophy, Psychiatry, and Psychology,* **8**(2,3), 89–100.

Coltheart, M. and Davies, M. (eds.) (2000). *Pathologies of Belief*. Oxford, Blackwell.

Daprati, E., Franck N., Georgieff, N., *et al.* (1997). Looking for the agent: an investigation into consciousness of action and self-consciousness in schizophrenic patients. *Cognition,* **65**, 71–86.

Davies, M., Coltheart, M., Langdon, R., and Breen, N. (2001). Monothematic delusions: towards a two-factor account. *Philosophy, Psychiatry and Psychology,* **8**(2,3), 133–158.

Decety, J. and Sommerville, J. A. (2003). Shared representations between self and other: a social cognitive neuroscience view. *Trends in Cognitive Sciences,* **7**(12), 527–533.

de Vignemont, F. and Fourneret, P. (2004). The sense of agency: a philosophical and empirical review of the "Who" system. *Consciousness and Cognition,* **13**, 1–19.

Dreyfus, H. (1987). Alternative philosophical conceptualizations of psychopathology. In *Phenomenology and Beyond: The Self and its Language* (eds. H. A. Durfee, and D. F. T. Rodier), pp. 41–50. Dordrecht, Kluwer Academic.

Eilan, N. (2000). On understanding schizophrenia. In *Exploring the Self* (ed. D. Zahavi), pp. 97–113. Amsterdam, John Benjamins.

Ellett, L., Freeman, D., and Garety, P. A. (2008). The psychological effect of an urban environment on individuals with persecutory delusions: the Camberwell walk study. *Schizophrenia Research,* **99**(1–3), 77–84.

Ellis, H. D. (1996). Delusional misidentification of inanimate objects: a literature review and neuropsychological analysis of cognitive deficits in two cases. *Cognitive Neuropsychiatry,* **1**, 27–40.

Ellis, H. D. and Young, A. W. (1990). Accounting for delusional misidentifications. *British Journal of Psychiatry,* **157**, 239–248.

Farrer, C. and Frith, C. D. (2001). Experiencing oneself vs. another person as being the cause of an action: the neural correlates of the experience of agency. *NeuroImage,* **15**, 596–603.

Farrer, C., Franck, N., Georgieff, N. Frith, C. D., Decety, J., and Jeannerod, M. (2003). Modulating the experience of agency: a positron emission tomography study. *NeuroImage,* **18**, 324–333.

Franck, N., Farrer, C., Georgieff, N. *et al.* (2001). Defective recognition of one's own actions in patients with schizophrenia. *American Journal of Psychiatry,* **158**, 454–459.

Freeman, D. and Garety, P. A. (2003). Connecting neurosis and psychosis: the direct influence of emotion on delusions and hallucinations. *Behaviour Research and Therapy,* **41**(8), 923–947.

Frith, C. (1992). *The Cognitive Neuropsychology of Schizophrenia.* Hillsdale, NJ, Lawrence Erlbaum Associates.

Gallagher, S. (2000a). Philosophical conceptions of the self: implications for cognitive science. *Trends in Cognitive Sciences,* **4**, 14–21.

Gallagher, S. (2000b). Self-reference and schizophrenia: a cognitive model of immunity to error through misidentification. In *Exploring the Self: Philosophical and Psychopathological Perspectives on Self-experience* (ed. D. Zahavi), pp. 203–239. Amsterdam and Philadelphia, PA, John Benjamins.

Gallagher, S. (2004a). Neurocognitive models of schizophrenia: a neurophenomenological critique. *Psychopathology,* **37**, 8–19.

Gallagher, S. (2004b). Agency, ownership and alien control in schizophrenia. In *The Structure and Development of Self-consciousness: Interdisciplinary Perspectives* (eds. P. Bovet, J. Parnas, and D. Zahavi), pp. 89–104. Amsterdam, John Benjamins.

Gallagher, S. (2006). Embodiment in multiple realities. Unpublished paper presented at the *Conference on "Presence".* Media and Film Science, University of Cophenhagen, June 6, 2006.

Gallagher, S. (2007). Sense of agency and higher-order cognition: levels of explanation for schizophrenia. *Cognitive Semiotics,* **0**, 32–48.

Garety, P. A., Kuipers, E., Fowler, D., Freeman, D., and Bebbington, P. E. (2001). A cognitive model of the positive symptoms of psychosis. *Psychological Medicine,* **31**, 189–195.

Garety, P. A., Bebbington, P., Fowler, D., Freeman, D., and Kuipers, E. (2007). Implications for neurobiological research of cognitive models of psychosis: a theoretical paper. *Psychological Medicine,* **37**, 1377–1391.

Georgieff, N. and Jeannerod, M. (1998). Beyond consciousness of external reality. A 'Who' system for consciousness of action and self-consciousness. *Consciousness and Cognition,* **7**, 465–477.

Gold, I. and Hohwy, J. (2000). Rationality and schizophrenic delusion. In *Pathologies of Belief* (eds. M. Coltheart, and M. Davies), pp. 145–165. Oxford, Blackwell.

Graham, G. and Stephens, G. L. (1994). Mind and mine. In *Philosophical Psychopathology* (eds. G. Graham and G. L. Stephens), pp. 91–109. Cambridge, MA, MIT Press.

Green, C., Garety, P., Freeman, D., *et al.* (2006). Content and affect in persecutory delusions. *British Journal of Clinical Psychology,* **45**(4), 561–577.

Heidegger, M. (1968). *Being and Time.* (Trs. J. Macquarrie and E. Robinson). New York, Harper and Row.

Heidegger, M. (2001). *Zollikon Seminars. Protocols- Conversations-Letters* (ed. M. Boss) (Trs. R. Askay and F. Mayr). Evanston, IL, Northwestern University Press.

Hohwy, J. (2004). Top-down and bottom-up in delusion formation. *Philosophy, Psychiatry and Psychology,* **11**, 65–70.

Hohwy, J. and Rosenberg, R. (2005). Unusual experiences, reality testing, and delusions of alien control. *Mind and Language,* **20**(2), 141–162.

Hurley, S. (1999). *Consciousness in Action.* Cambridge, MA, Harvard University Press.

James, W. (1890). *The Principles of Psychology.* New York, Dover, 1950.

Jaspers, K. (1913/1963) *General Psychopathology,* (Trs. J. Hoenig and M. W. Hamilton) Chicago, IL, University of Chicago Press.

Kafka, J. S. (1989). *Multiple Realities in Clinical Practice.* New Haven, Yale University Press.

Kapur, S. (2003). Psychosis as a state of aberrant salience: a framework linking biology, phenomenology, and pharmacology in schizophrenia. *American Journal of Psychiatry,* **160,** 13–23.

Klee, R. (2004). Why some delusions are necessarily inexplicable beliefs. *Philosophy, Psychiatry, and Psychology,* **11**(1), 25–33.

Kuipers, E., Garety, P., Fowler, D.,Freeman, D., Dunn, G., and Bebbington, P. (2006). Cognitive, emotional, and social processes in psychosis: refining cognitive behavioral therapy for persistent positive symptoms. *Schizophrenia Bulletin,* **32**(1), S24–S31.

Maher, B. (1999). Anomalous experience in everyday life: its significance for psychopathology. *The Monist,* **82,** 547–570.

Mundale, J. and Gallagher, S. (2009) Delusional experience. In *Oxford Handbook of Philosophy and Neuroscience* (ed. J. Bickle). Oxford, Oxford University Press.

Noë, A. (2004). *Action in Perception.* Cambridge, MA, MIT Press.

O'Regan, J. K. and Noe, A. (2001). A sensorimotor account of vision and visual consciousness. *Behavioral and Brain Sciences,* **24**(5), 883–975.

Pacherie, E., Green, M., and Bayne, T. (2006). Phenomenology and delusions: who put the 'alien' in alien control. *Consciousness and Cognition,* **15,** 566–577.

Parnas, J. and Sass, L. (2001). Self, solipsism, and schizophrenic delusions. *Philosophy, Psychiatry, and Psychology,* **8**(2/3), 101–120.

Passer, K. M. and Warnock, J. K. (1991). Pimozide in the treatment of Capgras' syndrome. A case report. *Psychosomatics,* **32**(4), 446–448.

Ramachandran, V. S. (1998). Consciousness and body image: lessons from phantom limbs, Capgras syndrome and pain asymbolia. *Philosophical Transactions of the Royal Society B: Biological Sciences,* **353,** 1851–1859.

Ratcliffe, M. (2004). Interpreting delusions. *Phenomenology and the Cognitive Sciences,* **3**(1), 25–48.

Raune, D., Bebbington, P. Dunn, G., and Kuipers, E. (2006). Event attributes and the content of psychotic experiences in first-episode psychosis. *Psychological* Medicine, **36**(2), 221–230.

Richardson, W. (1993). Heidegger among the doctors. In *Reading Heidegger: Commemorations* (ed. J. Sallis), pp. 49–66. Bloomington, Indiana University Press.

Sass, L. (1992). Heidegger, schizophrenia and the ontological difference. *Philosophical Psychology,* **5,** 109–132.

Sass, L. (1994). *The Paradoxes of Delusion: Wittgenstein, Schreber, and the Schizophrenic Mind.* Ithaca, NY, Cornell University Press.

Sass, L. (2004). Some reflections on the (analytic) philosophical approach to delusion. *Philosophy, Psychiatry, and Psychology,* **11**(1), 71–80.

Schutz, A. (1974). *Collected Papers Vol. 1. The Problem of Social Reality.* Dordrecht, Springer.

Sechehaye, M. (ed.) (1968). *Autobiography of a Schizophrenic Girl,* (Tr. G. Rubin-Rabson). New York, New American Library.

Sharpley, M. S., Hutchinson, G., Murray, R. M., and Mekenzie, K. (2001). Understanding the excess of psychosis among the African-Caribbean population in England: review of current hypotheses. *British Journal of Psychiatry,* **178,** S60–S68.

Singh, J. R., Knight, T., Rosenlicht, N., Kotun, J. M., Beckley, D. J., and Woods, D. L. (1992). Abnormal premovement brain potentials in schizophrenia. *Schizophrenia Research,* **8,** 31–41.

Spence, S. A., Brooks, D.J., Hirsch, S. R., Liddle, P. F., Meehan, J., and Grasby, P. M. (1997). A PET study of voluntary movement in schizophrenic patients experiencing passivity phenomena (delusions of alien control). *Brain,* **120,** 1997–2011.

Stephens, G. L. and Graham, G. (2000). *When Self-Consciousness Breaks: Alien Voices and Inserted Thoughts*. Cambridge MA, MIT Press.

Stone, T. and Young, A. (1997). Delusions and brain injury: the philosophy and psychology of belief. *Mind and Language*, 12, 327–364.

Thornton, T. (2008). Why the idea of framework propositions cannot contribute to an understanding of delusions. *Phenomenology and the Cognitive Sciences*, 7(2), 159–157.

Varela, F. J., Thompson, E., and Rosch, E. (1991). *The Embodied Mind: Cognitive Science and Human Experience*. Cambridge, MA., MIT Press.

Vogeley, K., Kurthen, M., Falkai, P., and Maier, W. (1999). The human self construct and prefrontal cortex in schizophrenia. *The Association for the Scientific Study of Consciousness: Electronic Seminar* (http://www.phil.vt.edu/assc/esem.html).

Wittgenstein, L. (1969). *On Certainty* (eds. G. E. M. Anscombe, and G. H. von Wright). (Trs D. Paul and G. E. M. Anscombe). Oxford, Blackwell.

Young, A. (1999) Delusions. *The Monist*, 82(4), 571–589.

Young, A. (2000). Wondrous strange: The neuropsychology of abnormal beliefs. In *Pathologies of Belief* (eds. M. Coltheart, and M. Davies), pp. 47–73. Oxford, Blackwell.

Section 6

Delusions and cognition

Chapter 14

Delusions: A two-level framework

Keith Frankish

Abstract

There is continuing debate about the nature of delusions and whether they are properly described as beliefs. This chapter argues that in order to make progress on this issue, we need to adopt a more complex taxonomy of psychological states and processes, building on recent work in philosophy of psychology and cognitive science. I distinguish two levels of belief, and argue that delusions, if they are beliefs at all, belong to the second of them. I go on to offer an account of second-level belief according to which it is a species of a broader mental type, sometimes called 'acceptance', which is dependent on attitudes at the first level. I then propose that delusions are acceptances, some of which fall within, and some without, the narrower class of second-level beliefs. I argue that this view explains our competing intuitions about delusions and that it has important implications for understanding deluded patients.

14.1 Introduction

Although well-documented, delusions have proved extremely hard to explain, and many important questions remain open, including the basic one of what kind of mental state a delusion is. The standard position is that delusions are beliefs (the *doxastic conception*); but there are difficulties for this view, and alternative characterizations have been offered. In this chapter, I shall propose a new framework for conceptualizing delusions, building on recent work in philosophy of psychology and cognitive science. There are good reasons for thinking that the term 'belief' is commonly used to refer to two different types of mental states, located at different levels. This view harmonizes with work in the psychology of reasoning, where many researchers now endorse some form of *dual-system* theory. I shall outline what is, I believe, the most attractive version of this two-level view and show how it offers an account of delusions that explains our competing intuitions about their status.

The chapter is in four sections. The first introduces the doxastic conception and its problems. The second distinguishes the two levels of belief, and argues that delusions, if they are beliefs at all, belong to the second. The third section offers an account of second-level belief according to which it is a species of a broader mental type, *acceptance*, which is dependent on attitudes at the first level. The fourth section proposes that delusions are acceptances, some of which fall within, and some without, the narrower class of second-level beliefs, and the chapter concludes with some reflections on the implications of this view. Throughout, I shall focus on monothematic delusions, rather than the elaborate polythematic kind, and use simple, schematic examples. This is not because I think it is unimportant to pay attention to the diversity of delusions and the detail of clinical observation (far from it). Rather, it reflects the modest aim of the chapter, which is to sketch a hypothesis for subsequent elaboration and evaluation.

14.2 **The doxastic conception and its problems**

People suffering from delusions make strange claims. To take three well-known examples, patients with the Cotard delusion claim that they are dead, those with the Capgras delusion claim that a loved one has been replaced by an impostor, and those with the Fregoli delusion claim that someone they know is disguising themselves as other people. Do they believe these things, as the doxastic conception has it? The standard view, enshrined in DSM-IV, is that they do: a delusion is defined as a false belief which is firmly held despite incontrovertible evidence and which is not shared by others in one's community (American Psychiatric Association, 2000, p. 821).

Prima facie, this is a plausible view. Deluded patients make their claims firmly and with apparent sincerity, and seem to understand the meanings of the words involved (Bayne and Pacherie, 2004a; Hamilton, 2007). Speech acts of this kind are standardly taken as expressions of belief, and the subjects themselves appear to take them that way. Moreover, it is precisely because deluded patients seem to believe their claims that we find their condition so bizarre and disturbing. Imagining or wishing that one is dead is not as strange a condition as believing that one is dead (though it might still be worrying). And although it is hard to see how a person could come to believe that they are dead, the content of such a delusion is not much stranger than that of some religious beliefs, which are widely accepted and therefore not considered delusional.

The doxastic conception has its difficulties, however, and many writers have stressed the differences between delusions and beliefs. Four stand out. First, delusions are often unsupported by reasons; deluded patients either offer no reasons for their claims or offer inappropriate ones (Campbell, 2001; Hamilton, 2007). Second, delusions tend to be relatively cognitively inert; deluded patients often fail to draw obvious conclusions from their delusions and are not bothered by the lack of consistency between them and their other beliefs (Breen *et al.*, 2000; Brett-Jones *et al.*, 1987). Third, delusions may be relatively behaviourally inert; many deluded patients do not consistently act on their delusions, and their assertions are often at odds with their non-verbal behaviour (Bovet and Parnas, 1993; Currie, 2000; Hamilton, 2007; Sass, 1994; Young, 2000). Some Capgras patients, for example, continue to live on friendly terms with the supposed impostor (for data, see Young, 2000, p. 53). Indeed, as Hamilton notes, in the case of some bizarre delusions, it will often be *impossible* to act on them (Hamilton, 2007). Finally, delusions often lack the emotional associations the corresponding beliefs would normally have (Sass, 1994).

These differences should not be overstated. It is arguable that some deluded patients *do* have evidence for their claims, in the shape of distorted perceptual inputs (e.g. Davies *et al.*, 2001; Maher, 1999; Stone and Young, 1997). And delusions are certainly not *completely* inert (Buchanan and Wessely, 1998). Deluded patients typically report their delusions, and they sometimes act on them in other ways – even with violence. (This is often what brings them to the attention of the medical services.) But it is widely agreed that delusions are somehow compartmentalized and not fully integrated into the subject's belief system. Jaspers, for example, noted that a patient's attitude to the content of their delusion is 'peculiarly inconsequent at times' (Jaspers, 1913/1997, p. 105), and Young refers to the 'curiously circumscribed quality' of delusions (2000, p. 49).

The issue here is not merely taxonomic, but bears on the question of whether we can make sense of delusions – whether deluded patients can be brought within the 'interpretive fold' (Bayne and Pacherie, 2004b). Even if we allow that deluded subjects do in some sense believe their claims, it is doubtful that we could form any empathic understanding of their state of mind if these beliefs are not subject to the usual rational constraints and do not have the usual sensitivity to evidence and influence on action.

Not everyone agrees that these considerations refute the doxastic conception, of course, even if they are granted. It is arguable, for example, that many non-delusional beliefs are also compartmentalized and held in violation of rational norms (Bortolotti, 2005). Some theorists, however, regard the doxastic conception as unsustainable, and propose alternatives to it. John Campbell argues that delusions express 'framework propositions', which are immune from questioning and set the context for reasoning and the interpretation of experience (Campbell, 2001). Greg Currie and his collaborators propose a *meta-cognitive* account, according to which delusions are imaginings which those experiencing them misidentify as beliefs: deluded patients believe that they believe their claims (which is why they assert them), but in fact only imagine them (which is why they do not act upon them) (Currie, 2000; Currie and Jureidini, 2001; Currie and Ravenscroft, 2002). Others take a more pessimistic line. Andy Hamilton argues that there is no fact of the matter about whether or not deluded patients believe their claims, since the verbal and non-verbal behavioural criteria for the ascription of belief do not cohere (Hamilton, 2007). German Berrios claims that delusional claims are simply 'empty speech acts that disguise themselves as beliefs' (Berrios, 1991, p. 8).

Now an important thing to note about this debate is that it is as much about belief as it is about delusion. The concept of belief is a folk-psychological one, defined by its role within our everyday practices of psychological explanation and prediction. But there is disagreement about what this role is, and different views on the matter have different implications for the doxastic conception. One basic contrast concerns the function of folk psychology itself. On an 'interpretivist' view, folk psychology has a rationalizing function, and ascriptions of beliefs and desires are made as part of an overall interpretation of a subject which aims to render their behaviour rationally intelligible in the light of their experience (e.g. Davidson, 1984; Dennett, 1987). Thus, in this view, to regard a person as the subject of mental states is precisely to bring them within the interpretive fold. This view does not harmonize well with the doxastic conception; if there are strict rational constraints on belief ascription, then we will not be warranted in ascribing beliefs that are unsupported, inconsistent, and partially inert. Indeed, given that interpretation is governed by a principle of charity, it is hard to see how we could ever be justified in interpreting a person as believing a very bizarre content, such that of Cotard's delusion, as opposed to merely believing (say) that it will help to *claim* to believe it.

In the 'theory–theory' view, by contrast, folk psychology is a rudimentary science of the mind, and mental-state concepts refer to internal states of our cognitive systems (e.g. Lewis, 1972). This approach is more compatible with the doxastic conception; when we consider the structure and limitations of the human cognitive system, the rational constraints on belief ascription appear weaker and the doxastic conception correspondingly more plausible (Bayne and Pacherie, 2005).

It is usually assumed that we must decide between these different views of the nature of belief, but this may be a mistake. There is a strong case for thinking that the everyday concept of belief picks out two distinct states with different properties. If so, this may go some way towards explaining and reconciling our competing intuitions about the function of folk psychology and, consequently, about the doxastic status of delusions. The next section outlines the case for this view.

14.3 Two types of belief

There are certain core elements to the concept of belief. Beliefs have propositional content; they have mind-to-world direction of fit (they represent their contents as obtaining, rather than as to be made to obtain); and they guide behaviour in a way that reflects their content and direction of fit. But there are also tensions within the concept of belief which suggest that it may not pick out a unitary state. I shall mention four of these. Note that what follows applies to *non-perceptual* beliefs; perceptual beliefs are a special case, and I shall not discuss them here.

The first tension concerns consciousness. On the one hand, we think of beliefs as part of the furniture of our conscious minds, to which we have direct introspective access. They are things we have thought about and endorsed, which we rely on in our conscious reasoning, and which we would avow if prompted. On the other hand, we also possess a mass of beliefs which we have never thought about, which operate silently, in the background, and which we are only indirectly aware of possessing. Think, for example, of the huge corpus of knowledge about the location and function of household objects which guides your behaviour around the house (where the cupboards are, how the taps work, which way the fridge door opens, and so on). Our behaviour shows that we have this knowledge, but we have no introspective awareness of it, and often the only way to access it is to imagine ourselves performing some relevant action (say, opening the fridge door), and noting how we do it (James, 1890, chapter 4).

The second tension relates to control. We often speak of ourselves as having a degree of direct control over our beliefs: we talk of *deciding* what to think and *making up* our minds. The idea is that we can consider a proposition, reflect upon the evidence for and against it, and then decide whether to give, or withhold, assent to it. (This is not to say that we can choose to believe anything we like; we can assent to a proposition only if we have good epistemic support for it; see Frankish, 2007.) Similarly, we can decide to revise or reject beliefs we no longer regard as warranted. Yet, not all beliefs are susceptible to this kind of reflective control; many are formed and modified automatically, by sub-personal processes over which we have no direct control.

The third tension concerns degree. We usually think of belief as a binary, or flat-out, attitude: we either believe something or we do not. Yet we also speak of people having degrees of confidence, which are continuously variable, and much of our behaviour can be interpreted as the upshot of probabilistic reasoning involving these states (e.g. Oaksford and Chater, 2007). Desire, too, can be thought of as either an on-off binary state or a matter of graded preference.

The final tension relates to the ontological status of belief, where, simplifying somewhat, we can distinguish functionalist and dispositionalist views. In the former, beliefs are functionally discrete states of the cognitive system, which are selectively activated in reasoning (e.g. Fodor, 1987; Ramsey *et al.*, 1990); in the latter, they are multi-track behavioural dispositions, which are holistically interdependent (e.g. Dennett, 1987; Ryle, 1949). By focusing on different aspects of folk-psychological practice, a strong case can be made for each view.

The importance of these tensions is often underrated. Typically, theorists assume that there is just one form of belief, and either dismiss one side of each tension or argue that it corresponds to a superficial variant of the core state. This is, I think, a mistake. I have argued elsewhere that the tensions are real and run deep (Frankish, 2004, 2009a). Moreover, the contrasting views of belief line up, suggesting that they correspond to two distinct forms of the state. The controlled/automatic contrast coincides with that between conscious and nonconscious; only our conscious beliefs are susceptible to direct reflective control. The binary/graded contrast also lines up with the conscious/nonconscious one. Conscious belief is typically binary: we either avow belief or withhold it, and our conscious reasoning usually proceeds from categorical premises to categorical conclusions. (Even when we form conscious beliefs about probabilities, such as that there is a 50% chance of rain, the *attitude* is unqualified.) Our degrees of confidence and preference, on the other hand, like our background knowledge, are unavailable to introspection and influence our behaviour at a nonconscious level. Finally, a functionalist view is required for conscious belief, whereas the intuitions supporting a dispositionalist position are best construed as relating to nonconscious belief. Conscious beliefs are functionally discrete (they can be selectively acquired, recalled, and lost), and they require activation in order to influence action (if we fail to recall a belief – if it *slips our mind* – then it has no effect on our behaviour). However, there is no reason to think that nonconscious beliefs have these properties, and indeed it seems unlikely. Implicit beliefs typically come in clusters, and they influence action in a holistic way – think of the mass of background knowledge that is relevant to even very simple everyday actions.

So we can tentatively distinguish two types of belief: one (call it *level 1*) that is a nonconscious, passive, graded, dispositional state, and another (*level 2*) that is a conscious, controlled, binary, functional state. (I shall say more, later, about why talk of levels is appropriate here.) A formally similar distinction can be made for desire.

There are precedents for this division within the category of belief. Daniel Dennett distinguishes between belief and opinion (Dennett, 1978, chapter 16), corresponding roughly to level 1 and level 2 belief, and some philosophers of science draw a distinction between belief and acceptance, which I shall discuss in the next section. The division also harmonizes well with recent work in both cognitive and social psychology, where many researchers have converged on some form of *dual-system* theory, according to which humans have two distinct systems for reasoning and decision making, often referred to as *System 1* and *System 2* (e.g. Evans, 2003; Evans and Over, 1996; Kahneman and Frederick, 2002; Sloman, 1996; Stanovich, 2004; see also Evans and Frankish, 2009). Theorists differ on the details, but the typical picture is as follows. System 1 is a collection of autonomous subsystems, many shared with animals, whose operations are nonconscious, automatic, fast, parallel, associative, heavily contextualized, and undemanding of working memory. System 2, by contrast, is a uniquely human system, whose processes are conscious, controlled, slow, serial, rule-governed, decontextualized, and demanding of working memory. Such theories were originally developed to account for well-documented conflicts between logical and non-logical processes in deductive reasoning tasks and between avowed attitudes and actual behaviour in social contexts, but they can also explain many other phenomena, including individual differences in reasoning, cross-cultural variation in cognition, and aspects of cognitive development (see the papers by, respectively, Stanovich, Buchtel and Norenzayan, and Klaczynski, in Evans and Frankish, 2009).

Dual-system theorists typically assume that the two reasoning systems have separate databases, and it is attractive to link the two types of belief we have distinguished with the two systems – level 1 belief with System 1 and level 2 belief with System 2. (Of course, if level 1 beliefs are behavioural dispositions, then we cannot identify them with the *inputs* to System 1 reasoning; that would be a category mistake. The inputs will be sub-personal informational states of some kind, which lie outside the purview of folk psychology. But level 1 beliefs can be seen as *manifestations* of System 1 activity and the associated sub-personal informational states.) This view is further bolstered by social–psychological work on persuasion and attitude change, where many theorists distinguish implicit and explicit memory systems, the former nonconscious, automatic, and slow-learning, the latter conscious, effortful, and fast-learning (e.g. Wilson *et al.*, 2000; Smith and DeCoster, 2000). Again, this distinction aligns well with that between the two types of beliefs; level 1 beliefs are typically slow to form and change, whereas level 2 beliefs can be formed and revised in one-off episodes. Consider, for example, what happens when normal background conditions suddenly change, as when a light bulb blows. We immediately form the level 2 belief that the bulb is blown and, consequently, that the light switch will not work; but on entering the room we still press the light switch, manifesting a level 1 belief that it will work.

This is, of course, only a sketch of the case for the level 1/level 2 distinction, and there is much more to be said about the relation between this distinction and related ones in scientific psychology (see my 2009b). But it is a useful working hypothesis and I now want to consider its implications for the doxastic conception of delusions.

Three points need to be made. First, although the two types of belief often go together, they are dissociable. We can believe something in a nonconscious way without consciously assenting to it, and we can consciously assent to something without it penetrating to the nonconscious level and affecting our spontaneous behaviour. (Strictly speaking, if level 1 belief is graded it would be better to say that we can believe something at a conscious level while believing it only *very weakly* at the nonconscious level; on Bayesian principles a rational agent will have some degree of confidence in every relevant proposition of whose falsity they are not certain. For simplicity's sake, however, I shall often speak as if level 1 belief were binary.) Indeed, we can harbour conflicting attitudes at the two levels. The light bulb case is an example, and the social–psychological literature contains abundant evidence of conflict between implicit and explicit evaluative attitudes. In such cases, the non-verbal behavioural criteria for belief may be seriously out of step with the verbal criteria.

Second, delusions fit the distinctive profile of level 2 belief better than that of level 1 belief. Delusional reports are conscious, and they manifest attitudes that are binary, discrete, and at least available to reflective control, however hard it may be for the subject to exercise it. Indeed, it is hard to make sense of the notion of an *implicit* delusional belief.[1] The relative behavioural inertia of delusions reinforces the classification of delusions at level 2, since level 2 beliefs have a more restricted influence on action than level 1 beliefs. In order to influence action, level 2 beliefs must be activated in episodes of conscious thought, whereas level 1 beliefs manifest themselves in spontaneous, unreflective behaviour.

Third, the distinction between level 1 and level 2 belief aligns with the two views of the function of folk psychology mentioned earlier. If we focus on level 1 belief, then an interpretivist perspective is called for. To have a level 1 belief with content p is to be disposed to behave in ways that would be rational if p were true; so, being consistently interpretable as possessing a given level 1 belief is both necessary and sufficient for possessing it. When we focus on level 2 belief, on the other hand, a theory–theory perspective is appropriate. These beliefs are functional states of the cognitive system, which can be selectively activated and which are subject to selective failures of activation (slips of mind). It follows, then, that the rational constraints on the ascription of level 2 beliefs are much weaker than those on the ascription of the level 1 kind. Thus the relative inertia of delusions tells strongly against their being level 1 beliefs, but much less strongly against their being level 2 beliefs.

The moral of this for the doxastic conception is obvious. Delusions may be beliefs of one type but not the other, and the evidence suggests they are not level 1 beliefs. So if delusional claims are believed, it will be at level 2 only. (Or at least, this is plausible

---

[1] Matthew Broome has pointed out to me that when patients are very ill, they may become mute and posturing, so that it is no longer easy to attribute delusions to them (though they themselves may later offer post-hoc delusion-related explanations for their behaviour). In so far as such behaviour is intentional, it is probably best seen as spontaneous and unreflective, manifesting non-delusional level 1 attitudes of some kind. This again suggests that delusions involve a higher level of cognitive activity, and that a patient can become, as it were, *too ill to be deluded*.

for the problematic monothematic delusions we have focused on; I do not wish to claim that *no* delusions are also believed at level 1.)[2] Of course, even if this is right, it does not end the debate; the objections to the doxastic conception may extend to the claim that delusions are level 2 beliefs. In order to make progress here, I want to outline a hypothesis about the nature of level 2 beliefs, which will open a further option for the classification of delusions, and may have far-reaching implications for our thinking about them.

The hypothesis is designed both to account for the distinctive features of level 2 belief and to address a problem raised by the level 1/level 2 distinction. The problem concerns the role of level 2 belief in the guidance of action. If level 1 beliefs are behavioural dispositions, which are ascribed on the basis of an overall interpretation of the agent's behaviour, then there seems no room for level 2 belief to influence action. All behaviour that is interpretable as intentional will be interpretable as a manifestation of graded, nonconscious, level 1 beliefs. (I have referred to this as the *Bayesian challenge*; Frankish, 2004.) Conscious, level 2 belief threatens to be behaviourally inert. Some writers are tempted by this conclusion. Dennett suggests that our opinions (roughly equivalent to level 2 beliefs) influence our verbal behaviour only (Dennett, 1978, chapter 16), and some cognitive scientists hold that conscious decision making is largely confabulatory, serving merely to rationalize intuitive responses generated by nonconscious processes (e.g. Gazzaniga, 1998; Wegner, 2002; Wilson, 2002). This view would also explain the inertia of delusions, on the assumption that they are level 2 beliefs. Nevertheless, it should be resisted. It may be that conscious thought has far less effect on behaviour than we ordinarily suppose, but it is highly implausible to hold that it has none, and in what follows I shall outline an account of level 2 belief which does not have this consequence. We shall then need a further explanation for the relative inertia of delusions.

14.4 **Level 2 belief and acceptance**

The account I propose builds on, and substantially modifies, existing accounts of what some philosophers of science refer to as *acceptance* – a psychological state that is often contrasted with belief. There are a number of independent versions of the belief/acceptance distinction, each addressing different concerns and fostering different conceptions of the two states (for a survey, see Engel, 2000). I shall focus on a version developed by Jonathan Cohen (Cohen, 1992). According to Cohen, belief is a disposition, which is involuntary, graded, and truth-directed. To believe *p* is to be disposed to feel it true that *p* when you consider the matter. Acceptance, on the other hand, is a policy, which can be actively adopted in response to pragmatic considerations. To accept *p* is to decide to *treat it as true* – to take it as a premise in one's conscious reasoning and decision making. For example, I might decide that, for the purposes of

---

[2] It is tempting to speculate that it is because delusions are believed only at level 2 that they lack the normal emotional associations. Level 2 belief is an intellectual form of belief, which is less intimately connected with behaviour and bodily responses, and it may be that the affective component of a level 2 belief depends on the existence of a corresponding level 1 belief.

deciding what food to buy, I shall take it as a premise that beef is unsafe to eat, even if I am not completely convinced that it is. Cohen also identifies a parallel conative state, goal adoption, which involves committing oneself to taking some outcome as a goal. (For convenience I shall use the term 'premising policy' for both acceptance and goal adoption.) Cohen's distinction between belief and acceptance clearly overlaps with that between level 1 and level 2 belief, particularly in the passive/active contrast, and I think his conception of acceptance offers a fruitful model for level 2 beliefs.

Cohen does not say much about what is involved in executing premising policies or what role such policies have in the guidance of action. In other work I have addressed these questions and developed a detailed account of the nature and function of acceptance (see Frankish, 2004, chapter 4). The key idea is that there is a level of human reasoning which is conscious and under intentional control – that is, which involves actively applying learned inferential procedures and problem-solving strategies, motivated by a desire to find a solution to some problem and a belief that the procedures employed may generate one. The activities involved – which will often employ inner speech – might include constructing deductive arguments, applying heuristics, running thought-experiments, imagining scenarios, or simply questioning oneself in order to stimulate spontaneous inference. I call this type of reasoning *personal reasoning*, in contrast to reasoning that is nonconscious and sub-personally controlled, and I have argued that System 2 reasoning, as described by dual-system theorists, is best understood as personal in this sense (see my 2009b). (We might think of System 2 as a *virtual* system, in the sense described in Dennett, 1991.) Because personal reasoning is under intentional control, we can commit ourselves to regulating it in various ways, and premising policies, I suggest, are just such commitments. In accepting a proposition or adopting a goal, we commit ourselves to taking it as an input to our personal reasoning.

Now it is attractive to think of level 2 beliefs as acceptances in this sense. Acceptance is by definition conscious and controlled. It is also a binary state: for any proposition, p, one either has or has not adopted a policy of premising that p. (It is true that we can have varying degrees of attachment to our premising policies, but so long as we hold on to a given set, our commitment to each of them will be the same.) Moreover, acceptance states are functionally discrete, in the way that level 2 beliefs are. Premising policies can be individually adopted and abandoned, and they can be selectively recalled and executed in personal reasoning (see Frankish, 2004, chapter 6). It is true that premising policies are not *brain* states – it is people who have policies, not their brains – but from a functional perspective, this is irrelevant.[3] Finally, this account offers a solution to the problem of how level 2 beliefs can influence action. This requires a little explanation, but will be important later.

The actions involved in forming and executing a policy are intentional ones, motivated by the desirability of adhering to the policy. We adopt policies because we think that following them will bring some long-term benefit, and we perform the

---

[3] To underscore the point that level 2 beliefs are formed and processed at a personal level, I have elsewhere dubbed them 'virtual beliefs' and 'superbeliefs'; see Frankish, 1998, 2004.

actions they dictate because we want to secure this benefit. (In the case of premising policies, I assume the benefit is that of having a settled knowledge base and goal structure to draw on in one's personal reasoning. The advantages of forming a premising policy are precisely those of *making up one's mind*.) Thus, when we take our premises and goals as inputs to personal reasoning, we do so because we believe our premising policies require us to do this. Of course, these beliefs will not normally be conscious ones. The attitudes that drive our premising activities will typically be of the nonconscious level 1 kind, which reveal themselves in our attitudes to our conscious premises and goals.

How does this explain how level 2 beliefs influence action? Well, suppose that premising policies also involve a tacit commitment to overt action. That is, suppose that in adopting a premise for use in personal reasoning we also commit ourselves to acting upon the results of that reasoning – adopting any derived conclusions as further premises or goals, and performing, or forming intentions to perform, any dictated actions. Then, if we believe that our premises and goals mandate a certain action, we shall be motivated to perform the action precisely because our policies dictate it – again the motivating attitudes being of the level 1 kind. Of course, we would not normally explain the resulting action by citing these meta-cognitive level 1 attitudes; we would simply cite the attitudes involved in our conscious personal reasoning. And this explanation would not be wrong, since those attitudes did play an important role; but it would be underpinned by another, more basic explanation, citing level 1 attitudes. This view again harmonizes with work by dual-system theorists, several of whom argue that conscious reasoning has only an indirect effect on behaviour, mediated by nonconscious reasoning processes (see Carruthers, 2006; Evans, 2009). Thus, if level 2 beliefs are acceptances, there is no conflict between the claim that all intentional actions have level 1 explanations and the commonsense view that level 2 attitudes influence behaviour; level 2 beliefs influence behaviour *in virtue of* our level 1 beliefs and desires about them. This dependency makes the terminology of levels particularly appropriate.

For all this, we cannot simply identify level 2 belief with acceptance. For, as writers on the subject emphasize, acceptance possesses properties that are alien to belief. Two in particular stand out. First, acceptance is responsive to prudential considerations – professional, ethical, religious, and so on. For example, a lawyer may accept that his client is innocent for the purposes of defending him, even though he does not believe it. Second, acceptance can be context-relative; we can accept something for reasoning in certain situations but not in others, as the lawyer does. Now, the first contrast here is not so clear. It is arguable that beliefs *can* be formed for pragmatic reasons, provided one also has good evidence for their truth (see Frankish, 2007). It is true, however, that belief formation is typically *sensitive* to evidential considerations in a way that acceptance is not. The second contrast is more straightforward: belief, as we commonly conceive of it, plays an open-ended role in deliberation. (This is connected with the first contrast; if rational, one will not be willing to rely on a proposition in an open-ended range of deliberations unless one has good evidence for its truth.) However, it remains possible that level 2 beliefs are a subset of acceptances, and this is the view I want to propose. Specifically, I suggest that level 2 beliefs are acceptances that are not restricted to particular contexts, and which are, therefore, typically evidence-sensitive. Again, there is more to be said in defence of this view (see Frankish, 2004, chapter 5), but I propose to adopt it as a working hypothesis and move on to consider how delusions might fit into this framework.

14.5 Delusions and acceptances

How does the hypothesis that delusions are level 2 beliefs fare in this model? Are delusions unrestricted acceptances? I think this is a possible view, though we still need to explain their relative inertia. In fact, an explanation of this falls out naturally from the proposed account of how level 2 beliefs influence action. For, we should expect the mechanism involved to break down in the case of delusions. Let me explain.

I suggested that our motivation for acting on our acceptances is essentially *meta-cognitive* – we act on them because we have a level 1 desire to adhere to our premising policies. But in some cases, other level 1 desires may outweigh that desire. We may consciously judge that, given our premises and goals, we ought to perform action A, and so become motivated to perform it by our level 1 desire to adhere to our premising policies. Yet, we may nonetheless refrain from performing A because we have a stronger level 1 desire not to do A, or to do something else. For example, I might conclude, on the basis of personal reasoning involving my chosen premises and goals, that I should refuse another slice of chocolate cake, yet take one anyway since my level 1 desire for chocolate cake is stronger than my level 1 desire to act in line with my premises and goals.

I have argued elsewhere that this is what occurs in cases of akrasia (Frankish, 2004, chapter 8), and something similar may happen with delusions. If we have – for whatever reason – adopted a premising policy which tends to dictate extreme or highly unusual actions, then our desire to adhere to the policy may be overridden by other level 1 desires making for caution and conformity. So, for example, a Capgras patient may conclude, from the premise that their spouse has been replaced by an impostor, that they should shun their current partner, and that they should search for their true spouse. Yet, they may fail to follow this course since their level 1 desire to act on their premises is weaker than their level 1 desire to remain with their current partner (perhaps because they have a strong level 1 belief that they are *not* in fact an impostor). (It is worth stressing that the claim here is not that level 2 attitudes are in *direct* competition with level 1 attitudes; if they belong to different systems this will not be the case. Rather, the conflict is between level 1 desires of different *orders*: a meta-cognitive desire to act on one's level 2 beliefs and a first-order desire to do something else.) Likewise, a Cotard patient has a level 2 belief (that is, a premise) which dictates that there is no point in their seeking food, shelter, companionship, and so on; but their level 1 desires for these things may outweigh their level 1 desire to act on their premises, rendering this particular level 2 belief largely inert. In such cases, a level 2 belief might continue to influence what a person *says* without affecting their non-verbal behaviour at all. In a similar way, level 1 desires may inhibit a person from using a premise freely in their personal reasoning, rendering it cognitively as well as behaviourally inert. This might happen, for example, because they fear the conclusions the premise may warrant, or because they are concerned that their adherence to it may be undermined by the discovery of inconsistencies with other important premises.

One option, then, is that delusions are atypical level 2 beliefs, whose atypicality is explicable in terms of their unusual content. Note that this view involves no specific commitments as to why delusional beliefs are formed and sustained, and it is compatible with most existing versions of the doxastic conception. It is, for example, neutral on the questions of whether delusions are grounded in abnormal experiences, whether they are the product of abnormal fixation processes, and whether they involve reasoning deficits. It does, however, require that these questions be recast as ones about *personal activities* – forming and executing premising policies – rather than sub-personal processes. In assigning a key role to meta-cognitive attitudes, the account also has commonalities with meta-cognitive accounts of delusions, such as that proposed by Currie.

This is not all, however. The proposed two-level framework also offers another option for conceptualizing delusions. This is that delusions fall into the class of acceptances that are not beliefs – *non-doxastic acceptances*. This would also explain our competing intuitions about them. On the one hand, non-doxastic acceptances are very like beliefs; they possess the core properties of propositional content, mind–world fit, and an action-guiding role (in certain contexts), together with all the distinctive properties of level 2 states (conscious, binary, etc.). And, like beliefs, we would – in the right context – avow them and defend them (they are our premises, to which we are committed). On the other hand, non-doxastic acceptances lack the sensitivity to evidence that is characteristic of belief (and characteristically absent in delusions), are effective only in certain restricted contexts, and may not be consistent with each other. (We can accept something for reasoning in one set of circumstances, and something quite different for reasoning in another.) All of this fits the profile of delusions very well.

We have then, two models of delusions, one doxastic and the other non-doxastic. In the former, delusions are atypical doxastic acceptances (level 2 beliefs), in the latter, they are typical non-doxastic ones. The models are broadly similar, and the differences between them concern motivation and sensitivity to evidence. Doxastic acceptances are typically formed for epistemic reasons and are sensitive to evidence, whereas non-doxastic acceptances are formed for pragmatic reasons and without reference to evidence. The distinction between the two models thus corresponds roughly to that between bottom-up and top-down models of delusions (Bayne and Pacherie, 2004a). (In bottom-up models, delusional beliefs are grounded in experience, whereas in top-down ones, they are the product of central, non-perceptual processes of some kind.) Indeed, non-doxastic acceptances are akin to Campbell's framework propositions, which structure reasoning but are immune from empirical scrutiny.

Of course, we may need both models; some delusions may belong to one class and some to the other, and some may shift from one category to the other over time. Moreover, from a theoretical perspective, the similarities between the models are more important than their differences; the key claim in both views is that delusions are acceptances. It is this inclusive position that I propose, and I shall conclude by looking at two important implications of it.

The first implication is that the search for the explanation of particular delusions should take a different route. If the present hypothesis is correct, then delusions are premising policies, whose adoption is motivated by level 1 desires. So the question is not simply 'Why is the patient in this mental state?', but 'Why are they *doing* this? What are their motives for pursuing this policy?' The *immediate* explanation will lie, not in abnormal psychological or neurological processes, but in the level 1 desire that motivates the pursuit of the policy. Of course, this desire may itself be the product of abnormal processes of some kind, but to skip straight to these would be to miss an important explanatory step. (I should stress that in claiming that delusions are the product of nonconscious mental states and processes, I am not endorsing a traditional psychodynamic theory. The level 1 mind is not the Freudian dynamic unconscious, but the modern cognitive unconscious; see e.g. Hassin *et al.*, 2005; Wilson, 2002.)

The motives for forming delusional beliefs might be epistemic ones – desires to adopt true premises for use in personal reasoning. A person might accept a delusional claim because it reflects or explains the content of their experience, as on bottom-up approaches. Equally, however, the motives might be pragmatic, and in non-doxastic cases they typically will be. The nature of these motives is a matter for empirical investigation, but as an illustration it may help to consider self-deception, which can be regarded as a type of mild, non-psychotic delusion. I have argued elsewhere that self-deception involves a form of general acceptance, borderline between doxastic and non-doxastic, which is motivated by a desire to shield oneself from disturbing truths (Frankish, 2004, chapter 8). The self-deceiver finds a certain view probable but highly disturbing, and has a strong level 1 desire to avoid consciously accepting its truth. This desire leads them to accept that the view is in fact false, thereby ending conscious deliberation on the matter and committing themselves to a view they find comforting. Psychotic delusions, too, may be formed and sustained in response to emotional influences of various kinds, perhaps pathological in origin. Even in cases where epistemic motives are operative, it is likely that emotional factors will have to be invoked to explain the unusual fixity of delusions, which in the proposed view will be a consequence of the strength of the supporting level 1 desires.

The second implication is that it will be possible to bring delusional patients within the interpretative fold, at least at level 1. Irrational and inconsistent level 2 attitudes can be rational manifestations of consistent level 1 attitudes. (Indeed, if we adopt a dispositionalist view of level 1, as I have proposed, then the attribution of the supporting level 1 attitudes will require an assumption of rationality at that level.) This may seem an unattractive consequence, given the notorious difficulties in understanding delusional patients. However, the sense in which delusions are understandable will not be the usual one. The claim is not that the actions of deluded patients are understandable as manifestations of their delusions *qua* level 2 beliefs; all the problems for that view remain. Rather, it is that they are understandable *qua* manifestations of the premising policies in which level 2 states consist, and interpreting a deluded patient will involve forming and testing hypotheses as to the character of these policies. And this may be a difficult task. Much of the activity involved in executing a premising policy is covert; it consists in pursuing a certain strategy in one's conscious personal reasoning, and although such reasoning is (I would maintain) squarely intentional, it is rarely publicly observable. Interpretivist theory usually ignores such covert behaviour, but if the present view is correct, it will be crucial to take it into account if we are to understand delusions (for defence of the claim that interpretivists can legitimately recognize the existence of covert behaviour, see Frankish, 2004, chapter 5). Fresh approaches may therefore be needed in order to uncover the relevant evidence. For example, 'talk-aloud' and 'think-aloud' protocols might be employed, in which subjects verbalize or explain their thought processes.

14.6 Conclusion

This chapter has offered a new hypothesis about the nature of delusions, which locates them within an expanded version of our commonsense mental taxonomy. I sketched a two-level view of the mind, supported by both analysis of folk psychology and experimental work on reasoning, and argued that delusions belong to the second level. I then outlined a model of level 2 belief based around the concept of acceptance developed by some philosophers of science, and proposed that delusions are acceptances – some doxastic, some non-doxastic. I argued that this view can reconcile our competing intuitions about delusions and explain their puzzling features. This does not, of course, amount to a conclusive case for the view, but I hope it establishes it as a serious hypothesis. Its fate will, of course, depend on whether it proves theoretically fruitful and clinically valuable.

Acknowledgements

I thank Lisa Bortolotti, Matthew Broome, and Maria Kasmirli for their comments on an earlier draft of this chapter. Work on the chapter was supported by a research leave award from the UK's Arts and Humanities Research Council.

References

American Psychiatric Association (2000). *Diagnostic and Statistical Manual of Mental Disorders, Fourth Edition, Text Revision.* Washington, DC, American Psychiatric Association Pub. Inc.

Bayne, T. and Pacherie, E. (2004a). Bottom-up or top-down? Campbell's rationalist account of monothematic delusions. *Philosophy, Psychiatry, and Psychology,* 11, 1–11.

Bayne, T. and Pacherie, E. (2004b). Experience, belief, and the interpretive fold. *Philosophy, Psychiatry, and Psychology,* 11, 81–86.

Bayne, T. and Pacherie, E. (2005). In defence of the doxastic conception of delusions. *Mind and Language,* 20, 163–188.

Berrios, G. E. (1991). Delusions as 'wrong beliefs': a conceptual history. *British Journal of Psychiatry,* 159, 6–13.

Bortolotti, L. (2005). Delusions and the background of rationality. *Mind and Language,* 20, 189–208.

Bovet, P. and Parnas, J. (1993). Schizophrenic delusions: a phenomenological approach. *Schizophrenia Bulletin,* 19, 579–597.

Breen, N., Caine, D., Coltheart, M. *et al.* (2000). Towards an understanding of delusions of misidentification: four case studies. *Mind and Language,* **15**, 74–110.

Brett-Jones, J., Garety, P., and Hemsley, D. (1987). Measuring delusional experiences: a method and its application. *British Journal of Clinical Psychology,* **26**, 257–265.

Buchanan, A. and Wessely, S. (1998). Delusions, action, and insight. In *Insight and Psychosis* (eds. X. F. Amador, and A. S. David) pp. 241–268. New York, Oxford University Press.

Campbell, J. (2001). Rationality, meaning, and the analysis of delusion. *Philosophy, Psychiatry, and Psychology,* **8**, 89–100.

Carruthers, P. (2006). *The Architecture of the Mind.* Oxford, Oxford University Press.

Cohen, L. J. (1992). *An Essay on Belief and Acceptance.* Oxford, Oxford University Press.

Currie, G. (2000). Imagination, delusion and hallucinations. *Mind and Language,* **15**, 168–183.

Currie, G. and Jureidini, J. (2001). Delusion, rationality, empathy: commentary on Martin Davies *et al. Philosophy, Psychiatry, and Psychology,* **8**, 159–162.

Currie, G. and Ravenscroft, I. (2002). *Recreative Minds.* Oxford, Oxford University Press.

Davidson, D. (1984). *Inquiries into Truth and Interpretation.* Oxford, Oxford University Press.

Davies, M., Coltheart, M., Langdon, R., and Breen, N. (2001). Monothematic delusions: towards a two-factor account. *Philosophy, Psychiatry, and Psychology,* **8**, 133–158.

Dennett, D. C. (1978). *Brainstorms: Philosophical Essays on Mind and Psychology.* Montgomery, VT, Bradford Books.

Dennett, D. C. (1987). *The Intentional Stance.* Cambridge, MA, MIT Press.

Dennett, D C. (1991). *Consciousness Explained.* Boston, MA, Little Brown and Co.

Engel, P. (2000). Introduction: the varieties of belief and acceptance. In *Believing and Accepting* (ed. P. Engel), pp. 1–30. Dordrecht, Kluwer.

Evans, J. St. B. T. (2003). In two minds: dual-process accounts of reasoning. *Trends in Cognitive Sciences,* **7**, 454–459.

Evans, J. St. B. T. (2009). How many dual process theories do we need? One, two, or many? In *In Two Minds: Dual Processes and Beyond* (eds. J. St. B. T. Evans, and K. Frankish), pp. 33–54.Oxford, Oxford University Press.

Evans, J. St. B. T. and Frankish, K. (2009). *In Two Minds: Dual Processes and Beyond.* Oxford, Oxford University Press.

Evans, J. St. B. T. and Over, D. E. (1996). *Rationality and Reasoning.* Hove, Psychology Press,.

Fodor, J. A. (1987). *Psychosemantics: The Problem of Meaning in the Philosophy of Mind.* Cambridge, MA, MIT Press.

Frankish, K. (1998). Natural language and virtual belief. In *Language and Thought: Interdisciplinary Themes* (eds. P. Carruthers, and J. Boucher), pp. 248–269. Cambridge, Cambridge University Press.

Frankish, K. (2004). *Mind and Supermind.* Cambridge, Cambridge University Press.

Frankish, K. (2007). Deciding to believe again. *Mind,* **116**, 523–547.

Frankish, K. (2009a). Partial belief and flat-out belief. In *Degrees of Belief: An Anthology* (eds. F. Huber and C. Schmidt-Petri), pp. 75–93. Dordrecht, Springer.

Frankish, K. (2009b). Systems and levels: dual-system theories and the personal-subpersonal distinction. In *In Two Minds: Dual Processes and Beyond* (eds. J. St. B. T. Evans, and K. Frankish), pp. 89–107. Oxford, Oxford University Press.

Gazzaniga, M. S. (1998). *The Mind's Past.* Berkeley, University of California Press.

Hamilton, A. (2007). Against the belief model of delusion. In *Reconceiving Schizophrenia* (eds. M. C. Chung, K. W. M. Fulford, and G. Graham), pp. 217–234. Oxford, Oxford University Press.

Hassin, R. R., Uleman, J. S., and Bargh, J. A. (2005). *The New Unconscious*. New York, Oxford University Press.

James, W. (1890). *The Principles of Psychology*. New York, Henry Holt and Co.

Jaspers, K. (1913/1997). *General Psychopathology: Volume 1* (Trs. J. Hoenig and M. W. Hamilton). Baltimore, MD, Johns Hopkins University Press.

Kahneman, D. and Frederick, S. (2002). Representativeness revisited: attribute substitution in intuitive judgement. In *Heuristics and Biases: The Psychology of Intuitive Judgment* (eds. T. Gilovich, D. Griffin, and D. Kahneman), pp. 49–81. Cambridge, Cambridge University Press.

Lewis, D. (1972). Psychophysical and theoretical identifications. *Australasian Journal of Philosophy*, **50**, 249–258.

Maher, B. A. (1999). Anomalous experience in everyday life: its significance for psychopathology. *The Monist*, **82**, 547–570.

Oaksford, M. and Chater, N. (2007). *Bayesian Rationality: The Probabilistic Approach to Human Reasoning*. Oxford, Oxford University Press.

Ramsey, W., Stich, S. P., and Garon, J. (1990). Connectionism, eliminativism and the future of folk psychology. In *Philosophical Perspectives, 4: Action Theory and Philosophy of Mind* (ed. J. E. Tomberlin), pp. 499–533. Atascadero, CA, Ridgeview Publishing Company.

Ryle, G. (1949). *The Concept of Mind*. London, Hutchinson.

Sass, L. A. (1994). *The Paradoxes of Delusion: Wittgenstein, Schreber, and the Schizophrenic Mind*. Ithaca, NY, Cornell University Press.

Sloman, S. A. (1996). The empirical case for two systems of reasoning. *Psychological Bulletin*, **119**, 3–22.

Smith, E. R. and DeCoster, J. (2000). Dual-process models in social and cognitive psychology: Conceptual integration and links to underlying memory systems. *Personality and Social Psychology Review*, **4**, 108–131.

Stanovich, K. E. (2004). *The Robot's Rebellion: Finding Meaning in the Age of Darwin*. Chicago, IL, University of Chicago Press.

Stone, T. and Young, A. W. (1997). Delusions and brain injury: the philosophy and psychology of belief. *Mind and Language*, **12**, 327–364.

Wegner, D. M. (2002). *The Illusion of Conscious Will*. Cambridge, MA, MIT Press.

Wilson, T. D. (2002). *Strangers to Ourselves*. Cambridge, MA, Belknap Press.

Wilson, T D., Lindsey, S., and Schooler, T. Y. (2000). A model of dual attitudes. *Psychological Review*, **107**, 101–126.

Young, A. W. (2000). Wondrous strange: the neuropsychology of abnormal beliefs. *Mind and Language*, **15**, 47–73.

Chapter 15

Explaining pathologies of belief

Anne M. Aimola Davies and Martin Davies

Abstract

The two-factor framework for explaining delusions is developed in a way that promises reasonable coverage without overgeneralization. We propose that heterogeneity in explanations of delusions can be conceived as parametric variation within the two-factor framework and we suggest several parameters. In three ways, we confront the fact that the second factor in the two-factor framework, a presumed impairment of belief evaluation, has been poorly specified in terms of cognitive function. First, an *a priori* task analysis suggests that belief evaluation involves working memory and executive processes of inhibition. Second, we review experimental and neuroimaging studies of the belief-bias effect in the context of dual-process accounts of reasoning. The results can be interpreted as supporting the proposal that the second factor in the explanation of delusions is an impairment of working memory or executive function with a neural basis in damage to the right frontal region of the brain. Finally, we present results from a study of cognitive impairments following stroke to support our proposal in the case of anosognosia considered as a delusion.

15.1 **Introduction**

In a case of delusion, belief goes wrong. A delusion is a belief that not only departs from the norms of truth and knowledge, but also is unresponsive to considerations of plausibility and evidence. A delusion is: 'A false belief . . . that is firmly sustained despite what almost everyone else believes and despite what constitutes incontrovertible and obvious proof or evidence to the contrary' (*DSM-IV-TR*, 2000, p. 821). Delusions are pathologies of belief.

This notion of a pathology of belief can usefully be distinguished from a conception of pathological belief or doubt, that figures in some recent work in epistemology (Pryor, 2004). Having evidence to doubt the proposition that there is an external world, for example, could undermine a subject's justification, based on perceptual experience, to believe the proposition that there is a table in front of him. In this context, it is important to distinguish between a doubt that is really supported by evidence and a doubt that the subject wrongly takes to be supported by evidence. It is also important – especially for the purposes of this chapter – to distinguish between a doubt that the subject takes to be supported by evidence (whether rightly or wrongly) and a pathological doubt – that is, a doubt that the subject knows to be unjustified but cannot help having. In a case of pathological doubt, the subject is beset by doubt but can offer no grounds for the doubt. Similarly, we can say that, in a case of pathological belief, the subject is *beset by belief* but can offer no grounds for the belief.

It is plausible that some cases of delusion are examples of pathological belief in this sense. Jaspers (1963) conceived of primary delusional beliefs in this way and these cases may be theoretically important. But there are surely other cases of delusion in which the subject does offer grounds for his or her belief, reasons that, at least from the subject's point of view, speak in favour of the belief. Conversely, there are imaginable cases of pathological belief that are not cases of delusion. A subject might, in principle, be beset by a belief that happens to be plausible, true, shared by other people, and consistent with available evidence. In short, when we say that delusions are pathologies of belief – that is, cases where belief goes wrong – we do not mean that delusions are pathological beliefs – that is, beliefs for which the subject can offer no grounds.[1]

15.2 **Anosognosia as a pathology of belief**

Anosognosia is a failure to acknowledge illness or impairment. Patients with anosognosia for their motor impairments following right-hemisphere stroke fail to acknowledge, and may outright deny, that they can no longer raise their left arm or move their left leg. Patients with anosognosia for the consequences of their motor impairments fail to appreciate their limited ability to carry out activities of daily living. They may insist, quite unrealistically, that they could live at home and care for themselves unaided.

Berti and colleagues (Berti *et al.*, 1998) describe the case of an 80-year-old woman, CC, who suffered left-side paralysis following a stroke that caused damage to fronto-parietal subcortical regions of the right hemisphere (1998, p. 27). When examined during the 2 months after her stroke, patient CC did not acknowledge her motor impairments, even when they were demonstrated to her. She not only insisted that she could move her left arm but also maintained that she was moving it in the period immediately after being asked to do so. She did, however, show some appreciation of the consequences of her impairments. When asked to rate how well she would perform

---

[1] Bortolotti and Broome (2008, in press) make use of the notion of *authorship* of a belief (Moran, 2001), conceived as 'the capacity to endorse the content of a belief and justify it with reasons' (2008, p. 822). They consider the question whether delusions are beliefs of which the subject is not the author and provide convincing examples of delusions that are not authored – cases in which the subject can offer 'no explanation or reason to believe that what they say is true' (*ibid.*, p. 829). But they also describe cases in which subjects with delusions are 'able to defend the content of the beliefs they report' (p. 829).

if she had to carry out an everyday task (such as lifting a glass) using her right hand or her left hand, she gave high scores for the right hand but low scores for the left hand.

House and Hodges (1988) describe the case of an 89-year-old woman who suffered left-side paralysis following a stroke that damaged the right basal ganglia but spared cortical regions. She was confined to a wheelchair and dependent on assistance for activities of daily living such as washing, grooming, and dressing. When examined 6 months after her stroke, she acknowledged some weakness, particularly when her impairments were demonstrated to her. But she insisted that 'she would be able to walk, feed, and dress herself unaided, and even drive a car although "the left side might be a bit awkward"' (1988, p. 114).

In a study by the first author (Aimola, 1999; Maguire and Ogden, 2002), patient M3 was a 59-year-old man who suffered severe left-side motor impairments following a right-hemisphere stroke that damaged the parietal, frontal, and temporal lobes and basal ganglia. Nine months after his stroke, he was confined to a wheelchair and would sometimes acknowledge his impairments. But he did not appreciate the consequences of his impairments. While at home alone, he repeatedly tried to get out of his wheelchair and injured himself. He had to be placed in a nursing home for his own safety. Patient M6, a 57-year-old man, also had severe motor impairments in the acute stage following a right-hemisphere stroke that caused extensive damage to the parietal, frontal, and temporal lobes and basal ganglia. Three months after his stroke he had made a relatively good recovery and was able to walk, although the weakness of his left leg was still evident as he needed to use a cane. Eight functional tests of hemiplegia (Gialanella and Mattioli, 1992) revealed that activities of daily living were possible for patient M6 only with difficulty. Nevertheless, he insisted that he could leave the rehabilitation hospital, live at home, and generally care for the family, even though this proved clearly beyond him when he made short visits home.

These patients failed to acknowledge their motor impairments or failed to appreciate the consequences of those impairments (or both). They overestimated their abilities to move their left-side limbs or their abilities to carry out activities of daily living and they maintained their false beliefs in the face of abundant evidence about their real situations. Anosognosia is a delusion, a pathology of belief. In the mid-twentieth century, it was common to explain anosognosia as a case of motivated denial. Weinstein and Kahn (Weinstein and Kahn, 1950, 1951, 1953, 1955; Weinstein et al., 1954) put forward an influential account of anosognosia as an expression of the drive to be well that is present in everyone. Since the drive is not expressed as anosognosia in everyone who suffers from motor impairments, they proposed that 'the occurrence of anosognosia is related to the pattern of the premorbid personality' (1950, p. 780).

In recent years, explanations of anosognosia as motivated denial have fallen from favour and explanations in terms of sensory, attentional, and cognitive deficits have been preferred. One factor in this change has been Bisiach and Geminiani's (1991) influential argument opposing interpretations of anosognosia as 'a defensive adaptation against the stress caused by the illness' (1991, p. 24).[2] More generally, the change

---

[2] For extended discussion of the possible role of motivation in anosognosia and other delusions, see Aimola Davies et al., 2009; Davies, 2009; Mele, 2009.

of approach is consistent with the development of cognitive neuropsychiatry – the use of the methods of cognitive neuropsychology for understanding disorders that were previously regarded as psychiatric phenomena.

15.3 Cognitive neuropsychology and cognitive neuropsychiatry

Research in cognitive neuropsychology has two complementary aims. One is to use data from people with acquired disorders of cognition to constrain, develop, and test theories of normal cognitive structures and processes. The other is to use theories about normal cognition to help understand disorders of cognition that result from stroke or head injury (Coltheart, 1985; Humphreys, 1991). It follows from the aims of cognitive neuropsychology that 'the underlying construct is . . . a model of normal performance in some cognitive domain or other' (Halligan and Marshall, 1996, pp. 5–6).

Language is arguably the cognitive domain in which cognitive neuropsychological research has been most highly developed. Beginning from two papers by Marshall and Newcombe (1966, 1973), the cognitive neuropsychology of reading has yielded theoretical accounts of acquired disorders of reading (dyslexias) in terms of a model of the cognitive structures and processes implicated in normal reading of words aloud (Coltheart, 2006a). The model is highly articulated and, at least partly, computationally implemented (Coltheart, 2006b). Some of the processes for reading aloud draw on orthographic and phonological information stored in the lexicon and can therefore only be applied to real words. Other processes make use of letter–sound (more accurately, grapheme–phoneme) correspondence rules and can be applied to pronounceable letter strings whether or not they are real words. Selective damage to some components of the model can thus explain impaired reading of irregular (exception) words (e.g. 'pint' pronounced to rhyme with 'mint') while reading of regular words (e.g. 'print') and non-words (e.g. 'slint') is spared. Selective damage to other components can explain impaired reading of non-words while reading of real words, both regular and irregular, is spared.

15.3.1 Cognitive neuropsychiatry

Hadyn Ellis is credited with the first public use of the term 'cognitive neuropsychiatry' for the application of the methods of cognitive neuropsychology to psychiatric disorders (in October 1991; see David, 1993, p. 4; Coltheart, 2007, p. 1042). In 1996, Halligan and Marshall's edited volume, *Method in Madness: Case Studies in Cognitive Neuropsychiatry*, was published and the journal, *Cognitive Neuropsychiatry*, was launched. The journal editors note some changes of approach attendant on the shift from the more familiar territory of cognitive neuropsychology (David and Halligan, 1996, p. 2): 'We need to think of excesses as well as deficits; transient rather than stable phenomena; distortions and biases rather than striking quantitative or apparent qualitative differences.' Young (2000) also reviews a 'catalogue of problems to be faced' and suggests that 'advances in cognitive neuropsychiatry will be hard won . . . [but] well worth the effort' (2000, p. 69).

An important early work in cognitive neuropsychiatry is Ellis and Young's paper, 'Accounting for delusional misidentification' (1990). One reason that this work was 'promising from the start' was that 'they [Ellis and Young] had a fairly simple yet well-substantiated model of face recognition based on studies of normal and clinical subjects including cases of prosopagnosia [Bruce and Young, 1986]' (David, 1993, p. 4; see also Ellis, 1998). A model of normal face recognition is clearly important for understanding delusions of misidentification, such as the Capgras delusion. But the 'underlying construct' that is required whenever the methods of cognitive neuro-psychology are applied to pathologies of belief is a model of the normal formation, evaluation, and revision of beliefs. Thus, one of the problems faced by cognitive neuropsychiatry – in comparison with the cognitive neuropsychology of reading, for example – is that we do not have an articulated, still less a computationally implemented, model of normal believing. Indeed, there may be reasons of principle why it is extremely difficult to understand belief formation in terms of the computational theory of mind (Fodor, 1983, 2000).

The lack of a model of normal belief presents a challenge for cognitive neuro-psychiatry. Halligan and Marshall display an optimistic and constructive spirit, saying (1996, p. 8): 'One would none the less hope that theories of normal belief-formation will eventually cast light on both the content of delusions and on the processes where-by the beliefs came to be held.' They also say that 'it is unlikely that a unified theory of delusions will be forthcoming' (ibid.). This latter idea is developed by Stone and Young in a seminal contribution to inter-disciplinary theorizing about delusions, 'Delusions and brain injury: The philosophy and psychology of belief' (1997). They draw on the analogy between the cognitive neuropsychology of reading and the cognitive neuro-psychiatry of delusions. Just as 'there can be different non-word reading deficits, resulting from the precise way in which spelling-to-sound conversion has been impaired', so also, 'there are different kinds of delusions. The precise nature of a delu-sion will depend, inter alia, upon the exact way in which the system supporting belief formation has been impaired' (1997, p. 331).

We agree that there are different kinds of delusions and that their explanations will be correspondingly different. Nevertheless, we propose that the explanations of a wide range of delusions exhibit a kind of unity. The explanations can be conceived in terms of parametric variation within a single explanatory framework, rather as natural languages can be conceived in terms of parametric variation within a single universal grammar (Chomsky, 1986).

15.3.2 The two-factor framework

Coltheart (2007, p. 1044) has proposed that, in order to explain any delusion, we need to answer two questions. First, where did the delusion come from? Second, why does the patient not reject the belief? This is the leading idea of the two-factor framework for explaining pathologies of belief. The first factor figures in the explanation of how the patient came to regard the false proposition as a salient and serious hypothesis and initially adopted the hypothesis as a belief. The second factor figures in the explanation of the patient's maintenance of the belief despite its implausibility and despite the evidence against it.

In line with the developing research programme of cognitive neuropsychiatry, the two-factor framework was initially presented as a schematic explanation for delusions of neuropsychological origin. In such cases, it is reasonable to expect that a first neuropsychological deficit will provide (at least part of) an answer to the question where the delusion came from and that a second deficit will explain why the patient does not subsequently reject the false belief. The explicitly neuropsychological development of the two-factor framework is thus a 'two-deficit account of delusional belief' (Coltheart, 2007, p. 1044).

The scope of the two-factor framework might gradually be extended from neuropsychological cases of monothematic delusion to include cases of delusion without apparent brain injury and, ultimately, the floridly elaborated delusional systems of some individuals with schizophrenia. But broader explanatory coverage requires less specific commitments concerning the nature of the explanatory factors. So there is a risk that the account will overgeneralize – perhaps, in the worst case, encompassing all false beliefs. Our aim is to develop the two-factor framework in a way that offers the prospect of reasonable coverage without overgeneralization.

15.4 The first factor: where did the delusion come from?

In most cases of delusion, the subject's false belief is new and also bizarre or exotic. The subject may say: 'This [the subject's left arm] is not my arm' (somatoparaphrenia; Halligan et al., 1995; Bottini et al., 2002) or: 'This [the subject's wife] is not my wife. My wife has been replaced by an impostor' (Capgras delusion; Capgras and Reboul-Lachaux, 1923; Edelstyn and Oyebode, 1999). The answer to the question where the delusion came from may appeal to the subject's explanation or interpretation of an anomalous experience (Maher, 1974, 1988, 1992). In the neuropsychological version of the two-factor framework, we assume that the anomalous experience arises from a first deficit. Coltheart describes it in this way:

> The patient has a neuropsychological deficit of a kind that could plausibly be related to the content of the patient's particular delusion – that is, a deficit that could plausibly be viewed as having prompted the initial thought that turned into a delusional belief.
>
> (Coltheart, 2007, p. 1047)

It is assumed that the first deficit varies from delusion to delusion and may also vary from patient to patient with the same delusion.

Neither a neuropsychological deficit nor an anomalous experience can provide a complete answer to the question where the delusion came from. A delusion is a belief, but having a deficit or experience is not yet having a belief; it is not even having a hypothesis that could be adopted as a belief. A complete answer to the question will have to appeal to a processing stage that leads from deficit or experience to belief. This is the idea that the two-factor framework is also a three-stage framework (Aimola Davies et al., 2009).

15.4.1 Endorsement or explanation

If an anomalous experience figures in the answer to the question where the delusion came from, then the representational content of the experience may be close to the content of the delusion itself or it may be very different. Suppose, at one end of the spectrum of possibilities, an experience *fully encodes* the content of the delusion. In this case, what is needed, to lead from anomalous experience to delusional belief, is just that the subject should take the experience at face value or *endorse* it (Bayne and Pacherie, 2004). That is, the subject should treat the experience as veridical. Plausibly, this is a default or prepotent doxastic response to perceptual experiences (Davies *et al.*, 2001, p. 153).[3]

Now suppose, at the other end of the spectrum of possibilities, that the representational content of an anomalous experience is *much less specific* than the content of the delusion to which it leads. For example, the experience might be a feeling of significance or a conscious sense that something has changed (Maher, 1999). There is a substantial gap between the inchoate sense that a limb lying beside my torso is different or not quite right and the belief that it is not my arm but someone else's, or between the sense that a person who looks like my wife is different or not quite right and the belief that she is not my wife but an impostor. In such cases, the processing stage that leads from experience to belief must involve substantive *explanatory* processes of hypothesis generation and confirmation.

Continuing with the explanationist option, suppose that E is the evidence provided by an anomalous experience and that an explanatory hypothesis, H, is generated. If the probability of the evidence E given the hypothesis H, *Pr*(E/H), is greater than the prior probability of E, *Pr*(E), then Bayes's theorem, in the form:

$$\frac{Pr(H/E)}{Pr(H)} = \frac{Pr(E/H)}{Pr(E)}$$

tells us that the probability of hypothesis H given the evidence E, *Pr*(H/E), is greater than the prior probability of H, *Pr*(H), in the same proportion. The evidence E raises the probability of hypothesis H; in short, E *confirms* H. Confirmation of a hypothesis by evidence warrants increased credence in the hypothesis, although it might not warrant changing the balance of credence between the hypothesis and an alternative. Evidence may confirm H without being *diagnostic* as between H and an alternative, H'.

15.4.2 Jumping to conclusions and attributional style

These explanatory processes of hypothesis generation and confirmation might, in principle, depart from normality although Maher says (1999, p. 550): 'The processes by which deluded persons reason from experience to belief are not significantly different from the processes by which non-deluded persons do.' Stone and Young (1997) note that normal belief formation is 'fallible' and 'subject to various biases' (1997, p. 332). They argue that a complete answer to the question where a delusion came from will need to appeal to 'a theory of the reasoning biases that lead to the delusional interpretation of the [anomalous experience]' (*ibid.*, p. 341).

As examples of these reasoning biases, Stone and Young mention the *jumping to conclusions* (JTC) bias studied by Garety and colleagues (for reviews, see Garety and Freeman, 1999; Fine *et al.*, 2007) and biased *attributional style*, particularly the

---

[3] The word 'doxastic' means pertaining to belief or opinion.

externalizing attributional style that seems to play a role in persecutory delusions (for reviews see Bentall *et al.*, 2001; Blackwood *et al.*, 2001; but see Freeman, 2007, p. 440, for the view that 'the empirical case for persecutory delusions being associated with an excessive externalizing style for negative events is unconvincing at present'). These are appropriate examples of biases that might be at work as a subject tries to explain an anomalous experience. The subject's attributional style might bias the generation and consideration of an explanatory hypothesis and the JTC bias might then lead the subject to consider a smaller-than-normal amount of evidence before regarding the hypothesis as adequately confirmed and proceeding to adopt it as a belief.

Stone and Young describe 'the reasoning style of people [with] delusions' as 'the second factor' (1997, p. 346) and they conceptualize this second factor in terms of biased resolution of a permanent tension in the processes of belief formation. It is important to note, however, that what Stone and Young call the second factor is conceived as playing a rather different role from the second factor in the two-factor framework. They are primarily concerned with the processing stage that leads from experience to belief so that their second factor provides part of the answer to the question where the delusion came from. It corresponds to the second stage in the two-factor/three-stage framework.

15.4.3 Observational adequacy, explanatory adequacy, and conservatism

Drawing on Fodor (1987, 1989), Stone and Young propose that there is (1997, p. 349): 'a tension between forming beliefs that require little readjustment to the web of belief (conservatism) and forming beliefs that do justice to the deliverances of one's perceptual systems [beliefs that are observationally adequate]'. In a case of delusion, the balance between these two requirements 'goes too far towards observational adequacy as against conservatism' (*ibid.*).

The idea that a delusion results from a bias towards 'do[ing] justice to the deliverances of one's perceptual systems' is easily appreciated in cases where perceptual experience encodes the content of the delusion and the processing stage that leads from experience to belief involves *endorsement*. Indeed, Stone and Young describe the requirement of observational adequacy as 'seeing is believing' (1997, p. 349). A similar idea also has clear appeal when the anomalous experience is less specific in content and the processing stage that leads from experience to belief involves *explanation*.

Maher proposes that feelings of significance arise from the operation of a comparator or 'detector of changes':

> Survival requires the existence of a detector of changes in the normally regular patterns of environmental stimuli, namely those that are typically dealt with automatically. The detector functions as a general non-specific alarm, a 'significance generator', which then alerts the individual to scan the environment to find out what has changed.
>
> (Maher, 1999, p. 558)

The normal operation of this device generates feelings of significance in daily life and its pathological operation may give rise to anomalous experiences:

> The origins of anomalous experience may lie in a broad band of neuropsychological anomalies. These include, but are not confined to . . . endogenous neural activation of the

feeling of significance normally triggered by pre-conscious recognition of changes in a familiar environment.

(ibid., p. 551)

From the subject's point of view, a feeling of significance demands explanation in terms of something that has changed.[4] The feeling may be general, occurring in many contexts and accompanying many perceptual experiences. If no change can be detected that would explain the persistent feeling of significance, then an apocalyptic hypothesis might be generated and considered. 'Everything must have changed in some fundamental way' (Maher, 1999, p. 560); perhaps the end of the world is coming (Arthur, 1964, p. 106). The feeling of significance may, however, attach only to particular experiences, such as the subject's experience of an arm (in fact, the subject's paralysed left arm) or of a person (in fact, the subject's spouse). The subject's experience is suffused with a feeling of significance and cries out for explanation in terms of change in the object, person, or situation perceived.

Whether the feeling of significance is general or more particular, trying to do justice to such an experience by postulating change will, inevitably, require adjustment to the preexisting web of belief. Explaining the experience in terms of global change – 'The end of the world is coming' – or in terms of local change in an arm or a person – 'This is not my arm', 'My wife has been replaced by an impostor' – is liable to take the subject far from the requirements of conservatism.

Stone and Young speak of a balance between 'two imperatives' of observational adequacy and conservatism (1997, p. 349). With the distinction between endorsement and explanation in place, we propose to add a third imperative of explanatory adequacy. The imperatives of observational adequacy and explanatory adequacy may both be in tension with the imperative of conservatism, which corresponds to the inertia exerted by a preexisting web of belief. The imperative of observational adequacy corresponds to the prepotent doxastic response of treating a perceptual experience as veridical (seeing is believing). The imperative of explanatory adequacy corresponds to a prepotent doxastic tendency towards acceptance of a hypothesis that explains a salient piece of evidence and is thereby confirmed.[5]

---

[4] Kapur (2003, 2004; Kapur *et al.*, 2005) proposes that, in schizophrenia, delusions arise as the patient attempts to make sense of experiences of 'aberrant salience' that result from dysregulated dopamine transmission. For discussion, see Broome and colleagues (Broome *et al.*, 2005b).

[5] For an earlier discussion of two ways of interpreting Stone and Young's (1997) suggestion about observational adequacy and conservatism, see Davies and Coltheart (2000, pp. 18–20). The imperative of explanatory adequacy might be conceived as an aspect of a 'theory drive' (Gopnik, 1998, p. 101): 'a motivational system that impels us to interpret new evidence in terms of existing theories and change our theories in the light of new evidence.'

In a study of orientation to uncertainty, Schuurmans-Stekhoven and Smithson (submitted) investigate two dispositions, need for discovery (a tendency to up-date existing beliefs) and need for certainty (a tendency to maintain incumbent beliefs). They show that it is quite possible for someone to have both inclinations to a strong degree, but unlikely that they will lack both of them, and they suggest that the scales may predict biases in belief formation and perhaps the onset or maintenance of delusions.

15.4.4 **Parametric variation**

The question whether any actual cases of delusion fit the endorsement, rather than the explanationist, model is contested. Fine, Craigie, and Gold (2005) raise problems for both styles of account of the Capgras delusion. Coltheart (2005) defends the explanationist account and says that the endorsement account 'requires much more fleshing out before it will be possible to decide whether it is a viable competitor to the "explanation" account' (2005, p. 153). In contrast, Bayne and Pacherie 'prefer the endorsement version' (2004, p. 4). Jeannerod and Pacherie (2004) provide a detailed account of experiences of agency that would complement an endorsement account of delusions of control in individuals with schizophrenia. Hohwy and Rosenberg (2005) offer an account of the alien control delusion that begins from the hypothesis that 'delusions arise when unusual experiences are taken as veridical' (2005, p. 144).

It seems likely that some cases of delusion will fit the endorsement model and others the explanationist model. If that is right, then the nature of the processing stage that leads from anomalous experience to delusional belief will be one locus of parametric variation within the two-factor framework for explaining pathologies of belief. In fact, the setting of the endorsement/explanation parameter is likely to be a matter of degree and when (or to the extent that) a case fits the explanationist model, there may be further variation amongst accounts of normal, biased, or impaired hypothesis generation and confirmation.

If the processing stage that leads from experience to belief is biased or impaired, then it might, in principle, yield a delusional belief by flawed explanation, or misinterpretation, of quite ordinary or perhaps ambiguous – but not anomalous – experiences. Since the two-factor framework is also a three-stage framework, it can allow for the possibility that there might be no departure from normality earlier than the second stage. This option for parametric variation within the two-factor framework may be relevant to the explanation of some persecutory delusions (Bentall *et al.*, 2001; Blackwood *et al.*, 2001; Freeman, 2007).

We have been assuming that the first deficit gives rise to an anomalous experience from which personal-level processes of endorsement or explanation lead to belief. But the neuropsychological version of the two-factor framework is officially neutral on the question whether the first deficit gives rise to an anomalous conscious experience. It may be that personal-level processes have no role to play and that the route from first deficit to belief lies wholly at the sub-personal level and involves wholly unconscious processes (Coltheart, 2007, p. 1044, footnote 4). This is a further example of parametric variation that is allowed by the two-factor framework. The route from first deficit to belief might lie mainly at the personal level or mainly at the sub-personal level. If the bottom-up psychological processes that lead to belief are opaque to the subject, then it seems likely that the belief will be pathological in the sense that we mentioned near the outset. The subject will be beset by a belief for which he or she can offer no grounds.

15.5 **The second factor: why does the patient not reject the belief?**

In any case of delusion, even when we have answered the first question – Where did the delusion come from? – there is a second question: Why does the patient not reject the belief? Suppose a patient has adopted a false proposition ('This is not my arm' or

'My wife has been replaced by an impostor') as a belief. Suppose the answer to the first question appeals to the patient's endorsement or explanation of an anomalous experience. The patient's initial adoption of the belief was a manifestation of a prepotent doxastic response to a perceptual experience or of a prepotent tendency towards acceptance of a confirmed hypothesis. Still, why does the patient not subsequently reject the belief on the grounds of its implausibility and its incompatibility with a mass of available evidence?

According to the two-factor framework, the answer to this question is that the patient has an impairment of belief evaluation. Coltheart proposes that the impairment 'is the same in all people with monothematic delusion' (2005, p. 154) although the impairment is 'very poorly specified' (*ibid.*). We do not yet have an account of the cognitive nature of the second factor in the two-factor framework. To say that the patient does not reject the belief because he or she has lost the ability to make appropriate use of evidence and plausibility in evaluating and revising beliefs (Davies *et al.*, 2001, p. 149) scarcely goes beyond reiterating the fact that the patient's belief is a delusion.

Although the second factor is poorly specified in terms of cognitive function, there are some suggestions that it is a neuropsychological deficit whose neural basis lies in damage to the right hemisphere. Coltheart describes the second deficit in this way.

> The patient has right-hemisphere damage (i.e. damage to the putative belief evaluation system located in that hemisphere).
>
> (Coltheart, 2007, p. 1047)

He goes on to review evidence that 'it is specifically *frontal* right-hemisphere damage that is the neural correlate of the impairment of belief evaluation' (*ibid.*, p. 1052).

15.5.1 Evidence and implausibility

Suppose (as before, section 15.4.1) that the evidence, E, provided by an anomalous experience confirms an explanatory hypothesis, H, which is initially adopted as a belief in response to the imperative of explanatory adequacy. In principle, the explanatory hypothesis may be subsequently evaluated in at least two ways. First, the support that the evidence E provides for H is defeasible. Although E confirms H, the totality of the available evidence, including E, may disconfirm H. Second, a hypothesis H that is confirmed by evidence E, and even by the totality of the available evidence, may still have a relatively low posterior probability if it has a very low prior probability.

Posterior probability depends on both degree of (dis)confirmation and prior probability. So the case for rejecting a hypothesis may sometimes depend primarily on the weight of disconfirming evidence and sometimes on the low prior probability of the hypothesis being true. The same grounds for rejection – evidence or implausibility – may apply to a false proposition that is initially adopted as a belief by way of endorsement, rather than explanation, of an anomalous experience.

Later in this chapter (section 15.9.3), we shall arrive at a proposal about the cognitive nature of the second factor that is somewhat informative but also suitably general. Nevertheless, we should be open to the possibility that the answer to the question why the patient does not reject the belief may vary in its details. Some patients may fail to reject their false belief because they do not make proper use of available disconfirming evidence, others because they do not take proper account of the belief's implausibility. This may be another locus of parametric variation within the two-factor framework.

In the Capgras delusion, the most obviously available evidence – the appearance of the patient's wife and her own statements – does not disconfirm the patient's false belief. After all, a good impostor would look like the patient's wife and would say that she was the patient's wife. The evidence confirms both the true hypothesis (that the person is the patient's wife) and the impostor hypothesis, but is not diagnostic as between them. The impostor hypothesis might be regarded as similar to sceptical hypotheses (such as Descartes's evil demon hypothesis) in being 'unfalsifiable'. What counts against the impostor hypothesis is primarily the fact that it is implausible, not only in the view of people without delusions, but also in the light of the patient's other beliefs.

In somatoparaphrenia, a patient's denial of ownership of the left hand may go against available evidence. Bisiach and Geminiani describe the case of patient LA-O:

> On request, she admitted without hesitation that her left shoulder was part of her body and *inferentially* came to the same conclusion as regards her left arm and elbow, given, as she remarked, the evident continuity of those members. She was elusive about the forearm but insisted on denying ownership of the left hand. . . . She could not explain why her rings happened to be worn by the fingers of the alien hand.

> (Bisiach and Geminiani, 1991, pp. 32–33)

Here, the presence of LA-O's own rings on the fingers of the hand confirms the hypothesis that the hand is hers and disconfirms her belief that the hand is alien.[6]

15.5.2 Subverting the role of evidence and implausibility

In some cases, a patient's initial adoption of a false belief subverts the disconfirmatory role of evidence. Young and Leafhead (1996) describe the case of a 29-year-old woman, JK, who claimed that she was dead (Cotard delusion; Cotard, 1882). They investigated whether patient JK regarded the fact that she had thoughts and feelings as evidence against her belief that she was dead:

> We therefore asked her, during the period when she claimed to be dead, whether she could feel her heart beat, whether she could feel hot or cold, and whether she could feel when her bladder was full. She said she could. We suggested that such feelings surely represented evidence that she was not dead, but alive. JK said that since she had such feelings even though she was dead, they clearly did not represent evidence that she was alive.

> (Young and Leafhead, 1996, p. 158)

Patient JK accepted that, in general, the probability that someone would have thoughts and feelings while dead was low. But she was convinced that she herself was dead and she regarded her own situation – a dead person experiencing bodily sensations – as unique. In contrast, McKay and Cipolotti (2007) present a case of the Cotard delusion in which evidence did play a disconfirmatory role.

A patient's initial adoption of an explanatory hypothesis as a belief may also subvert arguments for rejecting the hypothesis on the grounds of its implausibility. In somato-paraphrenia, a patient may deny ownership of his left hand and claim that it belongs to someone else. Patient PR (Bisiach, 1988) claimed that his left hand belonged to the

---

[6] Similar evidence might be presented to a patient with a misidentification delusion (Breen et al., 2002).

examiner and that the examiner had three hands – an implausible view. In an oft-quoted exchange, the examiner highlighted the implausibility of patient PR's belief, asking, 'Ever see a man with *three* hands?' (Bisiach, 1988, p. 469). The patient replied (*ibid.*): 'A hand is the extremity of an arm. Since you have three arms it follows that you must have three hands.' Patient PR believed that an arm – in fact, his own left arm – was not his. From his point of view, it was more plausible that the arm belonged to someone else, such as the examiner, than that it belonged to him. Given that starting point, it was not especially implausible that the examiner should have three hands.

15.6 The task of belief evaluation

In response to the power of a hypothesis to explain an anomalous experience, a patient may accept the hypothesis and regard competing hypotheses as correspondingly improbable. But, normatively speaking, the patient's acceptance of the hypothesis may be unwarranted. In a theoretical paper, Hemsley and Garety suggest (1986, p. 52): 'A normative theory of how people *should* evaluate evidence relevant to their beliefs can provide a conceptual framework for a consideration of how they do *in fact* evaluate it.' In the spirit of Hemsley and Garety's suggestion, we consider the task of belief evaluation in the light of the normative standards of probability theory.[7]

15.6.1 Alternative explanatory hypotheses

Suppose that hypothesis H adequately explains a patient's anomalous experience in the following sense. If E is the evidence provided by the experience then the probability of E given H, $Pr(E/H)$, is close to 1, and is higher than the prior probability of E, $Pr(E)$. According to Bayes's theorem, the evidence confirms the hypothesis. It raises the probability of the hypothesis in the same proportion as the hypothesis raises the probability of the evidence. But if the prior probability of H is very low then the posterior probability of H may still be low.

We have conjectured that, corresponding to the imperative of explanatory adequacy, there is a prepotent doxastic tendency towards acceptance of a confirmed hypothesis (section 15.4.3). But a patient who accepts H just because it is confirmed by evidence that it explains may, in effect, be underestimating the probability of that evidence given the negation of the hypothesis. The patient may be ignoring an alternative hypothesis, H', inconsistent with H, that has a higher prior probability than H and is no less adequate to explain the evidence.

Here, we should consider Bayes's theorem in the form:

$$\frac{Pr(H/E)}{Pr(H'/E)} = \frac{Pr(E/H)}{Pr(E/H')} \cdot \frac{Pr(H)}{Pr(H')}$$

Suppose that two competing hypotheses, H and H', are equally adequate to explain the evidence E; that is, suppose that $Pr(E/H) = Pr(E/H')$. Then the posterior probabilities of the hypotheses stand in the same ratio as the prior probabilities. The evidence is not

---

[7] In pursuing this strategy it is, of course, important not to lose sight of the distinction between the normative and the descriptive (see Stone and Young, 1997, p. 342).

diagnostic; it does not change the balance of probabilities between the competing hypotheses. Suppose, for example, that the prior probability of hypothesis H' is ten times that of H. Then the posterior probability of H' is also ten times that of H and so the posterior probability of H, $Pr(H/E)$, must be less than 0.091.

Hemsley and Garety describe a case of this kind:

> For example, one patient took the appearance of a police car in a busy thoroughfare as unequivocal evidence that the police were chasing him, neglecting the probability of this event occurring if the police had no interest in him.
>
> (Hemsley and Garety, 1986, p. 53)

The patient's hypothesis that the police were chasing him was, let us agree, adequate to explain the evidence of the police car's appearing on the street. But that evidence cannot shift the balance of probabilities in favour of the patient's hypothesis and against an alternative hypothesis if the alternative hypothesis is also explanatorily adequate. A suitable alternative hypothesis, with a higher prior probability than the patient's hypothesis, would be that the police were not chasing the patient but were chasing someone else in the area.

15.6.2 Alternative explanations, jumping to conclusions, and the confirmation bias

In common parlance, a subject who accepts a hypothesis just because it is adequate to explain a piece of evidence might be described as jumping to a conclusion. So it is important to consider the relationship between the phenomenon that we have been describing (in section 15.6.1) and the JTC bias studied by Garety and colleagues using the beads task (Huq et al., 1988; Garety et al., 1991). In the beads task, subjects are presented with two jars, one jar (A) containing (for example) eighty-five black beads and fifteen yellow beads and the other jar (B) containing eighty-five yellow and fifteen black beads. Subjects are told that initially each jar is equally likely to be chosen, that one will be chosen, and that beads will then be drawn, sequentially and with replacement, from the chosen jar. The subject's task is to decide whether the experimenter is drawing beads from jar A or from jar B. The typical finding is that, by comparison with clinical and non-clinical control participants, patients with delusions ask for fewer beads to be drawn before they reach a decision (which is usually correct). The JTC bias has also been found in individuals at high risk for psychosis (Broome et al., 2007), in relatives of patients with psychosis (Van Dael et al., 2006), and in delusion-prone members of the general population (Linney et al., 1998; Colbert and Peters, 2002).

Freeman and colleagues (Freeman et al., 2004) investigated whether patients with delusions were able to suggest any alternative explanation for their experiences, even if they thought the alternative very unlikely. They also assessed the JTC bias in these patients. About a quarter of the patients were able to suggest an alternative explanation and these patients showed a lesser JTC bias than those offering no alternative explanation. Freeman and colleagues suggest a causal connection between the JTC bias and failure to consider alternative explanations: 'Rapid acceptance of judgments is likely to limit consideration of alternative explanations' (2004, p. 672); 'It is plausible that a more cautious reasoning style may tend toward consideration of alternatives' (ibid., p. 678). Indeed, in the literature on delusions, the phenomenon of ignoring alternative explanations and the JTC bias are often presented as being closely linked (e.g. Stone and Young, 1997, p. 341). They seem, however, to be conceptually distinct.

The phenomenon that we have been describing involves three important features. First, the subject accepts a hypothesis with a relatively low posterior probability, $Pr(H/E)$. Second, the subject underestimates the probability of the evidence given the negation of the hypothesis, $Pr(E/not\text{-}H)$. Third, the subject ignores alternative explanations. In contrast, subjects in the beads task do not accept a hypothesis with a low posterior probability. The probability that jar A has been chosen is 0.85 given that the first bead presented is black and 0.97 given that the first two beads are black. Also, there is very little evidence that the JTC bias involves subjects underestimating the probability of the presented evidence given the negation of the favoured hypothesis. Furthermore, since it is explicit that only two hypotheses are relevant in the beads task, there is no possibility that subjects could ignore alternative explanations of the evidence presented to them. The nature of the connection between failure to consider alternative explanations and the JTC bias requires further theoretical and empirical investigation.

Failure to consider alternative explanatory hypotheses seems to be related to the confirmation bias (Wason, 1960; for a review, see Nickerson, 1998). In an interesting pilot study, Freeman and colleagues (Freeman et al., 2005) used Wason's (1960) 2–4–6 task to assess confirmatory reasoning in non-clinical individuals. In this task, participants are told that the experimenter has in mind a rule that classifies ordered triples of numbers. Participants are told that the triple 2–4–6 conforms to the rule and are asked to try to discover the rule by suggesting additional triples for which feedback will be provided. (Participants are told whether or not their suggested triple conforms to the rule.) The triple 2–4–6 suggests the rule 'successive even numbers' and the typical finding is that participants suggest many triples that conform to that hypothesized rule, such as 6–8–10 or 20–22–24. The feedback confirms their initial hypothesis and, because they do not try out triples that are inconsistent with the 'successive even numbers' rule (such as 3–5–7 or 1–2–3), participants may not discover that the actual rule is 'any three numbers in ascending order'.

In the study by Freeman and colleagues (2005), participants who suggested only triples that conformed to the rule that they (at that time) considered likely to be correct were said to show a confirmatory reasoning style. Participants who sometimes suggested triples that did not conform to the rule that they considered likely to be correct were said to show a disconfirmatory reasoning style. Intellectual and executive functioning, psychological symptoms, and delusional ideation were also assessed and participants completed a belief-evaluation task modelled on cognitive therapy.

The findings of the study were that individuals who adopted a disconfirmatory reasoning style in Wason's 2–4–6 task gathered more evidence before reaching a decision, and considered a greater number of hypotheses, than individuals with a confirmatory reasoning style. They had higher IQ scores and lower depression scores and, in the belief-evaluation task, they produced more evidence, both for and against their beliefs. Similar investigations of patient populations would appear to hold considerable promise for both theoretical understanding and therapeutic intervention.

15.7 **Acceptance and subversion**

A patient's acceptance of hypothesis H on the basis of evidence E is normatively not warranted if a competing hypothesis, H', also explains evidence E and has a higher prior probability than H. But, once the hypothesis H has been accepted, the power of the competing hypothesis to explain the evidence cannot shift the probabilities in favour of H' and against H since H is also explanatorily adequate. Having accepted H, the patient assigns a high probability to it and a correspondingly low probability to competing hypotheses.

An argument for rejecting an explanatory hypothesis on the grounds of its implausibility needs to be deployed while the patient still regards the hypothesis as somewhat improbable and when a more probable, and no less explanatory, hypothesis is also available. Thus, for example, there are potential benefits in providing clinical intervention for individuals identified as being in the 'at risk mental state' but before the first episode of psychosis (Broome *et al.*, 2005a). A patient's unwarranted acceptance of a hypothesis is apt to subvert an argument for rejecting it on the grounds of its implausibility, even if an alternative explanation is presented. In order to make proper use of considerations of implausibility when evaluating explanatory hypotheses, the patient needs to take a step back from his or her initial acceptance. The patient must, at least suppositionally, regard the question of the truth or falsity of the hypothesis as open. The patient must then attempt to settle the question whether the hypothesis is true or false by evaluating it alongside alternative explanatory hypotheses.

In his influential book on inference to the best explanation, Lipton (2004) describes the two-stage process of hypothesis generation and selection. First, a shortlist of explanatory hypotheses is generated; second, the best candidate on the shortlist is selected. When the mechanisms of hypothesis generation work well they favour 'those that are extensions of explanations already accepted' (2004, p. 151) and Lipton suggests that this may explain our normal conservatism (*ibid.*): 'Our method of generating candidate hypotheses is skewed so as to favor those that cohere with our background beliefs, and to disfavor those that, if accepted, would require us to reject much of the background.' In some cases of delusion, background beliefs do not adequately constrain hypothesis generation and, as a result, the best candidate on the shortlist is not good enough. This unsatisfactory situation is particularly difficult to rectify if the selection process is allowed to go ahead – if the best candidate on the shortlist is selected and is, so to speak, installed in the advertised position. That is, flawed hypothesis generation is difficult to rectify if, in accordance with a prepotent doxastic tendency, one hypothesis from the inadequately constrained shortlist is selected and adopted as a belief.[8]

We have been considering the task of belief evaluation from a theoretical perspective. On that basis, we can put forward an initial suggestion about cognitive processes that may be implicated in belief evaluation. First, the evaluation of competing hypotheses in the light of evidence and plausibility will involve working-memory resources for the maintenance and manipulation of information. Second, if there is a prepotent doxastic

---

[8] We are indebted to Tony Stone for drawing our attention to Lipton's (2004) discussion of hypothesis generation in normal inference to the best explanation.

tendency towards accepting a hypothesis that explains a salient piece of evidence and is thereby confirmed, then the step back from initial acceptance will involve executive processes of inhibition.

We now describe putative processes of belief formation and belief evaluation in the Capgras delusion, beginning from the assumption that an anomalous experience figures in the answer to the question where the delusion came from.

15.7.1 Considering alternatives in the Capgras delusion: the explanationist account

Ellis and Young (1990) propose that the anomalous experience in the Capgras delusion arises from disruption of the connection between the patient's face-recognition system and autonomic nervous system. In a development of this proposal, Ellis and Lewis (2001) suggest that '[an integrative device] would . . . compare the expected affective response [i.e. expected on the basis of the activity in the primary face-recognition system] with the actual affective response and some kind of attribution process would take place' (2001, p. 154). Coltheart makes a similar suggestion in terms of unconscious processes of prediction and comparison (2005, p. 155): 'the unconscious system predict[s] that when the wife is next seen a high autonomic response will occur, detect[s] that this does not occur, and report[s] to consciousness, "There's something odd about this woman"'.

These suggestions and Maher's (1999) proposals converge on the idea that, as the result of a neuropsychological deficit and the subsequent operation of a comparator system, the Capgras patient has an anomalous experience.[9] It is a perceptual experience of his wife that is suffused with a feeling of heightened significance, an experience that cries out for explanation in terms of change, or 'something odd', in the immediate environment and particularly in the woman perceived. The hypothesis, H, that the woman perceived is not really the patient's wife seems adequate to explain the patient's anomalous experience. The negation of that hypothesis – that is, the hypothesis, not-H, that the woman perceived is *not* an impostor and really *is* the patient's wife – does not seem to offer the same explanatory promise.

The patient underestimates the probability of the evidence given the hypothesis not-H and ignores – does not even consider – the alternative, more specific (and correct) explanatory hypothesis, H', that the woman is his wife *and he has suffered a brain injury*. The hypothesis H is, to some degree, confirmed by the evidence and, as the result of a prepotent tendency, is adopted as a belief. This woman, who looks like the patient's wife and says that she is the patient's wife, is not really his wife; she is an impostor.

If this initially adopted belief is to be evaluated and ultimately rejected, then the patient must step back from his acceptance of the impostor hypothesis. But stepping back is not

---

9 Here, we envisage abnormally reduced autonomic activity and normal operation of the comparator. Alternatively, an anomalous experience might be produced by abnormal operation of the comparator itself or perhaps by an abnormality that is causally downstream from the comparator (Maher, 1999, p. 551).

sufficient by itself since the false belief is liable to be reinstated by renewed demands for explanation each time the patient looks at his wife. The patient also needs to undertake an evaluation of the impostor hypothesis and alternative explanatory hypotheses, including the brain injury hypothesis, in terms of their plausibility and in the light of available evidence. The patient needs to inhibit a prepotent doxastic tendency and to undertake a cognitive task that is demanding of working-memory resources.

15.7.2 Considering alternatives in the Capgras delusion: the endorsement account

The same key features are also present according to the endorsement account. We now assume that the representational content of the Capgras patient's experience is more specific than 'This is someone who looks just like my wife *but there is something odd about her.*' It is, rather: 'This is someone who looks just like my wife *but it is not really her.*' The processes that determine this content of experience are not yet specified – the endorsement account, like much else in this area, needs 'fleshing out' (Coltheart, 2005, p. 153). We might conjecture that the generation of the content will – like the attribution process in Ellis and Lewis's (2001) account – involve a comparator system or integrative device that has access to both the primary face-recognition system and the autonomic nervous system.

The prepotent doxastic response to a perceptual experience with this content is to believe that this person, who looks just like the patient's wife, is not really her. This belief is subsequently elaborated into the belief that the patient's wife has been replaced by an impostor. We can conceive of this latter belief as an explanatory hypothesis that the patient has adopted. But it is important to recognize that what is being explained is the fact, as the patient believes, that the person who looks like his wife is not really her:

> The prior possibility that the spouse is an impostor of some sort is of course very low, but if this hypothesis best explains that (as the patient believes is true) the spouse is really a stranger that looks like the spouse, then it is very probable that the spouse is an impostor.
> (Hohwy and Rosenberg, 2005, p. 154)

As Hohwy and Rosenberg point out, what needs explaining, from the patient's point of view, is not adequately explained by the hypothesis that the woman is the patient's wife and the patient has suffered a brain injury (*ibid.*, p. 155): 'The brain pathology hypothesis would only be relevant if the patient could accept that what needs explaining is the mere *experience* that it is as if the spouse looks like a stranger.'

Thus, as before, in order to consider and evaluate alternative explanatory hypotheses, the patient first needs to take a step back. The patient must inhibit the prepotent doxastic response of treating a perceptual experience as veridical and, instead, treat the experience as standing in need of explanation.[10]

---

[10] We note that Hohwy and Rosenberg propose that 'it is intra- and inter-modal reality testing that can inhibit the pre-potent doxastic response to believe what we experience, and when such reality testing procedures are exhausted, nothing else will on its own inhibit the pre-potent response' (2005, p. 149). They also suggest that 'unusual beliefs arise when unusual

15.8 Interlude: hypotheses, beliefs, and evaluation

We have interpreted the question, 'Where did the delusion come from?', as asking how the patient came to adopt the false belief and we have considered belief evaluation under the assumption that, normatively, it is primarily supposed to take place after initial adoption of a belief. Thus, we have interpreted the question, 'Why does the patient not reject the belief?' as asking why the patient is not able to evaluate and reject the belief that has been initially adopted.

An alternative approach would be to interpret the first question as asking how the patient came to entertain or consider the false hypothesis. This may be what Coltheart intends when he glosses the first question as (2007, p. 1047): 'what is responsible for the *content* of the particular belief?' According to this approach, belief evaluation – really, hypothesis evaluation – begins earlier and the second question asks, in part, why the patient is not able to evaluate the hypothesis and reject it, instead of adopting it as a belief. (Since a delusion is a false belief that is maintained, the second question must also ask why the patient is not able to evaluate and reject the belief even after adopting it.)

The difference between these approaches seems to correspond to a difference between two accounts of normal believing. In a series of papers, Gilbert and colleagues (Gilbert *et al.*, 1990, 1993; Gilbert, 1991) have contrasted Cartesian and Spinozan views of belief and have presented experimental results in support of the Spinozan view.[11] Each view of belief can be summarized in terms of two stages, a representation stage and an assessment stage. On the Cartesian view, the representation stage involves *comprehension*, which 'precedes and is separate from assessment' (Gilbert, 1991, p. 108). A hypothesis is grasped and then, in the assessment stage, the hypothesis is either *accepted* as true and adopted as a belief, or else *rejected* as false. On the Spinozan view, in contrast, the representation stage involves both comprehension and *acceptance* (*ibid.*, p. 107): 'People believe in the ideas they comprehend, as quickly and automatically as they believe in the objects they see.' Then, in the assessment stage, the already adopted belief is either *certified* or else *unaccepted*.

Our approach in this chapter is influenced by the Spinozan view of belief as Gilbert presents it but recent experimental findings suggest that 'The relation between

---

experiences are taken as veridical because they occur in sensory modalities or at processing stages where application of the available reality testing procedures keeps giving the same result and where further intra- or inter-modal reality testing cannot be performed' (*ibid.*, p. 153). Their overall position is that in cases of delusion, such as the Capgras delusion or the alien control delusion, further reality testing is not possible. Consequently, they regard the transition from anomalous experience to delusional belief as unavoidable (p. 156) and reject the basic argument for a two-factor framework. That is, they reject the claim that there are patients who have the first factor that is implicated in a delusion – a particular kind of anomalous experience arising from a neuropsychological deficit – yet do not have the delusion.

11 We are grateful to Tony Stone for many conversations about the work of Gilbert and colleagues and we acknowledge the influence of his presentation, 'Delusions: Learning from Spinoza', at a workshop on delusion and self-deception held at Macquarie University in November 2004. We shall not engage with questions about the relationship between the two views that Gilbert contrasts and the historical philosophers for whom they are named.

comprehension and belief is a complex one' (Hasson *et al.*, 2005, p. 571). We acknowledge that the Cartesian view, or some hybrid, may provide a better account of normal believing. This acknowledgement might seem to pose a threat to our suggestion that belief evaluation involves inhibitory executive processes. If the processes of evaluation begin before any belief is adopted, then no 'step back' from initial acceptance of a hypothesis is required.

In fact, however, the suggestion is not threatened since the influence of prepotent responses and tendencies still needs to be inhibited; imperatives still need to be resisted. As Gilbert, Tafarodi, and Malone say, in a discussion of sceptical doubt:

> For Descartes, being skeptical meant understanding an idea but not taking the second step of believing it unless evidence justified taking that step. For Spinoza, being skeptical meant taking a second step backward (unbelieving) to correct for the uncontrollable tendency to take a first step forward (believing). Both philosophers realized that achieving true beliefs required that one subvert [inhibit, resist] the natural inclinations [prepotent tendencies, imperatives] of one's own mind; for Descartes this subversion was proactive, whereas for Spinoza it was retroactive.
>
> (Gilbert *et al.*, 1993, p. 230)

Stone and Young (1997) say that, in cases of delusion, the balance between imperatives goes too far towards observational adequacy – or, we have added, explanatory adequacy – and departs too far from conservatism. If this is where a delusion came from then, it may seem, evaluating and rejecting the belief involves inhibiting the natural inclinations towards observational or explanatory adequacy and restoring the influence of the imperative of conservatism. But merely allowing the preexisting web of belief to exert inertia, so that an observationally or explanatorily adequate hypothesis is not accepted, is not yet sufficient for belief evaluation. What is required is that the patient should assess competing hypotheses (by weighing evidence and plausibility) while also controlling and balancing (inhibiting or not) the influences of observational adequacy, explanatory adequacy, *and* conservatism. (In the case of anosognosia, the belief that needs to be rejected is part of the patient's preexisting web of belief.) Cognitive tasks with this structure – undertaking an analytic assessment while controlling heuristic influences – are the focus of dual-process accounts of reasoning.

15.9 Dual-process accounts of reasoning

Dual-process accounts propose that there are two quite different kinds of cognitive processes involved in reasoning – and also in judgement and decision-making (Evans, 2003). The two kinds of processes are sometimes referred to as 'System 1' versus 'System 2' processes although, as Evans (2007) says, 'the mapping of dual processes on to underlying dual systems is fraught with difficulties' (2007, p. 322) System 1 or *heuristic* processes are 'rapid, preconscious, and computationally powerful'; System 2 or *analytic* processes, in contrast, are 'slow, sequential, and effortful' (*ibid.*; see also Stanovich, 1999). System 1 processes underpin cognitive biases and are heterogeneous in their nature. Some may be evolutionarily ancient, but not all are. System 2 processes permit 'abstract hypothetical thinking that cannot be achieved by system 1' (Evans, 2003, p. 454). A central idea in dual-process accounts is that the two kinds of processes can come into conflict or competition.

In this section, our aim is to draw on research that is motivated by dual-process accounts in order to generate proposals about the cognitive nature and neural basis of belief evaluation. We shall connect the two areas by considering the imperatives of observational and explanatory adequacy and, particularly, conservatism as belonging with System 1 or heuristic processes and considering the assessment of competing hypotheses as belonging with System 2 or analytic processes. In a similar spirit, Freeman and colleagues suggest that 'belief evaluation may be partly understood by drawing upon the reasoning literature' (Freeman *et al.*, 2005, p. 243). They propose that cognitive therapy for clinical disorders, including the technique of 'encourag[ing] patients to evaluate their beliefs', may 'promote [System 2] analytic reasoning to modify particular conclusions derived from [System 1] processes' (*ibid.*, p. 244).

One important piece of evidence that supports dual-process accounts of reasoning is provided by the *belief-bias* effect (Evans *et al.*, 1983; for a review, see Klauer *et al.*, 2000). The belief bias is 'the tendency for people to judge the validity of an argument on the basis of whether or not they agree with its conclusion' (Evans, 2007, p. 322). Participants are asked to assess syllogistic arguments for logical validity. In some of the arguments, the conclusion is intuitively believable (e.g. Some highly trained dogs are not police dogs); in others, the conclusion is intuitively unbelievable (e.g. Some millionaires are not rich people). Validity of the arguments and believability of their conclusions can be varied independently to generate items of four types: Valid argument–Believable conclusion; Valid argument–Unbelievable conclusion; Invalid argument–Believable conclusion; Invalid argument–Unbelievable conclusion. In the second and third types of argument, there is a *conflict* between the response based on validity and the response based on believability; in the other two types of argument there is *no conflict*.

Participants are explicitly instructed to assume that the premises of the syllogism are true and to judge whether the conclusion necessarily follows from the premises. But the typical finding in these experiments is that participants' responses are influenced by the believability of the conclusion as well as by logical validity. Despite the explicit instructions, it is extremely difficult for healthy adult participants to inhibit the influence of their prior beliefs. The dual-process interpretation of the belief-bias effect is as follows:

> System 2 [analytic] thinking is both volitional and responsive to verbal instructions whereas System 1 [heuristic] thinking is not. Hence System 1 influences – in this case belief bias – can only be suppressed indirectly by asking people to make a strong effort to reason deductively.
>
> (Evans, 2003, p. 456)

As Stanovich (2003) says, there is a 'tendency to automatically bring prior knowledge to bear when solving problems' and this tendency is 'so ubiquitous that it cannot easily be turned off – [it is] a fundamental computational bias' (p. 292).

15.9.1 The role of working memory and inhibitory executive processes

Earlier (section 15.7), we suggested that belief evaluation may involve working mem-ory and inhibitory executive processes. Working-memory tasks are said to involve maintenance and manipulation of information but it is useful to make some distinc-tions among these tasks. Working-memory capacity is often assessed by span tasks of which the simplest require the subject to reproduce a list of digits or words. An exam-ple of such a task is Digit Span Forward, a subtest of the Wechsler Memory Scale–Revised (WMS-R; Wechsler, 1987). The subject is asked to reproduce successively longer lists of digits and the subject's digit span is the length of the longest list that the subject can reproduce correctly. In fact, these simplest span tasks, which involve maintenance but not manipulation of information (storage but not processing), would usually be described as testing attention or short-term memory rather than working memory. One way to introduce manipulation or processing of information is to ask the subject to reproduce a list of digits or words in reverse order, as in the Digit Span Backward subtest of the WMS-R.

In a more complex kind of span task, participants are asked to memorize a list of words while also carrying out simple arithmetical calculations. Each word on the list is preceded by an arithmetical problem, for example:

Is $(4 \div 2) + 3 = 6$? (yes or no) DOG

The number of words that can be recalled provides an estimate of working-memory capacity. This kind of working-memory span task requires both storage (of the words) and processing (for the calculations) and it also requires the participant to maintain task-relevant information (the words) in the face of distraction or interference (from the calculations). That is, the complex span task requires storage and processing of information and also executive processes of controlled attention – using attention to maintain or suppress information (Engle *et al.*, 1999; Engle, 2002). Working-memory capacity as assessed by the complex span task is inextricably linked to executive func-tion and is sometimes referred to as 'executive working memory'. Smith and Kosslyn say (2007, p. 259): 'The central executive is what does the "work" in working memory.'

In an experimental study, De Neys (2006) investigated an assumption of dual-process accounts concerning the role of working memory and inhibitory executive processes in cognitive performance that depends on System 2:

> [T]he two systems [System 1 = heuristic; System 2 = analytic] will sometimes conflict and cue different responses. In these cases, the analytic system will need to override the belief-based response generated by the heuristic system. *The inhibition of the heuristic system and the com-putations of the analytic system are assumed to draw on executive working memory resources.*
>
> (De Neys, 2006, p. 428; emphasis added)

This assumption yields the prediction that performance on conflict items will be bet-ter in participants with higher working-memory capacity and that performance on conflict items will be worse when participants have to perform a secondary task that burdens their executive resources. It is also predicted that neither working-memory capacity nor executive load will affect performance on no-conflict items, since heuristic (System 1) processes will generate the correct response.

In this study, the working-memory capacity of participants was assessed using a complex span task of the kind just described. The primary task was then a syllogistic reasoning task of the kind used in belief-bias experiments and a secondary executive load task required participants to remember a pattern of three (low load) or four (high load) dots in a 3-by-3 matrix. A dot pattern was presented before each syllogism and the participant had to reproduce the pattern after the syllogism had been assessed for logical validity.

This kind of dot-memory task involves maintenance but not manipulation of information and we might not expect that it would impose a load on executive function. Indeed, in the verbal domain, it has been shown that working-memory tasks that involve both storage and processing are more strongly related to executive functioning than tasks that involve storage alone. However, in a study of visuospatial working memory and executive functioning, Miyaki and colleagues (Miyaki *et al.*, 2001) showed that the situation is different in the visuospatial domain. There, both kinds of task, specifically including the dot-memory task, are strongly related to executive functioning.

The main findings of the De Neys (2006) study were these: greater working-memory capacity resulted in better performance on conflict items, while performance on no-conflict items was uniformly high. Executive load had a negative impact on performance on conflict items but did not affect performance on no-conflict items. These findings support the assumption that 'the inhibition of the heuristic system and the computations of the analytic system . . . draw on executive working memory resources' (2006, p. 428). The results of the study show that 'erroneous reasoning in the case of belief-logic conflict is not only associated with, but also directly caused by, limitations in executive resources' (*ibid.*, p. 432).

It is natural to suppose that belief evaluation involves both inhibition of heuristic systems – that is, inhibition of prepotent tendencies or resistance against imperatives – and computations of the analytic system – that is, assessment of competing hypotheses in the light of evidence and plausibility. So we interpret the findings of De Neys's (2006) study as providing some support for the suggestion that belief evaluation involves working-memory resources and inhibitory executive processes. Paraphrasing De Neys, we may also suggest that *erroneous* belief evaluation – maintaining a false belief – in cases where the normative requirements of belief evaluation *conflict* with the imperatives of observational adequacy, explanatory adequacy, or conservatism is *caused by limitations* in executive working-memory resources (that is, working memory and executive function).[12]

15.9.2 The neural basis of performance in a belief-bias experiment

Goel and Dolan (2003) used event-related functional magnetic resonance imaging (fMRI) to investigate the neural basis of performance by subjects in a belief-bias experiment. In particular, they measured neural activation as subjects responded to

---

12 It is of some interest to note that, in a study of individuals at high risk for psychosis (Broome *et al.*, 2007), the at-risk group performed significantly worse than healthy control participants on a test of working memory (a simple span task using coloured beads). Also, within the at-risk group, the degree of JTC bias was found to be correlated with the number of errors on the bead span task.

syllogisms in which there was a conflict between the response based on validity and the response based on believability (Valid argument–Unbelievable conclusion and Invalid argument–Believable conclusion). When subjects yielded to the influence of their prior beliefs and gave the logically incorrect response there was activation of ventromedial prefrontal cortex (VMPFC); when subjects inhibited the belief bias and gave the logically correct response there was activation of right inferior prefrontal cortex (2003, pp. B17, B19).[13]

Goel and Dolan say that 'the activation of VMPFC in incorrect trials highlights its role in non-logical, belief-based responses' (p. B19). Here it is of some interest to note the result of a study (Adolphs et al., 1996) using the Wason Selection Task (Wason, 1968). In this task, participants are asked which of four cards they need to turn over in order to decide whether a conditional statement is true or false. When the conditional statement is abstract (e.g. If there is a D on one side of any card then there is a 3 on its other side) very few healthy adult participants (fewer than 10%) make the logically correct response. When the conditional statement is deontic, realistic, and familiar (e.g. If you are in a bar drinking beer then you must be over 18 years old) and participants are asked which cards they need to turn over in order to decide whether anyone is breaking the rule, performance is much better (more than 75% of participants make the logically correct response).

In the study by Adolphs and colleagues (1996), the performance of patients with lesions of dorsolateral prefrontal cortex and control subjects with lesions outside the frontal cortex was facilitated by material that was deontic, realistic, and familiar by comparison with less familiar material. Patients with VMPFC lesions, in contrast, performed no better on the familiar than on the less familiar material. They were unable to make appropriate use of information about familiar situations.

Goel and Dolan also conjecture that 'the right prefrontal cortex involvement in correct response trials is critical in detecting and/or resolving the conflict between belief and logic' (2003, p. B19). One possibility is that this neural activation corresponds to controlled or executive attention that is required to facilitate the performance of the logical task of assessing the validity of the argument in the face of distraction from prior beliefs about the conclusion.

15.9.3 A proposal

We have said that it is natural to suppose that belief evaluation involves System 2 processes including processes of inhibiting the influence of prepotent responses and tendencies. Indeed, belief evaluation seems to be a fine example of the 'abstract hypothetical thinking that cannot be achieved by system 1' (Evans, 2003, p. 454). We now add that Goel and Dolan's (2003) finding of right prefrontal cortex activation when

---

[13] Goel and Dolan (2003) locate this activation in Brodmann's area 45 (p. B17). This area would be included in dorsolateral prefrontal cortex (DLPFC) on an inclusive use of that term. But, as Goel and Dolan's description 'right inferior prefrontal cortex' indicates, the area would be inferior to right DLPFC on a more restricted use of that term.

subjects give logically correct responses under conditions of conflict seems to be broadly consistent with the suggestion that belief evaluation has a neural basis in the right frontal region of the brain. A consequence of this suggestion would be that 'frontal right-hemisphere damage . . . is the neural correlate of the impairment of belief evaluation [the second factor]' (Coltheart, 2007, p. 1052).[14]

We are now in a position to make a proposal about the cognitive nature and neural basis of the second factor in the explanation of delusions. We can draw on our earlier task analysis (Sections 15.6 and 15.7), Coltheart's (2007) arguments, and the findings from behavioural experiments (De Neys, 2006) and neuroimaging (Goel and Dolan, 2003) using a task that is relevantly similar to belief evaluation. The proposal is that the second factor is an impairment of working memory or executive function with a neural basis in damage to the right frontal region of the brain.

15.10 **Anosognosia as a case study**

Patients with anosognosia for their motor impairments, or for the consequences of their impairments for activities of daily living, have false beliefs that are maintained against the evidence. In one respect, explaining this pathology of belief may be less complex than explaining other delusions, such as somatoparaphrenia or the Capgras delusion. In cases of anosognosia, there is a straightforward answer to the question where the delusion came from. The beliefs that constitute anosognosia are not new and exotic but old and commonplace (though there may seldom have been the occasion to articulate them explicitly). Patients with anosognosia have believed for many decades that they can raise their left arm and move their left leg, or that they can clap their hands and walk upstairs. What is new is that, in the dramatically changed circumstances following a right-hemisphere stroke, these beliefs are no longer true. The question that is pressing is: Why do these patients not reject their false beliefs in the light of the evidence available to them in their changed circumstances?

At this point, we can anticipate two problems. First, the question where the delusion came from has a straightforward answer that does not mention any anomalous experience or neuropsychological deficit. So how can anosognosia fit the two-factor framework for explaining delusions? Second, we have proposed that the second factor in the explanation of delusions is an impairment of working memory or executive processes with a neural basis in damage to the right frontal region of the brain. But how much working memory, and what executive processes, does a stroke patient need in order to recognize that his or her arm is paralysed?[15] We shall address these two problems in turn. But before that, we consider the change in a patient's beliefs when a right-hemisphere stroke causes motor impairments but not anosognosia.

---

[14] For a review of neuroimaging in individuals with delusions in the context of psychosis, see Broome and McGuire (2008).

[15] John Marshall asked us (personal communication): 'How much WM do I need to notice that my arm is paralysed?'

15.10.1 **Motor impairments without anosognosia**

Consider a hypothetical case of a patient with left-side paralysis following a right-hemisphere stroke and without anosognosia. The patient may intend and try to raise his left arm, but proprioception and vision will tell him that the arm is hanging by his side. The patient may direct his attention to the left side of his body and confirm that his left arm has not moved. Furthermore, when the patient tries to raise his arm, a comparator within the motor control system will detect a mismatch between the expected movement of the arm and what actually happens and the patient will be alerted to his paralysis (Heilman *et al.*, 1998, p. 1908). In short, the patient will have immediate bodily experiences of his paralysis – experiences with the representational content that his left arm does not move despite his trying. The prepotent doxastic response to experiences with this content is for the patient to believe that his left arm does not move. This may subsequently be elaborated into the belief that the patient's left arm is paralysed.

This belief, adopted in response to the imperative of observational adequacy, is implausible in the light of the patient's preexisting web of belief. But although adopting the belief goes against the imperative of conservatism, other evidence confirms the belief. The patient is unable to lift a glass with his left hand, unable to clap his hands, unable to tie a knot, to shuffle a pack of cards, or to type with both hands. Thus, the patient will be concurrently aware of his motoric failures, will acknowledge his impairments, and will appreciate their consequences for activities of daily living. His long-held but no longer true beliefs will be rejected and his newly adopted beliefs will be maintained.

The patient's change of belief is produced, in the first instance, by bodily experiences of motoric failure. The newly adopted belief is then maintained because of recurrent experiences of paralysis and other confirming evidence. If there were disconfirming, instead of confirming, evidence, then the patient might reject the belief. Suppose the patient were to discover that, despite his bodily experiences of his left arm apparently not moving, he could still lift a glass with his left hand, clap his hands, tie a knot, shuffle cards, and type. Then the patient would quite possibly conclude that he was suffering from anomalous and deeply disconcerting experiences as if he were paralysed but that he was not, in reality, motorically impaired.

15.10.2 **Anosognosia in the two-factor framework**

A patient who was concurrently aware of his motoric failures might still not acknowledge his motor impairments. This might happen if the patient were to have a memory impairment specific to information about the movements or positions of parts of his body (Carpenter *et al.*, 1995) or if, for some other reason, the information provided in bodily experiences were not consolidated into more lasting representations (House and Hodges, 1988; Marcel *et al.*, 2004). For example, Karnath and colleagues (Karnath *et al.*, 2005) report a neuroimaging study in which anosognosia was found to be associated with damage to the right posterior insula, a structure which 'seems to be involved in integrating input signals related to self-awareness and to one's beliefs about the functioning of contralateral body parts' (2005, p. 7137). Nevertheless, it is natural to suppose that concurrent *un*awareness of motoric failure may often be a factor in anosognosia for motor impairments. There are several proposals about neuropsychological deficits that would impair a patient's immediate experience of paralysis.

Levine (1990) has proposed that somatosensory loss is a factor in anosognosia and Vuilleumier (2004) that unilateral neglect is 'a notable suspect in anosognosia' (2004, p. 10). Heilman has proposed that paralysis is not detected as the result of an impairment to the intentional-preparatory systems involved in motor control (Heilman, 1991; Heilman *et al.*, 1998). Frith, Blakemore, and Wolpert (2000, pp. 1780–1782) suggest that, because of failure of a comparator within the motor control system, patients may experience illusory movements of their paralysed limbs (see also Feinberg *et al.*, 2000). Patients experience their limbs moving as intended when no movement actually occurs.[16] In patients with one or more of these impairments of sensation, attention, or motor control, long-held beliefs about their left-side limbs may remain somewhat credible.

These impairments are candidate factors in the explanation of anosognosia but they do not provide an adequate answer to the question why these patients maintain, rather than reject, their long-held but now false beliefs. Marcel and colleagues give vivid expression to this inadequacy:

> [I]t is not just that they fail *motorically*. The consequence of such [motoric] failures is that, in trying to get out of bed to go to the toilet or to lift an object, they fall over or incur a similar accident, often lying helpless or hurting themselves.
>
> (Marcel *et al.*, 2004, p. 35)

Even without the immediate bodily experience of paralysis, patients have a mass of other evidence of their motor impairments. Normatively, they should reject their false beliefs in the light of this evidence.

Furthermore, there are patients whose bodily experience suggests that they can still move their left-side limbs but who nevertheless acknowledge their motor impairments (Marcel *et al.*, 2004). Some patients who have recovered from anosognosia continue to describe bodily experiences of being able to move (Chatterjee and Mennemeier, 1996). One patient, when asked, 'Can you raise the left [arm]?', responded: 'It feels like it's rising, but, it's not' (1996, p. 229). Another patient, HS, reported that the idea that he could move his paralysed limbs still seemed credible even though he was able to reject it:

E: What was the consequence of the stroke?

HS: The left hand here is dead and the left leg was pretty much.

HS: (later): I still feel as if when I am in a room and I have to get up and go walking . . . I just feel like I should be able to.

---

[16] Berti and colleagues (Berti *et al.*, 2005) report a neuroimaging study in which anosognosia was found to be associated with damage to 'areas related to the programming of motor acts' (2005, p. 488), including dorsal premotor cortex. They interpret the findings as supporting the hypothesis that there is a degree of commonality in the neural substrates of motor control and awareness of action.

E: You have a belief that you could actually do that?

HS: I do not have a belief, just the exact opposite. I just have the feeling that sometimes I feel like I can get up and do something and I have to tell myself 'no I can't'.

(*ibid.*, p. 227)

We note, however, that the argument for a second factor in anosognosia might not apply in the first few days following a stroke if, because of sedation or lack of arousal, the patient did not try to engage in activities of daily living. In such a case, the evidence that Marcel and colleagues (2004) describe would not be available to the patient and anosognosia for motor impairments would arguably not be a delusion. We should expect that studies of anosognosia in the acute stage following stroke may focus on candidate factors that impair sensation, attention, or motor control. At that stage, neuropsychological deficits causing concurrent unawareness of motoric failure may be sufficient to explain the patient's false belief.

Still, anosognosia beyond the first few days following stroke fits the two-factor framework for explaining delusions. A first factor impairs the patient's concurrent awareness of paralysis. But the first factor is not sufficient; patients with the first factor may not have anosognosia. There must be a second factor that explains why the patient does not make appropriate use of a mass of available evidence. Levine (1990) proposed that, when a patient suffers somatosensory loss, paralysis is not phenomenally immediate. Knowledge of paralysis then requires a process of *discovery*. Anosognosia occurs when the first factor is accompanied by additional impairments that impact negatively on observation and inference so that the patient is 'unable to assimilate information from a variety of sources to form a consistent and accurate judgement' (1990, p. 254). Vuilleumier gives clear expression to a generalization of Levine's proposal (2004, p. 11; emphasis added): '*any* neurological dysfunction susceptible to alter the phenomenal experience of a defect might provide the ground out of which anosognosia can develop when permissive cognitive factors are also present'.

15.10.3 Impaired working memory and executive function in anosognosia

A patient with motor impairments but without impairments of sensation or attention, intentional-preparatory systems or comparator systems, memory or consolidation, would very probably recognize his or her paralysis and would do so relatively immediately, without depending heavily on working memory or executive processing. However, recognition of paralysis is more demanding when, as the result of one or more of these impairments, it is not phenomenally immediate. This is the leading idea of Levine's discovery theory and of our account of anosognosia within the two-factor framework.

It is theoretically useful to consider an analogy with the task of assessing a syllogism for logical validity in a belief-bias experiment. When there is no conflict between the response based on validity and the response based on believability, performance on the task is not affected by the availability of executive working-memory resources because heuristic (System 1) processes are adequate to generate the correct response. When there is a conflict, the task is demanding of executive working-memory resources. If those resources are unavailable – as in individuals with low working-memory capacity or under executive load – then performance on the task is degraded.

In the case of a patient with motor impairments, the fundamental conflict is between the reality of the patient's situation, for which there is a mass of evidence (particularly after the first few days), and the patient's long-held beliefs. If no first factor impairs the patient's concurrent awareness of paralysis, then the imperative of observational adequacy is set against the imperative of conservatism and is liable to lead to revision of those long-held beliefs. The conflict between the response based on available evidence and the response based on believability is thus reduced or eliminated. In such a case, the patient's ability to reach an accurate judgement should not depend on the availability of executive working-memory resources. The prepotent doxastic response to the patient's bodily experiences is already adequate to generate a true belief.

When there is a first factor, however, there is a severe conflict between the response based on available evidence and the response based on prior beliefs – and all the more so if illusory limb movements enter the battle on the side of the prior beliefs. In this kind of case, our earlier task analysis and the analogy with belief-bias experiments lead to a prediction. Limitations of executive working-memory resources (that is, working memory and executive function) may well have the consequence that prior beliefs that are now false may be maintained, rather than rejected.

In a study of persisting unilateral neglect, the first author investigated cognitive impairments, including impairments of working memory and executive function, in seven right-hemisphere stroke patients (Aimola, 1999; Maguire and Ogden, 2002).[17] All the patients suffered from unilateral neglect – a 'notable suspect' as a first factor in anosognosia – persisting at least 3 months following their stroke. Four of the seven patients (M1, M3, M5, and M6) demonstrated moderate or severe anosognosia for motor impairments and their consequences for activities of daily living – scores of 2 or 3 on the four-point (0–3) scale proposed by Bisiach (Bisiach et al., 1986; Bisiach and Geminiani, 1991). Two patients (F2 and M2) demonstrated at most mild anosognosia (score of 1)[18] and patient M4 frankly acknowledged his motor impairments and their consequences for everyday activities (score of 0). All the patients showed impairments in at least two of the following four areas: visual or verbal memory (recognition or recall), sustained attention, working memory, and executive function. Impairments of memory and sustained attention were doubly dissociated from anosognosia, but impaired working memory was associated with anosognosia.

One test of working memory was the Elevator Counting with Distraction subtest of the Test of Everyday Attention (TEA; Robertson et al., 1994). This requires the patient to respond to two types of auditory tones by counting the low tones and ignoring the high tones. Three patients (M3, M5, and M6), all with moderate or severe anosognosia, demonstrated problems on this test. The other patient with anosognosia (M1) scored in the normal

---

17 Nine patients were studied but two are excluded from the discussion: patient F1, following a left-hemisphere stroke, demonstrated no anosognosia; patient F3 had moderate-to-severe anosognosia but time issues prevented her from completing the full neuropsychological test battery.

18 We note that some studies use a three-point scale on which patients who acknowledge their impairment in response to a specific question (Bisiach's score of 1) are scored 0 and classified as not having anosognosia (Berti et al., 1996).

range on Elevator Counting with Distraction but demonstrated problems on another test of working memory, the Digit Span Backward subtest of the WMS-R (Wechsler, 1987).

The Elevator Counting with Reversal subtest of the TEA is also proposed to load on the working-memory factor. In this subtest, the patient is presented with tones in three pitches. The high and low tones indicate the direction in which the elevator is travelling, up or down, while the medium tones indicate floors that the elevator passes. The task is to calculate the final position of the elevator by counting the medium tones and using the high and low tones to indicate the direction of counting. Although most of the patients found it much too difficult to keep track of the number of tones while shifting direction of counting (see Robertson *et al.*, 1994), patient F2, with mild anosognosia, and patient M4, with no anosognosia, scored *above* the normal mean.

Executive function was assessed by a computerized version of the Wisconsin Card Sorting Test (WCST; Harris, 1988). The WCST is a demanding test involving several executive functions (Lie *et al.*, 2006) and it is acknowledged that poor performance on the test is difficult to interpret (Cinan and Öktem Tanör, 2002; Lezak *et al.*, 2004). It is, however, suggestive to observe that the only patient to score in the normal range on this test was patient M4, with no anosognosia. The Visual Elevator subtest of the TEA is proposed to load on the same attentional-switching factor as the WCST (Robertson *et al.*, 1994). The patient counts successive drawings of elevator doors. Along the way, large arrows pointing either up or down indicate the direction in which counting is to continue. Patient M4 again had the best performance on this task, scoring above the normal mean.[19] We also observe that all of the seven patients except M4 (following a right-basal-ganglia haemorrhage) had lesion locations that included right dorsolateral prefrontal cortex (Fig. 15.1).

In a subsequent statistical analysis,[20] we investigated whether patients' scores on fifteen tests of visuoperceptual function, memory, sustained attention, working memory, and executive function were predicted by their anosognosia scores (0–6, the sum of scores, 0–3, for upper and lower limbs). Only the scores on Elevator Counting with Distraction and the scores on the two measures commonly used to assess the WCST, Categories Achieved and Perseverative Errors, were significantly predicted by the anosognosia scores.

These findings are broadly consistent with the proposal that the second factor in the explanation of delusions, including anosognosia for motor impairments, is an impairment of working memory or executive function with a neural basis in damage to the right frontal region of the brain.

---

[19] In subsequent work, it will be important to separate out the inhibition of distraction and the attentional switching components of tasks such as Elevator Counting with Distraction and Visual Elevator.

[20] For a brief account of the statistical analysis, see Aimola Davies *et al.* (2009); for a more theoretical discussion, see Smithson *et al.* (submitted).

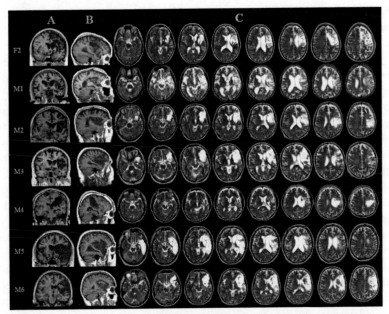

Fig. 15.1 Structural MRI scans: Column A represents a T1-weighted coronal section through the mid-temporal region; Column B represents a T1-weighted sagittal section on the side with the lesion (right in these patients); and Column C displays a series of axial T2-weighted scans in 7.5 mm steps. The right hemisphere is shown on the right.

15.11 **Summary and conclusion**

In this chapter, we have examined the two-factor framework for explaining pathologies of belief. According to the two-factor framework, we can explain a delusion by answering two questions. First, where did the delusion come from? Second, why does the patient not reject the belief?

We argued that the two-factor framework is also a three-stage framework and that answers to the question where the delusion came from may vary considerably from case to case. We proposed that this heterogeneity could be conceived as parametric variation within a single explanatory framework. There may or may not be abnormality in the first stage. If there is first-stage abnormality then the nature of the abnormality will vary from delusion to delusion and may vary from case to case of the same delusion. A first deficit may or may not give rise to an anomalous experience and the route from first deficit to belief may lie mainly at the personal or the sub-personal level. At the personal level, an anomalous experience may have a representational content close to or far from the content of the delusion itself and the route from experience to belief may be endorsement or explanation. The personal- or subpersonal-level processes of hypothesis generation and confirmation may be subject to one or another bias within the normal range, or to frank abnormalities.

We then confronted the fact that the second factor in the two-factor framework is poorly specified in terms of cognitive function. We noted that the case for rejecting a belief may sometimes depend primarily on the weight of disconfirming evidence and sometimes on the low prior probability of the belief being true. Thus, the answer to the question why the patient does not reject the belief may vary in its details and we suggested that this may be another locus of parametric variation. An *a priori* analysis of belief evaluation, drawing on the normative standards of probability theory, suggested that the task of evaluating an accepted hypothesis requires a step back from the initial acceptance, a step in the direction opposite to a prepotent response or tendency. We arrived at an initial suggestion that belief evaluation involves working memory and executive processes of inhibition.

Dual-process accounts of reasoning distinguish between heuristic (System 1) processes and analytic (System 2) processes and a central idea is that the two kinds of processes can come into conflict. We suggested that belief evaluation involves two kinds of analytic processes, assessment of competing hypotheses and inhibition of imperatives (the imperatives of observational adequacy, explanatory adequacy, and conservatism). Experimental and neuroimaging studies of the belief-bias effect were then interpreted as supporting the proposal that the second factor in the explanation of delusions is an impairment of working memory or executive function with a neural basis in damage to the right frontal region of the brain.

We began the chapter with examples of anosognosia considered as a delusion and we ended by addressing two problems – how can anosognosia fit the two-factor framework and how could recognition of paralysis depend on working memory or executive function? In response to the first problem, we argued that a first factor impairs the patient's concurrent awareness of paralysis and a second factor explains why the patient does not make appropriate use of a mass of other available evidence. We approached the second problem theoretically by drawing on the analogy between belief evaluation and the task used in belief-bias experiments. In the presence of a first factor, there is a conflict between the response based on available evidence and the response based on prior beliefs. Under these conditions, impairments of working memory and executive function may have the consequence that prior beliefs that are now false are maintained rather than rejected. Finally, we presented some results from a study of cognitive impairments in right-hemisphere stroke patients. These results support our proposal about the nature of the second factor.

We are still some way from having a satisfactory explanatory account of even one pathology of belief. Much more needs to be discovered about the specific ways in which working memory and executive function are impaired in patients with different delusions. There may be further parametric variation depending on which of the imperatives need to be resisted. Halligan and Marshall may be right that, given a demanding notion of unification, 'it is unlikely that a unified theory of delusions will be forthcoming' (1996, p. 8). But we maintain the hope that the two-factor framework can be developed so that, on the one hand, it is not hopelessly underspecified and, on the other hand, it reveals a common structure in our explanations of pathologies of belief.

Dedication

This chapter is dedicated to the memory of John C. Marshall (1939–2007) whose foundational contributions to cognitive neuropsychology and cognitive neuropsychiatry continue to guide research in those fields. We remember with gratitude, and also with sadness, our conversations with him on the topics of this chapter.

Acknowledgements

At many points in this chapter we have drawn on the work of Max Coltheart and Tony Stone and we acknowledge, with thanks, their influence on our thinking about delusions. Thanks also to Rebekah White, and to the editors, Lisa Bortolotti and Matthew Broome, for their comments on an earlier version and to Jerome Maller for preparing the figure.

References

Adolphs, R., Tranel, D., Bechara, A., Damasio, H., and Damasio, A. R. (1996). Neuropsychological approaches to reasoning and decision-making. In *Neurobiology of Decision-Making* (eds. A. R. Damasio, H. Damasio, and Y. Christen), pp. 157–179. Berlin, Springer-Verlag.

Aimola, A. M. (1999). *Dark Side of the Moon: Studies in Unilateral Neglect*. PhD Dissertation, University of Auckland.

Aimola Davies, A. M., Davies, M., Ogden, J. A., Smithson, M., and White, R. C. (2009). Cognitive and motivational factors in anosognosia. In *Delusions and Self-Deception: Affective Influences on Belief Formation* (eds. T. Bayne, and J. Fernández), pp. 187–225. Hove, East Sussex, Psychology Press.

American Psychiatric Association (2000). *Diagnostic and Statistical Manual of Mental Disorders, Fourth Edition, Text Revision (DSM-IV-TR)*. Washington, DC, American Psychiatric Association.

Arthur, A. Z. (1964). Theories and explanations of delusions: a review. *American Journal of Psychiatry*, **121**, 105–115.

Bayne, T. and Pacherie, E. (2004). Bottom-up or top-down? Campbell's rationalist account of monothematic delusions. *Philosophy, Psychiatry, and Psychology*, **11**, 1–11.

Bentall, R. P., Corcoran, R., Howard, R., Blackwood, N., and Kinderman, P. (2001). Persecutory delusions: a review and theoretical integration. *Clinical Psychology Review*, **21**, 1143–1192.

Berti, A., Bottini, G., Gandola, M., *et al.* (2005). Shared cortical anatomy for motor awareness and motor control. *Science*, **309**, 488–491.

Berti, A., Làdavas, E., and Della Corte, M. (1996). Anosognosia for hemiplegia, neglect dyslexia, and drawing neglect: clinical findings and theoretical considerations. *Journal of the International Neuropsychological Society*, **2**, 426–440.

Berti, A., Làdavas, E., Stracciari, A., Giannarelli, C., and Ossola, A. (1998). Anosognosia for motor impairment and dissociations with patients' evaluation of the disorder: theoretical considerations. *Cognitive Neuropsychiatry*, **3**, 21–44.

Bisiach, E. (1988). Language without thought. In *Thought Without Language* (ed. L. Weiskrantz), pp. 464–484. Oxford, Oxford University Press.

Bisiach, E. and Geminiani, G. (1991). Anosognosia related to hemiplegia and hemianopia. In *Awareness of Deficit after Brain Injury: Clinical and Theoretical Issues* (eds. G. P. Prigatano, and D. L. Schacter), pp. 17–39. Oxford, Oxford University Press.

Bisiach, E., Vallar, G., Perani, D., Papagno, C., and Berti, A. (1986). Unawareness of disease following lesions of the right hemisphere: anosognosia for hemiplegia and anosognosia for hemianopia. *Neuropsychologia,* **24**, 471–482.

Blackwood, N. J., Howard, R. J., Bentall, R. P., and Murray, R. M. (2001). Cognitive neuropsychiatric models of persecutory delusions. *American Journal of Psychiatry,* **158**, 527–539.

Bortolotti, L. and Broome, M. R. (2008) Delusional beliefs and reason giving. *Philosophical Psychology,* **21**, 821–841.

Bortolotti, L. and Broome, M. R. (in press). A role for ownership and authorship in the analysis of thought insertion. *Phenomenology and the Cognitive Sciences.*

Bottini, G., Bisiach, E., Sterzi, R., and Vallar, G. (2002). Feeling touches in someone else's hand. *NeuroReport,* **13**, 249–252.

Breen, N., Caine, D., and Coltheart, M. (2002). The role of affect and reasoning in a patient with a delusion of misidentification. *Cognitive Neuropsychiatry,* **7**, 113–138.

Broome, M. R., Johns, L. C., Valli, I., *et al.* (2007). Delusion formation and reasoning biases in those at clinical high risk for psychosis. *British Journal of Psychiatry,* **191**(suppl. 51), s38–s42.

Broome, M. R. and McGuire, P. K. (2008). Imaging and delusions. In *Persecutory Delusions: Assessment, Theory, and Treatment* (eds. D. Freeman, R. P. Bentall, and P. A. Garety), pp. 281–301. Oxford, Oxford University Press.

Broome, M. R., Woolley, J. B., Johns, L. C., *et al.* (2005a). Outreach and support in south London (OASIS): implementation of a clinical service for prodromal psychosis and the at risk mental state. *European Psychiatry,* **20**, 372–378.

Broome, M. R., Woolley, J. B., Tabraham, P., *et al.* (2005b). What causes the onset of psychosis? *Schizophrenia Research,* **79**, 23–34.

Bruce, V. and Young, A. W. (1986). Understanding face recognition. *British Journal of Psychology,* **77**, 305–327.

Capgras, J. and Reboul-Lachaux, J. (1923). L'illusion des 'sosies' dans un délire systématisé chronique. *Bulletin de la Société Clinique de Médecine Mentale,* **2**, 6–16.

Carpenter, K., Berti, A., Oxbury, S., Molyneux, A. J., Bisiach, E., and Oxbury, J. M. (1995). Awareness of and memory for arm weakness during intracarotid sodium amytal testing. *Brain,* **118**, 243–251.

Chatterjee, A. and Mennemeier, M. (1996). Anosognosia for hemiplegia: patient retrospections. *Cognitive Neuropsychiatry,* **1**, 221–237.

Chomsky, N. (1986). *Knowledge of Language: Its Nature, Origin, and Use.* New York, Praeger.

Cinan, S. and Öktem Tanör, Ö. (2002). An attempt to discriminate different types of executive functions in the Wisconsin Card Sorting Test. *Memory,* **10**, 277–289.

Colbert, S. M. and Peters, E. R. (2002). Need for closure and jumping-to-conclusions in delusion-prone individuals. *Journal of Nervous and Mental Disease,* **190**, 27–31.

Coltheart, M. (1985). Cognitive neuropsychology and the study of reading. In *Attention and Performance XI* (eds. M. I. Posner, and O. S. M. Marin), pp. 3–37. Hillsdale, NJ, Lawrence Erlbaum Associates.

Coltheart, M. (2005). Conscious experience and delusional belief. *Philosophy, Psychiatry, and Psychology,* **12**, 153–157.

Coltheart, M. (2006a). John Marshall and the cognitive neuropsychology of reading. *Cortex,* **42**, 855–860.

Coltheart, M. (2006b). Acquired dyslexias and the computational modelling of reading. *Cognitive Neuropsychology,* **23**, 3–12.

Coltheart, M. (2007). Cognitive neuropsychiatry and delusional belief. *Quarterly Journal of Experimental Psychology*, **60**, 1041–1062.

Cotard, J. (1882). Du délire des négations. *Archives de Neurologie*, **4**, 152–170, 282–295.

David, A. S. (1993). Cognitive neuropsychiatry. *Psychological Medicine*, **23**, 1–5.

David, A. S. and Halligan, P. W. (1996). Editorial. *Cognitive Neuropsychiatry*, **1**, 1–3.

Davies, M. (2009). Delusion and motivationally biased belief: self-deception in the two-factor framework. In *Delusions and Self-Deception: Affective Influences on Belief Formation* (eds. T. Bayne, and J. Fernández), pp. 71–86. Hove, East Sussex, Psychology Press.

Davies, M. and Coltheart, M. (2000). Introduction: pathologies of belief. *Mind and Language*, **15**, 1–46.

Davies, M., Coltheart, M., Langdon, R., and Breen, N. (2001). Monothematic delusions: towards a two-factor account. *Philosophy, Psychiatry, and Psychology*, **8**, 133–158.

De Neys, N. (2006). Dual processing in reasoning: two systems but one reasoner. *Psychological Science*, **17**, 428–433.

Edelstyn, N. M. J. and Oyebode, F. (1999). A review of the phenomenology and cognitive neuropsychological origins of the Capgras syndrome. *International Journal of Geriatric Psychiatry*, **14**, 48–59.

Ellis, H. D. (1998). Cognitive neuropsychiatry and delusional misidentification syndromes: an exemplary vindication of the new discipline. *Cognitive Neuropsychiatry*, **3**, 81–90.

Ellis, H. D. and Lewis, M. B. (2001). Capgras delusion: a window on face recognition. *Trends in Cognitive Sciences*, **5**, 149–156.

Ellis, H. D. and Young, A. W. (1990). Accounting for delusional misidentifications. *British Journal of Psychiatry*, **157**, 239–248.

Engle, R. W. (2002). Working memory capacity as executive attention. *Current Directions in Psychological Science*, **11**, 19–23.

Engle, R. W., Tuholski, S. W., Laughlin, J. E., and Conway, A. R. A. (1999). Working memory, short-term memory, and general fluid intelligence: a latent-variable approach. *Journal of Experimental Psychology: General*, **128**, 309–331.

Evans, J. St. B. T. (2003). In two minds: dual-process accounts of reasoning. *Trends in Cognitive Sciences*, **7**, 454–459.

Evans, J. St. B. T. (2007). On the resolution of conflict in dual process theories of reasoning. *Thinking and Reasoning*, **13**, 321–339.

Evans, J. St. B. T., Barston, J. L., and Pollard, P. (1983). On the conflict between logic and belief in syllogistic reasoning. *Memory and Cognition*, **11**, 295–306.

Feinberg, T. E., Roane, D. M., and Ali, J. (2000). Illusory limb movements in anosognosia for hemiplegia. *Journal of Neurology, Neurosurgery, and Psychiatry*, **68**, 511–513.

Fine, C., Craigie, J., and Gold, I. (2005). Damned if you do, damned if you don't: the impasse in cognitive accounts of the Capgras delusion. *Philosophy, Psychiatry, and Psychology*, **12**, 143–151.

Fine, C., Gardner, M., Craigie, J., and Gold, I. (2007) Hopping, skipping or jumping to conclusions? Clarifying the role of the JTC bias in delusions. *Cognitive Neuropsychiatry*, **12**, 46–77.

Fodor, J. A. (1983). *The Modularity of Mind*. Cambridge, MA, MIT Press.

Fodor, J. A. (1987). *Psychosemantics: The Problem of Meaning in the Philosophy of Mind*. Cambridge, MA, MIT Press.

Fodor, J. A. (1989). Why should the mind be modular? In *Reflections on Chomsky* (ed. A. George), pp. 1–22. Oxford, Blackwell.

Fodor, J. A. (2000). *The Mind Doesn't Work That Way*. Cambridge, MA, MIT Press.

Freeman, D. (2007). Suspicious minds: the psychology of persecutory delusions. *Clinical Psychology Review*, **27**, 425–457.

Freeman, D., Garety, P. A., Fowler, D., Kuipers, E., Bebbington, P. E., and Dunn, G. (2004). Why do people with delusions fail to choose more realistic explanations for their experiences? An empirical investigation. *Journal of Consulting and Clinical Psychology*, **72**, 671–680.

Freeman, D., Garety, P. A., McGuire, P., and Kuipers, E. (2005). Developing a theoretical understanding of therapy techniques: an illustrative analogue study. *British Journal of Clinical Psychology*, **44**, 241–254.

Frith, C. D., Blakemore, S.- J., and Wolpert, D. M. (2000). Abnormalities in the awareness and control of action. *Philosophical Transactions of the Royal Society of London B: Biological Sciences*, **355**, 1771–1788.

Garety, P. A. and Freeman, D. (1999). Cognitive approaches to delusions: a critical review of theories and evidence. *British Journal of Clinical Psychology*, **38**, 113–154.

Garety, P. A., Hemsley, D. R., and Wessely, S. (1991). Reasoning in deluded schizophrenic and paranoid patients: biases in performance on a probabilistic inference task. *Journal of Nervous and Mental Disease*, **179**, 194–201.

Gialanella, B. and Mattioli, F. (1992). Anosognosia and extrapersonal neglect as predictors of functional recovery following right hemisphere stroke. *Neuropsychological Rehabilitation*, **2**, 169–178.

Gilbert, D. T. (1991). How mental systems believe. *American Psychologist*, **46**, 107–119.

Gilbert, D. T., Krull, D. S., and Malone, P. S. (1990). Believing the unbelievable: some problems in the rejection of false information. *Journal of Personality and Social Psychology*, **59**, 601–613.

Gilbert, D.T., Tafadori, R. W., and Malone, P. S. (1993). You can't not believe everything you read. *Journal of Personality and Social Psychology*, **65**, 221–233.

Goel, V. and Dolan, R. J. (2003). Explaining modulation of reasoning by belief. *Cognition*, **87**, B11–B22.

Gopnik, A. (1998). Explanation as orgasm. *Minds and Machines*, **8**, 101–118.

Halligan, P. W. and Marshall, J. C. (eds.) (1996). *Method in Madness: Case Studies in Cognitive Neuropsychiatry*. Hove, East Sussex, Psychology Press.

Halligan, P. W., Marshall, J. C., and Wade, D. T. (1995). Unilateral somatoparaphrenia after right hemisphere stroke: a case description. *Cortex*, **31**, 173–182.

Harris, M. E. (1988). *Wisconsin Card Sorting Test Scoring Program (Version 2.0)*. Odessa, FL, Psychological Assessment Resources, Inc.

Hasson, U., Simmons, J. P., and Todorov, A. (2005). Believe it or not: on the possibility of suspending belief. *Psychological Science*, **16**, 566–571.

Heilman, K. M. (1991). Anosognosia: possible neuropsychological mechanisms. In *Awareness of Deficit after Brain Injury: Clinical and Theoretical Issues* (eds. G. P. Prigatano, and D. L. Schacter), pp. 53–62. New York, Oxford University Press.

Heilman, K. M., Barrett, A. M., and Adair, J. C. (1998). Possible mechanisms of anosognosia: a defect in self-awareness. *Philosophical Transactions of the Royal Society of London B: Biological Sciences*, **353**, 1903–1909.

Hemsley, D. R. and Garety, P. A. (1986). The formation and maintenance of delusions: a Bayesian analysis. *British Journal of Psychiatry*, **149**, 51–56.

Hohwy, J. and Rosenberg, R. (2005). Unusual experiences, reality testing and delusions of alien control. *Mind and Language*, **20**, 141–162.

House, A. and Hodges, J. (1988). Persistent denial of handicap after infarction of the right basal ganglia: A case study. *Journal of Neurology, Neurosurgery, and Psychiatry*, **51**, 112–115.

Humphreys, G. W. (1991). Review of Shallice, *From Neuropsychology to Mental Structure*. *Mind and Language*, **6**, 202–214.

Huq, S. F., Garety, P. A., and Hemsley, D. R. (1988). Probabilistic judgements in deluded and non-deluded subjects. *Quarterly Journal of Experimental Psychology*, **40A**, 801–812.

Jaspers, K. (1963). *General Psychopathology* (Trs J. Hoenig, and M. W. Hamilton). Manchester, Manchester University Press.

Jeannerod, M. and Pacherie, E. (2004). Agency, simulation and self-identification. *Mind and Language*, **19**, 113–146.

Kapur, S. (2003). Psychosis as a state of aberrant salience: a framework linking biology, phenomenology, and pharmacology in schizophrenia. *American Journal of Psychiatry*, **160**, 13–23.

Kapur, S. (2004). How antipsychotics become anti-'psychotic': from dopamine to salience to psychosis. *Trends in Pharmacological Sciences*, **25**, 402–406.

Kapur, S., Mizrahi, R., and Li, M. (2005). From dopamine to salience to psychosis. Linking biology, pharmacology and phenomenology of psychosis. *Schizophrenia Research*, **79**, 59–68.

Karnath, H-O., Baier, B., and Nägele, T. (2005). Awareness of the functioning of one's own limbs mediated by the insular cortex? *Journal of Neuroscience*, **25**, 7134–7138.

Klauer, K. C., Musch, J., and Naumer, B. (2000). On belief bias in syllogistic reasoning. *Psychological Review*, **107**, 852–884.

Levine, D. N. (1990). Unawareness of visual and sensorimotor defects: a hypothesis. *Brain and Cognition*, **13**, 233–281.

Lezak, M. D., Howieson, D. B., and Loring, D. W. (2004). *Neuropsychological Assessment*, 4th edn. New York, Oxford University Press.

Lie, C-H., Specht, K., Marshall, J. C., and Fink G. R. (2006). Using fMRI to decompose the neural processes underlying the Wisconsin Card Sorting Test. *NeuroImage*, **30**, 1038–1049.

Linney, Y. M., Peters, E. R., and Ayton, P. (1998). Reasoning biases in delusion-prone individuals. *British Journal of Clinical Psychology*, **37**, 285–302.

Lipton, P. (2004). *Inference to the Best Explanation*, 2nd edn. London, Routledge.

Maguire, A. M. and Ogden, J. A. (2002). MRI brain scan analyses and neuropsychological profiles of nine patients with persisting unilateral neglect. *Neuropsychologia*, **40**, 879–887.

Maher, B. A. (1974). Delusional thinking and perceptual disorder. *Journal of Individual Psychology*, **30**, 98–113.

Maher, B. A. (1988). Anomalous experience and delusional thinking: the logic of explanations. In *Delusional Beliefs* (eds. T. F. Oltmanns, and B. A. Maher), pp. 15–33. Chichester, Wiley and Sons.

Maher, B. A. (1992). Delusions: contemporary etiological hypotheses. *Psychiatric Annals*, **22**, 260–268.

Maher, B. A. (1999). Anomalous experience in everyday life: its significance for psychopathology. *The Monist*, **82**, 547–570.

Marcel, A. J., Tegnér, R., and Nimmo-Smith, I. (2004). Anosognosia for plegia: specificity, extension, partiality and disunity of bodily unawareness. *Cortex*, **40**, 19–40.

Marshall, J. C. and Newcombe, F. (1966). Syntactic and semantic errors in paralexia. *Neuropsychologia*, **4**, 169–176.

Marshall, J. C. and Newcombe, F. (1973). Patterns of paralexia: a psycholinguistic approach. *Journal of Psycholinguistic Research*, **2**, 175–199.

McKay, R. and Cipolotti, L. (2007). Attributional style in a case of Cotard delusion. *Consciousness and Cognition*, **16**, 349–359.

Mele, A. R. (2009). Self-deception and delusions. In *Delusions and Self-Deception: Affective Influences on Belief Formation* (eds. T. Bayne, and J. Fernández), pp. 55–70. Hove, East Sussex, Psychology Press.

Miyake, A., Friedman, N. P., Rettinger, D. A., Shah, P., and Hegarty, M. (2001). How are visuospatial working memory, executive functioning, and spatial abilities related? A latent-variable analysis. *Journal of Experimental Psychology: General*, **130**, 621–640.

Moran, R. (2001). *Authority and Estrangement: An Essay on Self-knowledge*. Princeton, NJ, Princeton University Press.

Nickerson, R. S. (1998). Confirmation bias: a ubiquitous phenomenon in many guises. *Review of General Psychology*, **2**, 175–220.

Pryor, J. (2004). What's wrong with Moore's argument? *Philosophical Issues*, **14**, 349–378.

Robertson, I. H., Ward, T., Ridgeway, V., and Nimmo-Smith, I. (1994). *The Test of Everyday Attention (TEA)*. Bury St Edmunds, Thames Valley Test Company.

Schuurmans-Stekhoven, J. and Smithson, M. (submitted). Orientation to uncertainty as a possible dual process.

Smith, E. E. and Kosslyn, S. M. (2007). *Cognitive Psychology: Mind and Brain*. Upper Saddle River, NJ, Pearson Prentice Hall.

Smithson, M., Davies, M., and Aimola Davies, A. M. (submitted). Additional methods for comparing cases with control samples and testing for dissociation.

Stanovich, K. E. (1999). *Who is Rational? Studies of Individual Differences in Reasoning*. Mahwah, NJ, Lawrence Erlbaum Associates.

Stanovich, K. E. (2003). The fundamental computational biases of human cognition: Heuristics that (sometimes) impair decision making and problem solving. In *The Psychology of Problem Solving* (eds. J. E. Davidson, and R. J. Sternberg), pp. 291–342. New York, Cambridge University Press.

Stone, T. and Young, A. W. (1997). Delusions and brain injury: the philosophy and psychology of belief. *Mind and Language*, **12**, 327–364.

Van Dael, F., Versmissen, D., Janssen, I., Myin-Germeys, I., van Os, J., and Krabbendam, L. (2006). Data gathering: biased in psychosis? *Schizophrenia Bulletin*, **32**, 341–351.

Vuilleumier, P. (2004). Anosognosia: the neurology of beliefs and uncertainties. *Cortex*, **40**, 9–17.

Wason, P. C. (1960). On the failure to eliminate hypotheses in a conceptual task. *Quarterly Journal of Experimental Psychology*, **12**, 129–140.

Wason, P. C. (1968). Reasoning about a rule. *Quarterly Journal of Experimental Psychology*, **20**, 273–281.

Wechsler, D. (1987). *Wechsler Memory Scale–Revised*. San Antonio, TX: The Psychological Corporation.

Weinstein, E. A. and Kahn, R. L. (1950). The syndrome of anosognosia. *Archives of Neurology and Psychiatry*, **64**, 772–791.

Weinstein, E. A. and Kahn, R. L. (1951). Patterns of disorientation in organic disease of the brain. *AMA Archives of Neurology and Psychiatry,* **65**, 533–534.

Weinstein, E. A. and Kahn, R. L. (1953). Personality factors in denial of illness. *AMA Archives of Neurology and Psychiatry,* **69**, 355–367.

Weinstein, E. A. and Kahn, R. L. (1955). *Denial of Illness: Symbolic and Physiological Aspects.* Springfield, IL, Charles C. Thomas.

Weinstein, E. A., Kahn, R. L., Malitz, S., and Rozanski, J. (1954). Delusional reduplication of parts of the body. *Brain,* **77**, 45–60.

Young, A. W. (2000). Wondrous strange: the neuropsychology of abnormal beliefs. *Mind and Language,* **15**, 47–73.

Young, A. W. and Leafhead, K. M. (1996). Betwixt life and death: case studies of the Cotard delusion. In *Method in Madness: Case Studies in Cognitive Neuropsychiatry* (eds. P. W. Halligan, and J. C. Marshall), pp. 147–171. Hove, East Sussex, Psychology Press.

Moral psychology and psychopathology

Chapter 16

Mental time travel, agency, and responsibility

Jeanette Kennett and Steve Matthews

Abstract

We have argued elsewhere (2002) that moral responsibility over
time depends in part upon the having of psychological connections
which facilitate forms of self-control. In this chapter we explore the
importance of mental time travel – our ordinary ability to mentally
travel to temporal locations outside the present, involving both
memory of our personal past and the ability to imagine ourselves in
the future – to our agential capacities for planning and control. We
suggest that in many individuals with dissociative disorders, forms of
amnesia, or other frontal lobe damage, our capacity for mental time
travel is impaired, resulting in commensurate losses to agency,
autonomy, and a forensic condition essential for holding persons
responsible: in legal terms, the capacity for *mens* rea.

16.1 Introduction

Our ability to remember, and to imagine how things will be in the future – the ability
for *mental time travel* – is familiar to most of us and taken for granted as something we
ordinarily do without much thought or effort.[1] We put this ability into the service of
our ends – again, almost without thought or effort – by, for example, remembering
past mistakes and planning for a future that avoids them. More generally, our capacity
for recalling the past and imaginatively rehearsing the future partly constitutes our
capacity for temporally extended agency in which we exercise forms of self control.

---

[1] When we say 'our' ability, we mean the human ability, and this may signal that mental time
travel is an exclusively human capacity. We do not wish to give that impression, and indeed
whether it is human-specific is of course an open empirical question. Recent research on
behavioural manifestations of some animals – non-human primates, some birds, and dol-
phins – suggests that they may '... have the capacity to remember personal experiences in
terms of what happened, where and when'. See Dere *et al.* (2006, p. 1206).

But what happens to individuals who lose the capacity to 'visit' the past or the future? There are real cases of dissociation, amnesia, or frontal lobe damage, in which those afflicted lose their internal 'time machines' – they, for example, cease to be able to remember events from their past in a way that goes beyond the ordinary tendency to forget the past. Since this ability is part and parcel of extended agency, its loss leads to commensurate losses to agency, autonomy, and a forensic condition essential for holding persons responsible: in legal terms, the capacity for *mens rea*. Here we define, and then outline the conceptual connections between mental time travel, agency, and responsibility.

16.2 **Autonomy and responsibility**

What capacities must agents possess in order to be candidates for moral or legal responsibility? R Jay Wallace argues for a widely shared view in moral philosophy and the law that responsible agents must possess the powers of reflective self-control (Wallace, 1994). This has two parts. First, the agent must have acquired moral concepts and be able to apply them in deliberation about what to do. Second, the agent must have the capacity to control their behaviour in accordance with their deliberative conclusions. If either of these is lacking, agents cannot be said to be fully responsible for their actions. We think these two criteria are not controversial; at any rate we will not argue directly for them here. What we want to focus on and make explicit are the ways in which both deliberation and self-control depend upon something more basic – our ability to mentally travel to times outside the present. Impairments to this ability are thus directly relevant to assessments of responsibility. We will elaborate on the notion of mental time travel in the next section. In the remainder of this section we show that (normative) autonomous agency is necessarily temporally extended agency.[2]

Autonomous agents are, intuitively, those with the capacity to shape, plan, and direct their own lives in accordance with their reflectively endorsed values. Agents typically value short-term pleasant experiences such as eating, sun-bathing, or listening to music as well as the fulfilment of longer-term projects such as a course of study, a career, marriage, or parenting, and participation in a range of cultural, religious, or political activities. While the longer-term projects seem most relevant to discussions of autonomy, note that even securing the more short-term needs or pleasures such as tonight's dinner or tomorrow's trip to the beach, requires the projection of oneself someway into the future.[3] A vast range of such everyday activities, as well as longer-term activities and projects, would be rendered impossible if we could not adequately

---

[2] *Normative* autonomous agency is here contrasted with a form of autonomous agency in which a being acts in a self-directed way from synchronic or non-reflective resources. The discussion here of autonomous agents should largely be taken to include the richer normative notion.

[3] Of course, a range of sensory goods might be secured for us by others as they are when we are children, or as they are for the mentally impaired; these goods are thus distinct from projects which require our *active* participation for their fulfilment, such as friendships and completing a degree. So, we think the second kind more central to autonomy.

conceive of or commit ourselves across time. I arrange to meet you for lunch tomorrow, confident that tomorrow I will remember, and (other things being equal) thereby feel bound by, our arrangement. Or I negotiate a contract to design and build a house for you, thereby committing my future self to a co-ordinated series of complex actions over an extended period of time. If we could not quite generally, and in these ways, commit our (future) selves, social and moral life would be made impossible.

There are a number of different ways in which an individual may fail to be autonomous. I cannot be said to be autonomous, to be shaping and directing my own life, if I do not have any overarching values or principles which guide my choices, that is, if I simply do not care about what I do, or if the plans and decisions I arrive at in deliberation are constantly undermined or overridden by the desires of the moment. In the first kind of case, I am a wanton rather than a person (Frankfurt, 1971); in the second kind of case, I am chronically weak-willed or compulsive. Likewise I am not an autonomous agent if I cannot make choices and decisions which commit my future self to certain courses of action, either because I am incapable of seeing into my personal future and evaluating future possibilities, or because I will not, when the time for action arrives, be able to remember or identify with the plans I make now. It is with these latter cases where the agent's temporal awareness and temporal identity is undermined by psychopathology that we will be primarily concerned. These cases threaten in the most fundamental way, the ability of the agent to meet the two conditions of responsibility – adequate deliberation and self-control.

16.3 **Mental time travel**

Our interest here is in mental time travel understood as a form of controlled activity undertaken by an agent usually for the purpose of evaluating the past or planning for the future. In mental time travel, the agent recalls and re-experiences episodes involving her past self, or alternatively imagines her self as taking part in some future episode. Mental time travel, then, includes what are sometimes called episodic, or personal memories, in the backward-looking cases, and what is sometimes called prospection, in the forward-looking cases. Episodic remembering is the familiar category of memory in which a person replays a past experience in which she was personally involved (Tulving, 1972/1983). Prospection involves the simulation of future events in which we mentally rehearse a situation in which we ourselves are involved. As with episodic memory, prospection is often qualitatively rich, across two main dimensions. In 'experiencing' the past or the future we simulate a world with at least some of its sensory detail: the softness of the bed, the warmth of the sun, the smile of one's beloved, the sarcasm of one's boss, the applause of the audience. In addition, and since it is self-involving, we respond emotionally to the simulation. In memory, these responses lead to reflection upon and judgements about how we acted, or how we were treated and so on, and in prospection, we may think about the consequences of what would happen if we acted in a certain way and respond accordingly.

As we have just stated, there are two aspects to mental time travel. First, there is what might be called an executive control aspect. Irving Koch points out that, central to a story about self-control, is 'the ability to flexibly adapt to changing situations, realize new intentions, or schedule intended actions'.[4] This plainly depends upon the capacity to voluntarily attend to past and future scenarios involving myself. In remembering, for example, I *direct* my attention to an episode in the past, and in doing so exercise control over this representation of my past self. But in addition, I must respond to this representation as of being *my* past self. The sense that this is *me*, the sense of myself as thus persisting across time, is referred to in the literature as *autonoetic awareness (sometimes 'autonoesis')*. This is the second aspect of mental time travel. The underlying sense I have of myself as a creature with a past and a future – as travelling through time – does not appear to be voluntary but it is essential to the capacity for the directed mental time travel in which we are interested, and thus for self-control.[5]

There is in the literature a tendency to use the expressions 'autonoetic awareness' and 'mental time travel' interchangeably, but we think this is a mistake. While mental time travel is a complex *capacity* – it combines an executive function with a sense of self-awareness – it is better to understand autonoesis as simply that sense of oneself across time that forms a part of the complex that is mental time travel.[6] We will thus avoid reference to autonoesis as a capacity, though it does make sense to talk about a noetic or autonoetic process. The former is one in which we come to know of some item in the world, or know some proposition about the world – perhaps even a proposition about ourselves – and that we know it without necessarily remembering ourselves outside the present acquiring that knowledge; an autonoetic process is one in which the method of knowing essentially requires the subject to be conscious of themselves at a different moment from the present. Thus the distinction between noesis and autonoesis forms the basis for what is called the remember/know test in psychology.[7]

---

[4] See Irving Koch, available at http://www.mpipf-muenchen.mpg.de/CA/RESEARCH/ exec_control_e.htm (accessed October 2008). Self-regulatory disorder is seen in patients with right ventral frontal pathology pointing to the importance of the frontal cortex for executive control and goal-directed activity.

[5] Autonoetic awareness usually refers to a temporally displaced awareness of self. We will later suggest a broader understanding which includes an awareness of oneself that need not entail the temporal connectedness element.

[6] We confess that the origins of 'noesis' suggest it to be an ability – it is a kind of conscious knowing, and as such does seem to imply something that a mind *does*. And so autonoesis might strictly etymologically suggest something like the ability for self-knowledge. Thus the reader should take our definition of 'autonoetic awareness' as stipulative, as motivated by the argument we have presented.

[7] In the remember/know test, clinical subjects are presented with items – say lists of words – and then later asked, of a second set of items that contains the same items, as well as some novel ones, to state whether they episodically recall an item from the first set, or whether they recognize it in the same way they recognize items based on semantic knowledge. If the source of the recognition is nominated as the first learning event, it is a remembered pathway; otherwise it is a knowledge pathway.

According to Levine *et al.* (1998), the right ventral frontal cortex and underlying white matter is hypothesized to mediate retrieval of events from one's personal past.[8] Individuals with frontal pathology may use non-episodic processes to attain normal test performance without the phenomenal experience of remembering.

The self-awareness that occurs in mental time travel has a particular character: in becoming aware of myself in the past, I re-experience some past event as it occurred then. In becoming aware of myself in the future, I picture my future self as taking part in some putative set of events, by imagining now what those events would be like for me then. Thus, mental time travel requires a particular form of subjective experiencing now in which a representation of oneself is displaced in time; it requires in addition the sense that this temporally displaced self is *identical* with the currently remembering or imagining self; and it requires further the sense that these temporally up-or-downstream selves be *connected* to the present self. In the backward-looking case the experiences of the earlier self must be taken to causally explain, in the right kind of way, the present awareness; in the forward-looking case, at least where one is seriously deciding what to do, one must take the future self to be, in the right kind of way, a potential causal descendant of the present.[9]

We have said that mental time travel requires both a sense of identity and a sense of connectedness. This raises many tricky issues, but we address three main ones here.

First, consider the requirement that mental time travel preserve a sense of personal identity. This is ambiguous because 'personal identity' can mean (numerical) personal identity, or it can mean retaining a sense of who you really are. Thus, a person with an identity delusion,[10] say someone who believes he is Jesus Christ, may have a continuing sense that he is Jesus Christ, with accompanying episodic memories and future plans.[11] In these cases, as those with such delusions later report, the memories

---

[8] The arrival of episodic memory coincides with the development of frontal cortex and more extensive connections between frontal and posterior areas. See Gerrans and Kennett (ms) for discussion.

[9] We add the clause 'in the right kind of way' to acknowledge a difficulty arising in cases of deviant causal chains. So, for example, it is at least logically possible I might seem to remember an incident from my childhood, the seeming memory might have the quality of a veridical episodic memory, and the incident might have really happened just as I seem to remember it; yet, what causes my seeming to remember it this way is something my parents tell me as a result of witnessing this same incident. We do not think this counts as mental time travel, roughly because the formation of the memory occurs in the wrong way, and its qualitative likeness to the incident is an extreme fluke. Martin and Deutscher (1966) famously pointed out the insufficiency of mere causal dependence, identifying the problem of such cases.

[10] In bipolar disorder, such delusions are termed 'grandiose delusions'. We use the term 'identity delusion' because it picks up a broader set of cases. We have argued elsewhere (Kennett and Matthews, 2003) that the alter states of dissociative identity disorder (DID) patients where they, for example, believe they are a child, a member of the opposite sex etc., are akin to delusional states.

[11] Mondimore (1999, p. 12), writing about the manic phase of bipolar disorder, says 'Feelings of religious inspiration are very common. Patients may feel that they are a modern prophet, the founder of a new religion, a reincarnation of Christ, even a new god.'

and plans have mixed veridical and non-veridical content. Craig Hamilton (2005), for example, remembers the period during which he sincerely believed he was Jesus Christ. Hamilton was a sports journalist about to attend the Sydney Olympic Games. Reflecting on the day he was hospitalized he wrote:

> *In my mind I had become Jesus Christ reincarnate* . . . The Jesus notion hadn't struck me like a lightning bolt but, rather, taken shape as a result of an escalating mania throwing off grandiose delusions . . . All the events of my life to that point had been readying me for this occasion, or so I thought. In the two days before arriving at the railway station my Olympics planning had changed. I had a new assignment. It was perfectly clear: I was going to change the world. My gospel for the global audience was disarm, feed the hungry and love one another.

> (Hamilton, 2005, p. 2)

Hamilton then goes on to describe the event immediately after at which the police came to remove him from the train station. He remembers what happened, where it happened, and when it happened. He has a robust set of psychological connections back to his delusional self. Patients such as Hamilton satisfy, during the delusional period, the conditions for numerical identity over time.[12] Yet, they do not adequately satisfy the condition of knowing who they really are. So, do they satisfy the identity requirement on mental time travel? We think they do to a significant extent, because, first, they have an awareness of themselves as a person with a past, present, and future, tracing out a trajectory across time, and second, the basic brute capacity to voluntarily reach back or go forward in personal time seems intact. However it might be said that, as a result of their delusional beliefs about which historical individual they in fact are, their upstream and downstream selves are not *cognitively connected* in the right kind of way to their present self.[13] Their memories and interpretations are distorted by their delusions such that they are not properly in touch with their true historical selves. The failure of the right kind of cognitive connection means that such agents are impaired with respect to interpreting the past and planning for the future as the excerpt from Hamilton's biography makes plain.

Second, it might be thought that in episodically remembering an experience from yesterday, my brute capacity to be aware of it makes redundant the need to claim that mental time travel should also include a sense of connectedness over time. How could

---

[12] There is clearly no doubt about this claim. First, a patient with such a delusion is obviously regarded by his family, friends, and doctor as the same person. Second, such delusions typically do not undermine the retention of many non-delusional memories the patient may have that are identity-preserving (in both senses of identity) as well. In a sense such delusions have a single theme, with some initial degree of predictable elaboration, and so the patient may think his 'true' identity as Jesus Christ has only recently been revealed to him, though of course he bears a robust enough psychologically continuous link to who he was prior to such 'revelations'.

[13] Thus we have now described two apparently different categories of deviant connections: causally deviant connections, and cognitively deviant connections. We acknowledge the theoretical possibility that cognitively deviant connections may be reducible to causally deviant connections, all occurring inside the head. In the philosophy of mind, functionalists will regard this as theoretically inevitable.

my view of yesterday through memory, as mediated by my *experiencing* self then, not give rise to a sense now of my being temporally connected to that experience? In many cases, we acknowledge that episodic remembering does give rise to a distinct feeling of there being a continuous experiential 'worm' connecting the current rememberer with the remembered self, even though we typically never have a complete view of the worm (in say a memory from last week there just isn't time!). But in some cases, the identity and connectedness features may come apart. Sometimes, 'memories' from long ago, contain mere snapshots of events that now seem isolated from one's sense of a continuous world. These are 'memories' that form islands situated away from one's sense of a continuing life. They certainly have the feel of personal identity about them but as detached episodic fragments they cannot be fitted into an overarching sense of a narrative life. We think we do experience 'memories' such as these, and so they count as identity-preserving even though they do not give rise to a sense of connectedness.

The question, though, is whether such 'memories' preserve a sense of oneself. Since we have claimed that the capacity for mental time travel requires both a sense of identity and a sense of connectedness we can imagine someone objecting, in the light of the kinds of case just mentioned, that the connectedness feature may be important in central cases, but is not strictly speaking required. In response we would not argue too strongly against this; it is surely appropriate that it remain sensitive to some degree of looseness. The *sense* of connectedness is something that comes to us in degrees of psychological intensity, and so our understanding of mental time travel should be likewise sensitive to these degrees.

Finally, consider the reverse case of alleged mental time travel in which a sense of temporal connectedness is preserved but not a sense of personal identity. Are there such cases? What should we say about them? We believe there are such cases and that it is straightforwardly psychologically possible to experience a form of awareness in which a person now has a sense of being connected to a timeslice of a person from the past, and yet no sense of personal identity. In cases of dissociative identity disorder (DID), some patients experience something called the 'looking-on phenomenon' during which, in an altered state, the patient views 'from the outside' experiences that befell one of her other personality states. (See Kennett and Matthews (2003, p. 37).) The patient may later, when under the control of the personality state that had been looking on, recall the experience. She thus does have a sense of being connected to these events but without the sense of identity, and therefore without the sense that during this previous experience she was the controlling agent. Similarly, in depersonalization disorder, the patient may experience her thoughts, activities, and emotions as an observer; though in these cases she *knows* that the actions are hers she lacks the sense of identity and control that we will argue is required for full moral responsibility.[14]

16.4 The limits of mental time travel and broad autonoesis

We said mental time travel requires a very specific understanding of the capacity for mentally placing oneself outside the present via some controlled conscious process.

---

[14] *DSM-IV*, p. 500.

This is because there is another sense in which a person may have temporally extended self-knowledge which does not depend on this very specific capacity. Persons develop an understanding of their character, their *trait* self-knowledge, as some psychologists call it, via a mechanism that appears to be neuro-anatomically separable from that which permits autonoetic awareness. There is empirical evidence that this trait self-knowledge is generated from a mechanism that is independent of episodic memory.[15] Klein *et al.* (2003) describe the case of KR, who had Alzheimer's dementia. The patient had difficulty retrieving 'mundane' facts about the world, but retained accurate knowledge of her own personality as she was before the onset of the dementia. However, she was unable to update her trait self-knowledge. This, Klein notes, contrasts to other neuropsychological patients who can update their self-knowledge even with damage to the episodic and semantic memory systems. '[These] results add to the growing body of literature suggesting that semantic memory contains a sub-system devoted to the acquisition and representation of trait self-knowledge'(p. 157).

This last point does not affect our main thesis that mental time travel is a critical requirement for planning and control, yet it is important for two reasons. First it reminds us that our sense of an autobiographical self emerges from a variegated and dissociable set of systems all implicated in its formation.[16] Second, it shines a light on the specific nature of our main thesis: our claim is that self control can be derailed if we lose the capacity for mental time travel. It seems from the literature that this capacity may be lost or damaged while trait self-knowledge is preserved. The point here is that agents with insights into their character may nonetheless have no access to their past and future actions, thoughts, and feelings. In a forensic context, a display of self-knowledge that is the result of an intact sub-system within the semantic memory system should not, therefore, be taken as sufficient evidence that the agent satisfies the conditions of responsibility.

It is worth qualifying the notion of mental time travel when thinking about the way it applies to the forward-looking cases. In the backward-looking cases, we can invoke autonoetic awareness unproblematically since we can indeed mentally travel to the one and only experience that is fixed in the past. There is a single, fixed, and historically true point within our past for us to 'visit', and thereby be aware of. For, memory, as opposed to some apparent recollection such as a confabulation, is a success verb. I cannot be said to remember an event that never occurred. But mentally travelling to 'the' future is misnamed in a deliberative context since in deciding what we will do, we must necessarily presuppose at least two possible futures; yet we will travel to only one of them if the deliberative process is successful. It might, in the light of this, be thought that the asymmetry between the backward-looking and forward-looking cases shows there is not a single capacity for mental time travel. But it does make sense to speak of a general capacity to direct self awareness outside the present moment.

The difference between the forward- and backward-looking cases brings to the fore the importance of the distinction between autonoesis and mental time travel, the latter being a complex capacity which includes autonoesis. In the forward-looking

---

[15] See, e.g. Klein *et al.* (2003), and Wheeler and Stuss (2003, p. 828).
[16] See Klein *et al.* (2004).

cases, strictly speaking, we mentally travel to *possible* futures, albeit often for the purpose of deciding what we will do at some quite specific future time. But autonoetic awareness arguably supports other activities which do not strictly involve mental time travel. It supports the general capacity to simulate ourselves in what we might call an *offline* context. For example, daydreaming may not be temporally indexed and is not undertaken for any particular purpose, yet often these self-involving excursions can inform our deliberative activities. We think that mental time travel, then, is a subset, albeit a very important subset, of the range of self-involving thoughts in which human beings replay or rehearse certain experiences or actions.

In canvassing the cognitive resources available to us in practical reasoning, it is important to acknowledge these other cases. Take, for example, occasions where we knowingly, in imagination, re-write the past – we use our episodic memories as a take-off point. So we might re-imagine question time from a presentation we delivered, removing the bad answers we gave and improving the others. This is the kind of activity we engage in as a matter of course, and it serves an important learning purpose. It is one of many strategies of offline processing in which the self we entertain is not indexed to any particular time. Thus, we often think about not only what we did and will do, but also what we might have done, and about what we would have done in somewhat different circumstances; we think also about what we might do if, say, faced with a diagnosis of cancer or an armed gunman, or about the kinds of things we should do if we wish to live up to our ideals and principles. In mentally rehearsing a dance routine or a guitar solo, we have a more radically de-contextualized awareness of self. We think, then, in the light of these thoughts, that a broader understanding of autonoesis is both possible and theoretically sensible.[17] There may even be support within the cognitive science literature for the broad construal.[18] If the same neurocognitive mechanism is invoked in both the temporal and atemporal cases, this would seem both a more elegant interpretation, and one that is better supported empirically.

We claimed that autonoesis is a sense or process, and that mental time travel is an effortful action under conscious control in which a subject *utilizes* this sense. Indeed the fact that we can utilize the sense is at the heart of our concern with it. It is not just an interesting phenomenological feature of our existence; it is essential to our lives as agents. Similarly, a temporally unindexed awareness of oneself can be brought under the conscious control of the agent and exercised for a variety of purposes. The more broadly autonoeis is construed, the broader the implications for the agency and thus for the responsibility of those in whom it is impaired or absent.

Nevertheless, we do emphasize that although this broader notion is required for a full understanding of the processes of deliberation, mental time travel is the more central deliberative tool because it is more tightly constrained by the facts about what we have done, and about which of the futures we imagine are actually available

---

[17] The temporally indexed notion has been dominant till now. See, for example, Wheeler *et al.*, (1997, p. 335).

[18] See Klein *et al.* (2004, p. 469).

to us. Moreover it is, after all, the central capacity we have for our taking responsibility for what we have done, for it allows us to respond appropriately to our past deeds as our own. We now consider the relation between mental time travel and the moral emotions.

16.5 **Mental time travel, emotion, and planning**

At first glance it might be thought that planning requires the invocation of forward-looking connections to future selves and that is all. On the contrary, planning is a complex human activity often requiring both episodic memories and imaginative rehearsal for what is to come, as well as emotional tagging of past events and future events. How does this complexity arise and function?[19]

Episodic recall involves the re-experiencing of a past event, or acting in the past, together with an automatically held belief that a person represented within the recollection is oneself.[20] The generation of this reflexive belief may be put down to several features. First, there is a kind of automated inductive response we make to the having of an episodic memory: this is an episodic memory; so this really happened *to me*. We almost never labour through such an inference, though there are occasions when we sometimes wonder whether the state we are in is a remembering state or the recollection of, say, a mere dream; on such occasions we might well decide that the state we are in feels more like remembering states we have experienced in the past, and on that basis conclude that it is. Second, as earlier discussed, the content of episodic memories contains a *me-ness* feature, and we mean by this, an awareness of this self now as experiencing or doing something in the past. Thus we do not mean here a sense of identity in the historically true sense we spoke of earlier, but rather the sense of being aware of oneself as the kind of thing with a temporal trajectory.

There is a very interesting aspect to the way in which this feature comes to be represented. In *field-formatted* remembering, we recall experiences as they came to us first hand – we replay the experience just as it occurred from the same perspective as before. It is this mode which preserves the me-ness feature. By contrast, in *observer format* we re-view an event from, as it were, the third person perspective, looking at ourselves in the way we might imagine others do. Thus, in field format we identify ourselves directly, but in observer mode, the identification contains an additional element – that is how I *would* have looked to a third party. This difference in mode of access raises questions of self-knowledge, and self-interpretation. For example,

---

[19] For a recent description of the mechanisms for prospection, see Gilbert and Wilson (2007, p. 1352)

[20] That one automatically believes a personal memory recalls *oneself* emerges in a different guise in Shoemaker (1968). He described an epistemic feature of certain I-statements by saying that they are 'immune to error through misidentification relative to the first person pronouns.' First person memory reports are paradigms of such statements. Part of the idea is that our first person knowledge of ourselves in the past, as delivered by memory, is direct; the ability to make such memory statements can be learned without the need to use criteria of identity. Shoemaker argued explicitly for this in his work (1963).

in observer format it does seem that one loses immunity to error through misidentification because of the real possibility one might seem to remember the actions of someone else, say one's identical twin.[21] The difference in mode of access also leads to a difference in the moral emotions triggered in response to memories. If I remember an episode in observer format, I see myself as if through others' eyes, and this might lead me to a realization of just how rude I was. But this realization will normally only trigger shame and embarrassment if I can also see this person as *me* rather than as my twin, or my alter personality, or as someone wholly unconnected to me. And this requires the availability of the memory in field format.

To return to the role mental time travel plays in planning, we think the first step is the identification *with* oneself that field-formatted memories provide. Such identification, *ceteris paribus*, gives rise to appropriate emotional responses; a recollection of my having acted in a way that I now judge to be bad would normally give rise to self-directed emotions of guilt, shame, or regret and this may prompt reflection on what I need to do to make amends, or on how I need to change my behaviour in the future. The key point is that awareness of a past self must contain more than just the semantic or cognitive understanding that this was an action of mine if it is to support planning. If the memory is not available in the right mode, I cannot get myself to take experiences and actions performed as my own; it will thus not trigger the appropriate self-directed emotions, and so it will not provide a sufficient basis upon which I can project myself into the future.

To get a sense of the importance of mental time travel for planning, consider a case where it is lost. Levine *et al.* (1998) report the case of M.L. which we now summarize. M.L. suffered a severe brain injury and was in the immediate post-injury period amnesic both for events and persons as well as suffering impairments in semantic knowledge. He made a good recovery from his semantic deficits and he re-learned significant facts about his own past. However, his recall of events from his personal past remained fragmentary. Moreover and significantly, M.L. was unable to episodically re-experience *post*-injury events to the same extent as control subjects, although he could use familiarity or other non-episodic processes to distinguish events he had experienced from those he had not experienced. He continued to report a feeling of subjective distance from recall of events occurring *after* his recovery. He displayed errors of judgement and failures to understand his responsibilities as a parent that required supervision of his behaviour and structured routines. He was unable to secure paid employment and 'socially he reported difficulty knowing how to behave around family and friends and had to be taught socially acceptable behaviour' (p. 1956). Cases such as M.L. bring out the importance of the kind of access we have

---

[21] Indeed, this *kind* of mistake – though not just involving twins – is a real possibility. In earlier work (2003, p. 45) we discuss cases of looking-on in DID which we think are facilitated precisely via the slide from field-formatted to observer-formatted memory links. This slide might also explain the shift one might make from memories that support *de re* beliefs to ones supporting *de se* beliefs. As a sufferer of the mirrored self-misidentification delusion, one might remember 'seeing that man in the mirror', and later update one's interpretation of the very same memory with 'seeing myself in the mirror'. (For discussion of this delusion see Breen *et al.* (2001).)

to past episodes for the purposes of planning and deliberation. Merely semantic access deprives an agent of the right kind of emotional engagement with his past and future selves to be able to effectively guide behaviour.

In normally functioning human beings, the process of deliberation and planning is typically accompanied by an act of imaginary 'dress rehearsal'. We imagine our putative future selves acting in a variety of scenarios, we imagine the consequences of our actions, and we respond emotionally to the whole simulation. The information we gain via such simulations, along with our emotional and evaluative responses to them, guides our choice-making present selves in forming a preference about what we should do. I imagine myself eating a third helping of pie, the resulting sore stomach, and the thinly veiled disapproval of my gluttony from those around me, and rightly decide to stop now. So, again, in the future-oriented case, the capacity to see myself in possible future scenarios, to respond appropriately, and to choose from among them is critical to planning and control of one's personal future.[22]

Yet, there is a further connection between memory and planning, and not just the relatively trivial requirement that in order to carry out a plan I must remember what plan I have resolved to take on. A consideration that often informs my choice about what to do tomorrow is a reflection on past experiences of a similar type where things may have gone a certain way. In this way, effective planning typically requires both forward and backward-looking autonoesis. In strategic planning, for example, reviewing past mistakes cues negative emotional responses. If an imagined future contains a scene likely to give rise to a similar mistake, it can be vetoed. This form of deliberation is thus unavailable to agents who are unable to 'visit' the mistakes of the past. If I cannot remember my drunken car accident last month, then I have lost a critical consideration just before ordering 'one more for the road'.

In the next section we elaborate this kind of deliberation by noting that mental time travel supplies the basis for two important ingredients of planning: coordination and reflection.

16.6 **Mental time travel and the elements of reflective self-control**

In this section we undertake a more detailed examination of the foundational role mental time travel plays in the capacity for self-control across time and thus with the role it plays in establishing and securing responsive and responsible agency. We suggest there are two, often overlapping dimensions to the exercise of self-control: the normative and the operational. First, temporally extended self-awareness seems to be a necessary condition of the kind of reflection – on the type of person we want to be and on the worth of our future plans – that provides us with *normative* reasons, including moral reasons. These are reasons which extend across time and whose force

---

[22] This is not to say of course that the information, either about the consequences of our actions or our emotional responses will be accurate. We can be quite wrong about how we would react to certain events. Nevertheless, it seems essential that we have some sort of conception of how the future will be for us in order to prepare for it.

is thus independent of, and in a position to compete with, our immediate wants. What John Locke called continuity of consciousness permits the normative connections between different person stages that motivate exercises of self-control, and seem essential to accountability. Second, mental time travel operationally underpins self-control in two distinct ways; it facilitates the co-ordination necessary for carrying out temporally extended projects, and it makes available important techniques of self-regulation which prevent us being thrown off course by immediate temptations and distractions.

Let us consider in more detail the role of mental time travel in normative reflection. In imagining possible future *selves* I weigh up which of these best enacts my values and I may select the future that shapes me and my values in the ways I want to be shaped. Perhaps I am considering which area of the law to practice in. In projecting myself into possible futures, I come to worry that the pressures and environment of corporate law might lead to a corruption of my concerns for social justice and so reject that option. Would being a barrister for hire lead to my developing a taste for the high life, and would a win-at-all-costs mentality override my concern for the truth? Or would undertaking high-profile law suits and celebrity divorces provide me with the kind of income that allows me to take deserving *pro bono* cases and thus better serve my goal of securing justice for the disadvantaged than I could as a family solicitor or lowly paid employee at a community legal centre? What kind of person am I and what kind of person do I want to be? A more everyday example of normative practical reflection might be reflection on whether to put my demented mother into a nursing home or to let my career take a back seat and care for her at home. This case clearly has both backward- and forward-looking aspects. I might recall her tender care for me when I suffered depression in my early twenties, her often-expressed fear of nursing homes, and promises I have made to her. I might rehearse the difficulties and expense of providing adequate care for her and keeping her safe at home as she deteriorates and wonder whether a good nursing home and daily visits is after all compatible with my duty to her and my conception of myself as a loving son or daughter. It would seem that good decision making in these cases requires normative reflection which necessarily invokes mental time travel.

Mental time travel also facilitates reflective endorsement and disendorsement of actions and sub-actions being considered as part of a *plan*. This role is one of quality control – in deliberation we often select from a range of different possible ways to the completion of a project, doing so on the basis of a set of normative considerations. In thinking, for example, about how to structure a lecture series, I might remember the way the lecture on Hume went badly last year and imagine myself giving an alternative version this year. My temporal travels to last year lead me to reflectively endorse an imagined different, and improved, lecture this year. This form of deliberation is enabled only because of a complex piece of reasoning that makes use of a visit to the past, and then a visit to a possible future, in order to best plan for it.

This leads then to a consideration of the second dimension of mental time travel: how it (operationally) facilitates *co-ordination*. Once we have chosen a goal or course of action with which we can normatively identify, we need to implement it. Planning for the future often involves setting out a series of steps, which must be undertaken in a particular temporal order, that constitute the means to various sub-goals which themselves serve an overarching goal. The goal of health might require attention to the sub-goals of improved diet (education, shopping, cooking), exercise (scheduling gym visits, training for the triathlon in September), and relaxation (regular saving for a trip to Thailand in January, the taking up of salsa dancing). Clearly, we need the capacity to assign ourselves to 'be on duty' at the required times in order to fulfil this complex of means to our adopted ends. Mental time travel is critical to our being able to situate our temporally indexed future selves in relation to a project that stretches out in time. Here, it is important to note a fundamental distinction between such self-generated and self-governed long-term projects on the one hand, and ongoing patterns of behaviour which might merely *seem* to be the product of a capacity to extend one's agency across time. Thus, there might be cases in which a person regularly attends some ongoing activity, or in which the acquisition of semantic (impersonal) knowledge facilitates the completion of some task. So, for example, Tulving (2002, p. 15) reports the case of three young children who despite a severe impairment to their episodic memory function successfully attended school and in so doing '. . . acquired normal, or near-normal semantic knowledge of the world.' In such cases as these, we think the 'agency' involved critically depends on external scaffolding, presumably in this case significant logistical support from parents and teachers. The planning is all done for, and not by, the children and so the pattern of behaviour we see is the product of a kind of colonial arrangement.

In contrast, examples of self-governed projects invoking mental time travel include writing a paper, completing a day-long shopping trip, taking a week's vacation with one's family, running a business, or coordinating a weekend of athletics for one hundred school children.[23] In these cases, the logistics are taken care of via the agent's sense of how to 'position' her various temporal stages in relation to the overarching project. An effective agent is the true author of the project, fully invested in its completion, and above all she has a knowledge of it that is part and parcel of her self-knowledge. The theme of self-knowledge becomes important in connection with the forensic issue of responsibility and *mens rea* in the legal sphere. As we discuss below, we think mental time travel as described here is just what John Locke had in mind in his famous discussion of personal identity. Locke too had in mind a forensic notion of 'person' because he thought that in order to take responsibility for one's deeds, one needed a certain kind of self-knowledge that derived from an internal perspective.

Finally mental time travel is also required for exercises of *self-regulation*.[24] Self-regulation is argued by psychologists to be the capacity '. . . by which the human psyche exercises control over its functions, states, and inner processes. It is an important key to how the self is put together.' (Baumeister and Vohs, 2004, p. 1). More specifically,

---

[23] We hope these examples are not controversial. Someone might argue that someone lacking the ability to mentally time travel could complete some of these. Couldn't someone use external props – a notebook with instructions for example – to complete a shopping trip? Well, perhaps they might. The point of course is that if they did manage to pull it off we would not describe this as a case of ordinary agency.

[24] We are indebted to Cordelia Fine for pointing us to work done in psychology on self-regulation, and to many of the quotations in this section on that topic.

Levine *et al.* (1998), talk about a sub-function in which normal individuals are able to fashion and then make operational their ends, in the absence of environmental cues and structures. In this way, individuals generate from within, the psychic materials they need to complete tasks without the kinds of social scaffolds that might be required in their absence, such as we saw in the case of Tulving's schoolchildren.

One prominent kind of model of such self-regulation has been put forward by Ayduk and Mischel, (2002, 2004), and (independently) MacCoon, *et al.*, (2004). These writers emphasize the capacity for *attentional control*. MacCoon *et al.* (2004, p. 422), for example, define self-regulation as the 'context-appropriate allocation of attentional capacity to dominant and non-dominant cues.' Self-regulation requires an individual to attenuate her response to cues that would otherwise derail her projects. A typical situation which calls for the exercise of attentional control is one in which we are required to delay or eschew gratification. Those who are successful in resisting temptation find ways to focus their attention away from the immediate consummatory qualities of the chocolate mousse, cigarettes, second beer, or what-have-you. One important way of doing so is to attend instead to the negative consequences of such indulgence in terms, say, of ill-health or loss of reputation; another is to generate and focus on some future reward for abstinence such as shopping for a new dress or spending the money saved on a holiday. These kinds of self-regulatory strategies, then, would appear to involve mental time travel.[25] Certainly, some psychologists have explicitly said as much. Levine (2000, p. 200), for example, claims:

> Autonoetic awareness supports the ability to project oneself into the future [i.e., mentally time travel], to cast oneself as a player in scenarios emerging from the various choices available at any given moment. Put to practical use, this capacity facilitates the self-regulation of behaviour necessary for the achievement of personally relevant goals.
>
> (Levine, 2000, p. 200)

Mental time travel, then, is relevant to synchronic self-regulation and control – that is, self-control exercised under conditions of immediate temptation – as well as to diachronic self-control. If we foresee that our future valued plans and commitments could be derailed because of some expected future temptation we may plan ahead by, say, leaving the car keys at home, by making some public commitment or bet, or by undertaking some kind of cognitive therapy that will make future temptations easier to resist when they arrive. Diachronic self-control requires both co-ordination strategies and the employment of self-regulatory strategies and is predicated upon autonoetic awareness.

Of course not every failure of self-control turns upon an absence of autonoetic awareness or an impaired capacity for mental time travel though they all do threaten extended agency. Persons afflicted by compulsive desires may perfectly well be able to foresee the consequences of their actions and to evaluate their worth but the strength of their desires means that their efforts at self-control are unsuccessful.

---

[25] Not all strategies of attentional self-control rely on mental time travel. One might for example count to 100, or as Mischel reports, choose a cold ideation of the rewards on offer, e.g. 'The marshmallows are puffy like clouds' rather than 'the marshmallows taste yummy and chewy' (Mischel 1981, pp. 226–227).

Autonoesis is a necessary but not sufficient condition of reflective self-control and so, we claim, of responsibility.

16.7 **Mental time travel, autonomy, and responsibility**

John Locke accounted for personal identity by regarding the self-knowledge delivered by continuity of consciousness as the source of its forensic content. To be held accountable for one's actions, one needed to know they were one's own in a certain sense, and this could be so only if one could appropriate those actions by reaching back in subjective time to their occurrence. As Locke (1690/1984, p. 148) put it:

> This personality extends it*self* beyond present existence to what is past, only by consciousness, whereby it becomes concerned and accountable, owns and imputes to it*self* past actions, just upon the same ground, and for the same reason, that it does the present.

We think it highly suggestive that the right theoretical role for continuity of consciousness is mental time travel. It captures intuitively the Lockean sense of self-ownership, but in addition builds in a forward-looking dimension. It plays a significant role as enabling *extended* agency, and so provides a link between this influential account of personal identity and some well-known accounts of extended agency.[26]

Although our main conclusion in this chapter is that the absence or impairment of the capacity for mental time travel, as seen in some of the neuropsychiatric cases we identify here, provides a condition of exemption from responsibility for alleged wrongdoing, our central theoretical point is that mental time travel just *is* the central means by which normal human agents extend their agency over time and gain authorship over their lives. One way to see this is to contrast accounts of autonomy that make no essential reference to the notion of extended agency, with accounts like Christine Korsgaard's that make this a constitutive feature. Our point is that one might fulfil the requirements of the former in the absence of mental time travel.[27] Yet, if this capacity were absent altogether there would be no sense in which the individual might be said to be shaping their own life or acting on the basis of reasons over enough time so as to be regarded as morally autonomous. And if one cannot grasp and apply normative reasons in this way, including moral reasons, one cannot satisfy the conditions of responsibility.

Some humans never develop the capacity for mental time travel or develop it to only a limited extent; others may suffer the loss or impairment of such a capacity, and

---

[26] See Christine Korsgaard (1988, 1996, 1999), Michael Bratman (2000), and Neil Levy (2003). Bratman explicitly notes a connection between his account of extended agency and Locke's account, though his purpose there is not same as ours.

[27] We assume here the possibility of an individual who has moral concepts, and the relatively synchronic ability to endorse first-order desires. Such an individual may experience severe amnesia, but there is time within the span of working memory to reflect upon the desire of the moment, reflection that moves the synchronic individual all the way to action. That such an individual fails to meet the conditions of normative agency and responsibility suggests that accounts of moral autonomy need to build in the condition of mental time travel. (See Kennett and Matthews (2008) for an account of why we think it highly unlikely that agential connections could be anything other than normative connections.)

experience such losses in varying combinations with other cognitive impairments. What should we say about these different kinds of cases with respect to the capacity for *mens rea*, the guilty mind, and hence our warrant for holding them responsible where a crime has been committed? We will consider here the implications of our argument for attributions of responsibility in some representative cases.[28]

First, we consider the most extreme cases of absence or disruption to the memory connections between different person stages. In DID, the subject has only limited and selective awareness of those of her prior actions, thoughts, and decisions that occurred when she was in as we term it, an alter state. She will either have no memory of actions performed while in an alter state or her memories of them will be in observer format. She will have no sense of being the author of those actions, joined to them by a series of narrative and normative links such that they constitute part of her self-knowledge. Moreover her capacity to plan for and control her activities into the future is severely impeded by the unavailability of the normal assumption that she will in the future remember and feel bound by decisions she makes now. It seems clear that DID sufferers should not be held responsible and punished for bad actions committed when in an alter state. There are two grounds for this claim. First, the lack of the right kind of memory connections to the event means that the central purposes of punishment – reform, rehabilitation, and retribution – cannot be met.[29] Reform and rehabilitation would seem to require self-acknowledgement of wrongdoing and the possibility of experiencing the appropriate moral emotions. In the retribution case, surely we wish to punish the agent who committed the crime. In the normal case, the agent at the point of account and the crime-committing agent are the same, and this link is facilitated because the former retains the capacity to, as Locke might have said, extend himself to what is past and to thereby become accountable for it. Where this capacity is absent we are not justified in punishing.[30]

Second, on any conception of moral responsibility that relies on the possession of the capacity for autonomy, DID sufferers cannot count as responsible even at the time

---

[28] We exclude from consideration, cases where the capacity never develops at all since such an individual could no more be considered a candidate for moral responsibility than an infant or a dog.

[29] It may, however, succeed in serving the purpose of general deterrence.

[30] We acknowledge a well-known difficulty arising here due to Geach (1969, p. 4) who thought Locke's account 'repugnant' since it implied that forgetting one's crime excused it. This objection could be extended: if I take a pill that removes the memory of having committed the crime, am I thereby excused? Well, obviously not. However, we think this an objection only to a naïve reading of the function of mental time travel in moral responsibility. For taking the pill that removes the memory does not thereby disable autonoetic awareness as such, or my *general* capacity for mental time travel. The point is that memory failures have to go beyond ordinary forgetfulness in order to be excused, and they cannot be cynically engineered precisely to avoid responsibility. After all, taking a pill is an action designed to remove the possibility of one's crime being discovered (since a guilty person tends to give himself away in, for example, lie detector examinations), and so is akin to removing possible evidence of one's guilt.

of action, if they are in an alter state. As we have pointed out elsewhere (2002, p. 520) their autonomy is impaired since, as a result of falling into this state, they are either incapable of remembering their prior rational decisions and commitments, or they are incapable of buying into or being appropriately affected by, the reason-giving force of them. The normative connections between person stages which are essential to self-control rely upon autonoetic awareness – the sense that the decisions and commitments I am remembering are *mine*. A sufferer's capacity for normative reflection is further reduced since they do not, when in an alter state, know who they really are, and thus do not have access to the full range of considerations which a robust and veridical self-awareness would provide.[31] As Braude notes, '. . . [T]he multiple as a whole cannot judge actions in a suitably integrated and comprehensive way' (1996, p. 51).

Next, consider again the case of M.L. It seems clear from the foregoing discussion that M.L., or others in his position, cannot now be held to account for any wrong actions performed prior to injury of which they now have no memory, even if we can safely assume that they satisfied the conditions of responsibility for those actions at the time at which they performed them. But what about M.L's responsibility for actions performed post injury? We think that M.L's post-injury failure to form memories with a robust subjective sense of me-ness means that he is impaired in his capacity to adequately reflect upon even his recent past self or to feel constrained by the decisions of that self. M.L's failures in planning and self-regulation may be in part the result of an inability to inhibit thoughts and behaviour generated from habit (procedural memory), or from environmental stimuli. But M.L. also appears to be impaired in his capacity to engage in evaluative reflection by his relative inability to represent his past and future selves and to manipulate those representations in imagination as described in the previous section. That is, he is *both* normatively and operationally impaired. From the description given by Levine it appears that to the extent that M.L. engages in activities or projects that extend over time, his engagement is not governed by an internally generated plan. It relies upon habit or external props.

However M.L and others like him may appear to satisfy at least one of the conditions of reflective self-control. It is possible that such a person may possess moral concepts and be able to apply them appropriately to their present situation. If M.L. knows that stealing is wrong then surely, the argument might go, he can be held responsible if he shoplifts because he knows *at the time* at which he acts that the action is wrong and he acts intentionally at that time. He satisfies the conditions for *mens rea*. His incapacity to reach forward into the future and evaluate the consequences of his shoplifting is largely irrelevant. The seriousness of the offence might be mitigated by the fact that it was not premeditated but that is all. Provided he can remember the incident, albeit without a clear sense of ownership, are not we justified in punishing him for it? Indeed, the argument might continue, is not punishment an appropriate trigger for generating aversive responses that could guide his behaviour in the future?

---

[31] In our (2002) we argue that cases of DID can be usefully assimilated to, e.g. cases of bipolar disorder for the purposes of responsibility. In our (2003), we argue that alter states are relevantly similar to delusional states. The sufferer believes against the evidence that they are a child, or of the opposite gender etc.

There are a number of things to be said in response to this argument. First, we would need to know more about the sense in which such a person 'knows' something is wrong. Mere semantic knowledge of the moral rules might not meet Wallace's (or the law's) requirement of moral understanding.[32] Second, even if we conclude that someone with these impairments does have more than merely semantic knowledge of the moral rules, their incapacity to reach forward into their personal future and represent and evaluate the consequences of their action does deprive them of an important means of self-control. We think therefore that their responsibility is significantly diminished even in simple cases of wrongdoing. It is clear that they will not be able to satisfy the conditions of responsibility where premeditation is an integral part of the wrong act or where it involves a series of coordinated acts, for example, cases involving fraud or deception. Where a person with significant deficits in mental time travel is involved in such wrongdoing, a likely explanation for their behaviour is that they have been duped by another.

More difficult for an account of responsibility are cases of damage to the prefrontal cortex which result in so-called 'acquired sociopathy', and cases of developmental psychopathy, where patients appear to have some capacity to visit the past but in whom the usual normative connections between person stages are absent. In this connection, consider an example from Grant:

> I always know damn well I shouldn't do these things, but they're the same as what brought me to grief before. *I haven't forgotten anything.* It's just that when the time comes I don't think of anything else. I don't think of anything but what I want now. I don't think about what happened last time, *or if I do it just doesn't matter.* It would never stop me.
>
> (Grant, 1977, p. 60, our emphasis)

On one natural reading of this case it would appear that moral understanding is preserved along with the capacity to remember and foresee the consequences of the action but as a result of his neural condition the patient is unable to inhibit impulse by exercises of attentional control, including those that involve mental time travel. He is either incapable of directing his attention to non-dominant cues or doing so is ineffective. Such cases highlight that autonoetic awareness and the capacity for mental time travel are necessary but not sufficient for the exercise of reflective self-control and the effective extension of one's agency across time.

But another salient possibility, especially in the case of developmental psychopathy, is that made famous by Frankfurt (1971). *Persons* are capable of wanting their desires to be different from how they are. They are capable of evaluating their desires and forming attitudes of approbation or disapprobation towards them. But the wanton, according to Frankfurt is the individual who is moved indifferently by his strongest desire. Unlike the rest of us, he simply does not care (and is incapable of caring) which of his desires moves him to action. Wantons have no overarching principles to govern their choices and can engage in no secure planning since any plans they make will be abandoned with every shift in desire. It seems clear that the wanton is not conatively connected in

---

[32] See Fine and Kennett (2004) for an extended discussion of the requirement of moral understanding in the law.

the right kind of way to their past and future stages, set against the standards of normative agency. The interests of past and future selves seem as remote to their present concerns as those of strangers. These interests are incapable of providing any reasons which could compete with present desires. The wanton is not a moral agent (Frankfurt thinks they are not persons) and so is not appropriately subject to moral assessment. We suggest the same is true of psychopaths. We want briefly to suggest one further point and that is that if psychopathy is a real-life example of wantonness, it calls into question the assumption that their capacity for mental time travel *is* unimpaired.[33]

The wanton, as Frankfurt describes him, has a vastly impoverished sense of self. He has no principles, no goals, no ideals, no values, and no attachments. He is just a cluster of desires and impulses, likings, and aversions. He can thus have no genuine self-directed emotions such as pride or shame, since they require a sense of how one has or has not lived up to one's values and principles. A background assumption of the discussion of the role of mental time travel in practical reflection and moral responsibility is that we take a normatively rich sense of self to the kind of deliberation on our personal past and future that supports exercises of planning and self-control. And such acts of deliberation and planning further shape and enrich this normative sense of self. But psychopaths have no such sense of self to guide their travels to past and future. It is unsurprising then to find, as Hare tells us, that psychopaths' thoughts and ideas are 'organized into rather small mental packages and readily moved around' (1993, p. 136). Their attention shifts rapidly, they go off track, they confabulate, and they have trouble maintaining a narrative thread (1993, p. 138). They are also unlikely, he says, to spend time considering the consequences of their actions; rather their aim is 'immediate pleasure, satisfaction, or relief' (1993, p. 58). The diagnostic criterion of a lack of a realistic long term-goal also suggests that mental visits to the past and future engaged in by psychopaths tend to be haphazard and relatively unconstrained by the facts: they are not the controlled activity essential to planning, autonomy, and self-control which we have focussed on here. We do not mean to suggest that these deficiencies in mental time travel are the psychopath's primary impairment;[34] rather, we think the case of the psychopath highlights the role played by normative self-awareness – which includes trait self-knowledge as well as the endorsement of some guiding concerns and principles – in the effective utilization of the brute capacity to reach back and forward in subjective time.

16.8 **Conclusion**

The central claim we make here is that the capacity for mental time travel is necessary for reflective self-control and therefore for responsible, autonomous agency. Moral autonomy requires the extension of agency across time in order that individuals can plan, shape, and direct their lives in accordance with their values, and exercise control

---

[33] It also calls into question the assumption that psychopaths possess the required level of moral understanding for moral responsibility. For more detailed discussion of moral understanding and self-regulation in psychopathy see Kennett (2006) and Fine and Kennett (2004).

[34] The primary deficit of the psychopath is commonly taken to be affective. Nevertheless psychopaths clearly also have problems with self-regulation.

over their actions, and this in turn depends upon their having mental access to both their past and to their possible futures. The neural basis of mental time travel is complex relying on the availability of a sufficient database of episodic memories as well as on frontal systems which access and manipulate the data in the executive processes central to self-control.[35] We have argued that individuals who are severely impaired in their capacity for mental time travel as a result of brain damage or mental disorder, are not only unable to effectively exercise control over their behaviour across time, they are also unable to develop a stable deliberative nature, and without this, they lose an effective source of normative connections over time. If they cannot view their past actions as their own, or exercise control over prospective actions, they cannot meet the conditions for moral or legal responsibility. Finally, it is worth reflecting that mental time travel, though central to extended agency and responsibility, forms part of a suite of meta-cognitive capacities important to deliberation. We touched on this in discussing a broader concept of autonoesis. A full account of our deliberative natures awaits a complete exploration of the ways in which these meta-cognitive capacities function and interact.

References

American Psychiatric Association (1994). *Diagnostic and Statistical Manual of Mental Disorders*, (*DSM-IV*). Washington, DC, American Psychiatric Association.

Ayduk, O. and Mischel, W. (2002). When smart people behave stupidly: inconsistencies in social and emotional intelligence. In *Why Smart People Can Be So Stupid?* (ed. R. J. Sternberg) pp. 86–105. New Haven, CT, Yale University Press.

Ayduk, O. and Mischel, W. (2004). Willpower in a cognitive–affective processing system: the dynamics of delay of gratification. In *Handbook of Self-Regulation: Research, Theory, and Applications* (eds. R. F. Baumeister, and K. D. Vohs), pp. 99–129. New York, Guilford.

Baumeister, B. J. and Vohs, K. D. (2004). *Handbook of Self-Regulation*. New York, Guilford Press.

Braude, S. (1996). Multiple personality and moral responsibility. *Philosophy, Psychiatry and Psychology*, **3**(1), 37–54.

Breen, N., Caine, D., and Coltheart, M. (2001). Mirrored-self misidentification: two cases of focal onset dementia. *Neurocase*, **7**(3), 239–254.

Dere, E., Kart-Teke, E., Huston, J. P., and Souza Silva, M. A. (2006). The case for episodic memory in animals. *Neuroscience and Behavioural Reviews*, **30**(8), 1206–1224.

Fine, C. and Kennett, J. (2004). Mental impairment, moral understanding and mitigation: psychopathy and the purposes of punishment. *International Journal of Law and Psychiatry*, **27**(5), 425–443.

Frankfurt, H. (1971). Freedom of the will and the concept of a person. *Journal of Philosophy*, **68**, 5–20.

Geach, P. (1969). *God and the Soul*. London, Routledge and Kegan Paul.

Gilbert, D. T. and Wilson, T. D. (2007). Prospection: experiencing the future. *Science*, **317**, 1351–1354.

---

[35] Shallice *et al.* (1994) report a PET study which showed that acquisition of episodic memory was associated with activity in the left prefrontal cortex and the retrosplenial area, whereas retrieval was associated with activity in the right prefrontal cortex and the precuneus.

Grant, V. (1977). *The Menacing Stranger.* New York, Dover.

Hamilton, C. (2005). *Broken Open.* Sydney, Bantam.

Hare, R. D. (1993). *Without Conscience: The Disturbing World of the Psychopaths Among Us.* New York, Pocket Books.

Kennett, J. (2006). Do psychopaths really threaten moral rationalism? *Philosophical Explorations,* **9**, 69–82.

Kennett, J. and Matthews, S. (2002). Identity, control and responsibility: the case of dissociative identity disorder. *Philosophical Psychology* **15**, 509–526.

Kennett, J. and Matthews, S. (2003). Delusion, dissociation and identity. *Philosophical Explorations,* **VI**, 31–49.

Kennett, J. and Matthews, S. (2008). Normative agency. In *Practical Identity and Narrative Agency* (eds. K. Atkins, and C. Mackenzie), pp. 212–231. New York, Routledge.

Klein, S. B., Cosmides, L., and Costabile, K. A. (2003) Preserved knowledge of self in a case of Alzheimer's dementia. *Social Cognition,* **21**, 157–165.

Klein, S. B., German, T., Cosmides, L., and Gabriel, R. (2004). A theory of autobiographical memory: necessary components and disorders resulting from their loss. *Social Cognition,* **22**(5), 460–490.

Korsgaard, C. (1988). Personal identity and the unity of agency: a Kantian response to Parfit. *Philosophy and Public Affairs,* **18**, 101–132.

Korsgaard, C. (1996). *The Sources of Normativity.* Cambridge and New York, Cambridge University Press.

Korsgaard, C. (1999). Self-Constitution in the ethics of Plato and Kant. *Journal of Ethics,* **3**, 1–29.

Levine, B. (2000). Self-regulation and autonoetic consciousness. In *Memory, Consciousness and the Brain: The Tallinn Conferences* (ed. E. Tulving,), pp. 200–214. Philadelphia, PA, Psychology Press.

Levine, B., Black, S. E., Cabeza, R., *et al.* (1998). Episodic memory and the self in a case of isolated retrograde amnesia. *Brain,* **121**, 1951–1973.

Levy, N. (2006). Autonomy and addiction. *Canadian Journal of Philosophy,* **36**, 427–448.

Locke, J. (1690/1984). *An Essay Concerning Human Understanding.* Glasgow, Collins.

MacCoon, D., Wallace, J. F., and Newman, J. P. (2004). Self-regulation: context-appropriate balanced attention. In *Handbook of Self-Regulation Research* (eds. R. F. Baumeister, and K. D. Vohs), pp. 422–447. NY, Guilford Press.

Martin, C. B. and Deutscher, M. (1966). Remembering. *The Philosophical Review,* **75**, 161–196.

Max Planck Institute for Human Cognitive and Brain Sciences. Irving Koch's *Cognition and Action: Learning of Sequential Structures.* Available at http://www.mpipf-muenchen.mpg.de/CA/RESEARCH/sequence_e.htm (accessed October 2008)

Mischel, W. (1981). Metacognition and the rules of delay. In *Social Cognitive Development* (eds. J. H. Flavell, and L. Ross), pp 240–271. Cambridge, Cambridge University Press.

Mondimore, F. M. (1999). *Bipolar Disorder: A Guide for Patients and Families.* Baltimore, MD, John Hopkins University Press.

Shallice, T., Fletcher, P., Frith, C. D. *et al.* (1994). Brain regions associated with acquisition and retrieval of verbal episodic memory. *Nature,* **368**, 633–635.

Shoemaker, S. S. (1963). *Self-Knowledge and Self-Identity.* New York, Ithaca.

Shoemaker, S. S. (1968). Self-reference and self-awareness. *Journal of Philosophy,* **65**(19), 555–567.

Tulving, E. (1972). Episodic and semantic memory. In *Organization of Memory* (ed. E. Tulving), pp 381–403. New York, Academic.

Tulving, E. (1983). *Elements of Episodic Memory*. Oxford, Clarendon.

Tulving, E. (2002). Episodic memory: from mind to brain. *Annual Review of Psychology,* **53**, 1–25.

Wallace, R., J. (1994). *Responsibility and Moral Sentiments*. Cambridge, MA, Harvard University Press.

Wheeler, M. A. and Stuss, D. T. (2003). Remembering and knowing in patients with frontal lobe injuries. *Cortex,* **39**(4–5), 827–846.

Wheeler, M. A., Stuss, D. T., and Tulving, E. (1997). Toward a theory of episodic memory: the frontal lobes and autonoetic consciousness. *Psychological Bulletin,* **121**(3), 331–354.

Chapter 17

Motivation, depression, and character

Iain Law

Abstract

It has been noted by philosophers that depression involves not being motivated to act virtuously. Some, for example, Michael Smith, assert that since depression involves a split between cognitive appraisal of one's situation and one's motivation, knowledge cannot motivate, and so virtue cannot be knowledge. In this chapter, I aim to refute the claim that depression provides evidence against virtue being knowledge. Depression does involve altered beliefs as well as altered desires. I provide a cognitivist account of the way in which depression interferes with normal moral motivation. The beliefs of someone with depression will interfere with the normal process of being motivated by their moral beliefs. I thus acknowledge that someone with depression will lack virtue. This should not be understood as moral criticism of the depressed however, since someone may lack virtue without having failed to do anything that morality obliges them to do.

17.1 Depression and motivation

This chapter investigates two related but distinct issues. The larger issue concerns what it is to be a good or virtuous person. One important strand in the history of moral philosophy sees virtue as a matter of doing one's duty as a result of having correct beliefs about what one's duty is, with desire and emotion under the control of reason. A rival strand takes the opposite view: virtue consists in having appropriate feelings and desires and being moved by them. Bernard Williams identifies these strands as Kantian and Humean, respectively, distinguishing 'the basically Kantian enterprise of trying to elicit altruism from certain structural conditions on rational practical thought' from 'the basically Humean claim that it is not such conditions, but rather a certain desire or sentiment that constitutes the vital step in the direction of altruism' (Williams, 1973, p. 253). Both strands go farther back than Hume and Kant, of course. Elements of each can be found in ancient Greek ethical thought, but more intertwined with each other. We may hope for a reconciliation of the two strands if we accept the Aristotelian view that appropriate desire accompanies correct belief. If that is true, the 'Kantian' thought that morality consists in acting on correct beliefs about duty can be accepted, and so can the 'Humean' thought that acting well consists in having the right feelings and desires.

This leads us to the second, narrower issue discussed here. Another position commonly dubbed 'Humean' threatens the possibility of the Aristotelian reconciliation sketched above. The Humean account of motivation asserts that beliefs and related states cannot be motivating. Only with the addition of a separate desire or related desire-like state can an agent be motivated to act.

Depression is relevant to both these issues. It prompts questions arising from the way in which depression interferes with normal motivation. Taking the second issue first, it appears to lend support to the Humean account of motivation, exemplifying the way in which feelings and desires can come adrift from beliefs. In relation to the larger issue, the same depression-related phenomenon of belief and desire coming apart forces us to confront the case in which the agent acts according to her beliefs about what she should do but fails to feel any independent inclination to do so. Should we consider such an agent virtuous? The Kantian view would say 'yes'. The Humean would say 'no'. The Aristotelian appears to have to side with the Humean, if such a person is even possible on the Aristotelian account. On the other hand, if such a person is not possible on the Aristotelian account, we may think that this is evidence against that account.

In what follows, I will in Section 17.1.1–3 set out the Aristotelian position, and deal immediately with the objection to it based on the Humean account of motivation. I will appeal to empirical data about actual depression to refute one major argument for Humeanism about motivation, purportedly based on depression, and go on to argue that in fact depression provides support for an anti-Humean, cognitivist account of motivation. This means that the Aristotelian view of virtue remains viable, and in Section 17.2, I explore implications for that account, considering depression again.

17.1.1 Virtue as knowledge and the Humean challenge

What is it to have good character? A trivial answer would be that it is to possess the virtues, but this answer merely raises the question of what it is to possess virtue. Many suggestions have been made, but here I want to focus on a major strand of thought about virtue: that virtue is a species of knowledge. This was a central feature of ancient Greek thinking about virtue, and has more recently been defended by John McDowell.[1] According to this conception of virtue, to be virtuous is to possess (or to be disposed to possess) a cognitive state that also motivates. The way in which the virtuous person conceives of (or perhaps perceives) her situation also functions as her motivation to act virtuously. She is moved to act as she does just in conceiving of the situation this way. We might ask many questions of such an account: what is the nature and content

---

[1] See, for example, McDowell (1978, 1979).

of this knowledge? Can it be learned, and if so, how? How can such an account accommodate people who possess virtue imperfectly? All of these questions must be deferred until we have addressed a challenge to the very possibility of such an account of virtue. The dominant account in philosophy of how action is motivated denies that cognitive states such as belief and knowledge can be motivating states. If this is correct, the understanding of character that I have begun to sketch would be cut off.

The so-called 'Humean' view of motivation is pretty standard in the philosophy of mind. Even its most prominent contemporary defender, Michael Smith, calls it a 'dogma' (Smith, 1994, p. 92). Humeans believe in a strict divide between beliefs and desires. Beliefs have no intrinsic motivating force: I may believe anything at all, but only with the contribution of a separate desire will I be motivated to act. This claim should be broadened out to include all cognitive states. The Humean claim is that cognitive states are wholly lacking in conative power, i.e. they have no direct influence on the agent's desiring or willing. If some beliefs seem to us to motivate action, that can only be due to a contingent association with a separate conative state such as a desire.

Humeans do not deny that such contingent connections between belief and motivation occur. They are very commonplace: if you were to acquire the belief that the building you are in is on fire, you would immediately be motivated to do various things: to call the fire service, to warn others, to leave the building. Humeans are happy to accept contingent connections between belief and motivation. These connections may be sufficiently powerful and immediate that it would be very difficult for an agent to break the connection. This poses no problem for the Humean, since they merely want to insist that the belief is not necessarily linked to the motivation; that for an agent to be motivated there must be a separate mental state present – a desire. Smith says that the Humean's claim is '. . . that it is always at least *possible* for agents who are in a belief-like state to the effect that their ϕ-ing is right to none the less lack any desire-like state to the effect that they ϕ; that the two can always be pulled apart, at least modally' (Smith, 1994, p. 119).

The argument between Humeans and anti-Humeans comes to place curious stress on the phenomenon of depression.[2]

17.1.2 **The depressive**

Smith employs the character of 'the depressive', whose example is intended to demonstrate that there can be no necessary connection between belief and motivation. He borrows this character from Michael Stocker who discusses the sort of case in which:

> . . . one may feel less and less motivated to seek what is good. One's lessened desire need not signal, much less be a product of, the fact that, or one's belief that, there is less good to be

---

[2] It is only fair to point out that Smith has another argument for Humeanism, based on the claim that belief states and desire states have different and incompatible 'directions of fit' with the world (Smith 1994, pp. 111–118). I argue against this argument elsewhere. It has received considerable critical attention, with counterarguments including Humberstone (1992) and Little (1997). The depression argument has received comparatively little attention.

> obtained or produced. . . Indeed, a frequent added defect of being in such 'depressions' is that one sees all the good to be won or saved and one lacks the will, interest, desire or strength.
>
> (Stocker, 1979, p. 744)

Smith concludes that 'various sorts of "depression". . . can leave someone's evaluative outlook intact while removing their motivations altogether' (Smith 1994, 120). In other words, the depressive may have exactly the same set of cognitive states representing how the world is as the virtuous person; and yet fail to be motivated as the virtuous person is. This is, he asserts, conclusive evidence in favour of Humeanism. The anti-Humean cannot accommodate this (supposed) fact about the depressive's desires coming apart from his beliefs, but the Humean can. 'The anti-Humeans' view must therefore be rejected in favour of the Humeans.' (Smith, 1994, p. 121). How should we understand this argument? We must decide between two ways of interpreting the figure of the depressive. One interpretation is that in introducing this figure, Smith intends to appeal to real phenomena associated with actual depression as it is experienced by sufferers. The alternative interpretation is that he is using 'depression' as a term of art, divorced from its meaning in psychiatry, intending only to pick out a phenomenon he claims occurs – this coming apart of beliefs and desires.

I think that we must assume that the second interpretation is incorrect, since it would rob the argument of its force. If 'depression' means nothing more than the phenomenon of belief and desire coming apart in the way that Smith and Stocker describe, it would be nothing but an instance or an illustration of the claim he is arguing for – that the cognitive and conative are never necessarily connected. If this were so, the claim that there could be such instances cannot serve as evidence for Humeanism, since Humeanism is nothing more than the claim that there are such instances. To put it another way, the matter in dispute is whether it is always possible for belief and desire to be pulled apart, to use Smith's own words. Smith, being a Humean, wants to say that this is possible. But the claim cannot be its own evidence, and that's what would be happening if 'depression' is being used merely as a term of art picking out an occasion of such 'pulling apart'.

I therefore take it that Smith's claims about depression should be read as claims about what actual depression is like – that someone who becomes depressed retains the cognitive outlook that they had before becoming depressed, but is no longer motivated in line with that outlook. My discussion will therefore address how well Smith's account matches actual depression.

There is some plausibility in his view. Certainly, we would not want to say that the depressive who ceases to be moved as he once was has simply changed his mind about what there is value in doing. That would entirely fail to capture the depressive's experience – indeed, it would be worth asking why such a change of mind should be labelled depression. That said, it seems to me to be equally wrong to say that the depressive's cognitive view of the world, or of any particular situation, is identical with that of the non-depressed person, that in becoming depressed, his motivations have changed but his beliefs and perceptions remain unaltered.

My own experience of being depressed is not like this at all. In depression, everyday tasks take on an aspect of impossibility. I do not see, say, replying to an email, as an easy task I am peculiarly lacking in motivation to perform. Rather, I see it as far more difficult than it actually is, or, I see myself as not being up to the task. When I'm depressed, every job seems bigger and harder. Every setback strikes me not as something easy to work around or get over but as a huge obstacle. Events appear more chaotic and beyond my control: if I fail to achieve some goal, it will seem that achieving it is forever beyond my abilities, which I perceive to be far more meagre than I did when I was not depressed.

But perhaps that is just a personal peculiarity. Just because in my case desire has not come apart from belief, that does not mean that it cannot. My case may be contingent, leaving open the possibility that belief and desire can be pulled apart. If my case is unusual, if we can find cases of depression that match the Stocker/Smith description, the argument for Humeanism will remain intact. Looking at psychiatric literature suggests, however, that my experience of depression is by no means idiosyncratic.

17.1.3 The cognitive account of depression

In recent years, an approach to depression which treats it as essentially cognitive has become both popular as a treatment and well-supported by research as an account of depression's nature. This cognitive approach was pioneered by Aaron Beck. According to Beck, people who are depressed have negative cognitions about themselves, the world around them, and the future (Beck *et al.*, 1979, p. 11). This set of negative thoughts is known as the 'cognitive triad'. A good example of such thinking is 'I am worthless, everyone hates me, and nothing will ever go well for me' (McIntosh and Fischer, 2000, p. 153). The mere fact that such altered beliefs are present in depression would cast doubt on the Stocker/Smith model, but Beck and other cognitivists go further. They claim that not only are negative thoughts and beliefs associated and correlated with depression, but also that these negative thoughts and beliefs are the root of the depression.[3] The depressed person does not think poorly of themselves, their situation, and their future because they are depressed; they are depressed because they think in this negative way. 'The cognitive model views the other signs and symptoms of the depressive syndrome as consequences of the activation of the negative cognitive patterns' (Beck *et al.*, 1979, p. 11). Cognitive therapy, which Beck pioneered, aims to alleviate the sufferer's depression by changing their cognitions ('cognitive restructuring'). If the subject can alter what they think, and what they believe about themselves, the world and the future, they will also alter how they feel and what they want to do.

---

[3] Some cognitivists take this even further: they say that the distorted cognitions are the depression. For this reason, they claim that there is no point in pursuing research into neurological causes or other biological approaches to the problem. This strong position is not only much stronger than I need for the purposes of the present argument, it seems too strong altogether. I can see no good reason to rule out in advance the possibility that both distorted cognition and depressed mood, etc. are caused by some third factor. And to adopt the strong position would rob us of the ability to make the sorts of claims that the more moderate cognitivists want to make. Typically, the studies cited in support of the cognitivist hypothesis identify depressed and non-depressed people, and find that there are higher rates of negative cognition among the depressed people (see Clark, *et al.* (1999) for examples). If, however, we must identify the depressed people with those who have negative cognitions, how could such research even be done?

The cognitivist account of depression is not merely an armchair theory. It has been subjected to a great many empirical tests. Understandably, the majority of these focus on the efficacy of cognitive therapy rather than on the accuracy of the account *per se*. If cognitive therapy is successful, that would provide evidence in favour of the cognitivist account of depression. If, on the other hand, cognitive therapy is only partially successful, that would not by itself disprove the cognitivist account, for the following reason. There are two ways in which cognitive therapy might fail. One would cast doubt on the cognitive account: the cognitive restructuring might succeed, so that the patient no longer thinks negatively about himself, his surroundings, and his future, and yet he might continue to be depressed – to lack motivation, to have low mood, etc. The other would not: it might be that the attempt to restructure the subject's thoughts fails. The subject may resist the restructuring, or the habit of thinking negatively may be too strong to break despite their best efforts. If cognitive therapy were to perform poorly for this second reason, it would be evidence against the efficacy of the therapy, but not evidence against the account of depression upon which the therapy is based.

In fact, there is considerable empirical evidence for the efficacy of cognitive therapy: while it is not universally effective, one survey of the evidence says that 'numerous studies have demonstrated the efficacy of cognitive therapy for depression' (Sanderson and McGinn, 2001, p. 263). If depressed people can be treated successfully by cognitive restructuring that indirectly supports a cognitivist account of the nature of depression. Only indirectly, however: 'Whereas there has been widespread agreement that cognitive *therapy* of depression is effective . . . there has been less consensus on the validity of cognitive *theory* ...' (Haaga *et al.*, 1991, p. 215). Haaga *et al.* note that little research on the theory has been done and set out to remedy this – to 'review empirical work relating to the entire theory as described by Beck.' (Haaga *et al.*, 1991, p. 215). Their study concludes that 'the idea that all subtypes of depression are associated with increased negative thinking has been consistently supported' (Haaga *et al.*, 1991, p. 226). They do suggest that Beck is incorrect in his views about the cognitive triad, however: 'the triad refers to views of the self as a whole and two aspects of the self, not three completely distinct entities' (Haaga *et al.*, 1991, p. 218). This suggestion is supported by further empirical research suggesting that a single 'self-relevant negative attitude' can be found in subjects with depression (McIntosh and Fischer, 2000, p. 156). For our current purposes, however, whether a single factor is at work rather than three is less important than the accuracy of the fundamental claim that depression is strongly associated with negative cognitions.

This claim, as we have seen, is borne out by empirical studies. This strongly suggests that affective and conative states are not disconnected from cognitive states in the way that the Humeans believe. Certainly, it would mean that Humeans should hesitate to invoke depression as evidence in support of such a disconnection, and should especially refrain from referring to such putative evidence as 'the facts of ordinary moral experience' (Smith, 1994, p. 124). Any depiction of depression that has it that the depressed person's 'evaluative outlook [remains] intact' (Smith, 1994, p. 120) is simply not faithful to the facts.

If this is correct, the dispute between Humeans and anti-Humeans at least remains open. Indeed, the phenomena associated with depression may even suggest that the anti-Humean is on stronger ground, as I will go on to discuss.

17.2 Depression and character

17.2.1 Motivation in the virtuous person

According to McDowell's view of virtue, to be virtuous is to have a certain sensitivity deployed in how you perceive the situations you encounter. This perception brings with it appropriate motivation. 'To a virtuous person, certain actions are presented as practically necessary . . . by his view of certain situations in which he finds himself' (McDowell, 1978, p. 14). Other motives are 'silenced' (McDowell, 1978, p. 26). McDowell gives the example of being able to see that someone else is 'shy and sensitive' (McDowell, 1978, p. 21). The virtuous person perceives things around them which those who are not virtuous do not, and it is in this ability to perceive that their virtue consists. There is a difficulty with this suggestion, though, which is that it seems possible for someone to see the same situation in the same way and yet not be kind (McDowell, 1978, p. 16). Socrates denied this possibility, saying that anyone who failed to be virtuous did so through ignorance. Aristotle suggested that while there was a sense in which a kind and an unkind person could perceive the same things, the difference would be that the unkind person's perception of them would be in some way clouded or imperfect. This is a suggestion that I will pursue in relation to depression below.

This sort of account of virtue makes the following sort of story tempting. Virtue is a matter of noticing ethically salient features of the world, but noticing them will not lead to right action unless the agent has general knowledge of what to do in such circumstances. The sensitivity needed for kindness is useless unless the agent knows what to do when kindness is called for. This sort of story can be modelled by an Aristotelian practical syllogism: Distress is to be comforted (general knowledge); this person is in distress (sensitivity); I'll comfort this person. Tempting as this picture is made by an account of virtue in terms of knowledge, McDowell thinks that it must fail. The reason is that it is impossible to discover moral principles such as the first premise that are always correct. Morality is, he thinks, uncodifiable (McDowell, 1979). Practical wisdom is the master-virtue.

Jonathan Dancy has pursued similar ideas (Dancy, 1993). He too insists that there are no general moral principles that the virtuous person grasps (Dancy, 1993, pp. 73–108). Instead, knowing what to do is a matter of perceiving the situation correctly: perceiving its ethically salient features (Dancy, 1993, pp. 111–116). Virtue both enables us to perceive these features properly and respond properly to them. Without virtue, I will of course be able to see the non-moral features of the situation upon which the moral features supervene, but I will not be able to see the supervenient moral properties, and nor will I even be able to understand how the sub-venient properties are related to each other. Unable to see that they go together to make up a morally salient feature of the situation, I will not see that they go together in any way at all: they will be 'shapeless' (Dancy, 1993, pp. 76, 79).

Thus the virtuous person and the non-virtuous person will see the same scene, and be able to pick out equally accurately its non-moral features. But the virtuous person will also be able to perceive an ethical demand inherent in the situation, and they will in virtue of that perception, or that way of conceiving of their situation, also be motivated to respond to that demand. Opponents of virtue-as-knowledge will point out that there is nothing about the situation expressible in non-ethical propositions that they know and that the non-virtuous person does not (e.g. Smith, 1994, pp. 123–124). Friends of virtue-as-knowledge will retort that this does not show that the difference between the two is not that the virtuous person knows something that the non-virtuous person does not.

This leaves a puzzle, even if we are willing to accept the cognitivist account. For it appears to leave us facing one of the 'Socratic paradoxes', namely that anyone who fails to do the right thing does so out of ignorance. For, if they knew what the situation called for, they would, just in virtue of possessing that knowledge, be motivated to act accordingly. McDowell appears to embrace this conclusion: he thinks the virtuous person's conception of the situation is one that is sufficient to motivate them to act. And, he reasons, if it is sufficient in one case, it must be sufficient in all (McDowell, 1979, pp. 333–334). Dancy explains why:

> The virtuous person's conception of the circumstances is one which could not be shared by someone who does not see exactly the same reason to act. For where opposing reasons are silenced, all who share the silencing conception must surely act in the same way; they have no reason left to do anything else.
>
> (Dancy, 1993, p. 53)

One way to respond to this problem is to note that being motivated to act in a certain way is not the same as acting in that way. I may be motivated to do something to some degree, but not do it because stronger motivations against performing the deed prevail. In McDowell's terms, this would amount to sharing the virtuous person's conception of the situation up to a point: I might see (along with him) the salient features of the situation that called for action on my part, but there might be interfering elements in my conception of the situation that prevented all other motives and reasons from being silenced. I think that this may be what is going on in the case of depression.

Consider the example (expanding from McDowell, 1978, p. 21) of being at a party and perceiving that someone you do not know very well, or perhaps at all, is shy and sensitive, and standing by themselves feeling uncomfortable. In the virtuous person, this perception is accompanied by being motivated to go and talk to the shy and sensitive party guest. It is quite likely that the depressive will fail to do this – not being motivated as (they think) they should be is after all one feature of depression that all sides agree on. The depressed person's failure to act need not occur, I would suggest, because they fail to perceive anything that the virtuous person perceives, but because they have additional thoughts or background beliefs that get in the way. Recall that according to the cognitivist account of depression, the depressive is plagued by negative thoughts about himself and by extension about his circumstances and his future. One obvious example of such thinking would be the thought that even though the party guest is uncomfortable, he wouldn't want to talk to *me*. Such self-denigrating thoughts are highly characteristic of someone with depression. Another potential block to action is the depressive person's habitual indecision and self-doubt. The inability to make decisions is one symptom of depression. One reason for it may be the tendency to have too little confidence in one's own perceptions and judgements. So, although the depressive sees the other guest's discomfort, they may be insufficiently confident in that assessment to feel able to go up and talk to them, thinking: 'What if he is not really uncomfortable – perhaps he will just be annoyed to be accosted by someone he doesn't know.'

If this is a plausible account of what's going on in one case of the difference between the virtuous and the non-virtuous person (in this case a depressed person), then something which has been said to be a major problem for the anti-Humean (Smith, 1994, pp. 123–124) has been accounted for in entirely cognitivist, anti-Humean terms.

17.2.2 Depression and lack of virtue

People who are depressed commonly see themselves as deficient in various ways. It is very common for them to doubt whether there is anything medically wrong with them. Students suffering from depression, for example, often tell me that they feel that they do not merit the sort of mitigation that would be appropriate to someone with a straightforwardly physical illness affecting academic work. They see their condition as a character flaw rather than as an illness. This is usually taken to be a symptom of the condition, and something that the depressed person is incorrect in thinking. Some of the foregoing thoughts indicate, however, that the depressed person is in part correct: in being depressed, they lack virtue. This is not to say that they are correct to blame themselves for this state, nor to lend support to any tendency the depressed person may have to accept their suffering as just punishment.

Depression is something that prevents someone from being motivated in the way that they would otherwise be. This extends to their moral motivations, in perhaps two ways: (1) They believe that they ought to φ and yet do not feel motivated to φ. (2) They feel no motivation to φ other than feeling that they ought to. Activities that they would hope to participate in gladly become unattractive: I do not want to play with my children, but I muster the energy to do so anyway because I think that morality requires it of me. Good deeds are performed only out of duty.

Both of these phenomena can be interpreted as ethical deficiencies. The first must be considered a lack of virtue if we accept that the virtuous person is motivated to do what she should. Allying my comments on the way in which depression produces altered perceptions of the world with McDowell's view of virtue, we can say more: the depressed person lacks virtue because they are no longer able to see the world in the way which is constitutive of virtue. Or, if they can in some sense see the world in this way, their vision is clouded by interfering negative beliefs about themselves.

The second phenomenon looks very similar to a character trait recently dubbed a 'fetish or a moral vice' by Michael Smith (Smith, 1994, p. 75): having what Williams calls 'one thought too many'. Bernard Williams set out to show that being motivated by duty, or even considering the moral status of one's action may be the wrong thing to do. He illustrates this claim like this. Suppose you somehow you find yourself in a situation in which both your wife and a complete stranger appear to be drowning. Although you are a strong swimmer, it is clear that you will not be able to save both of them. Someone who checks the moral status of his actions before performing them will, in this situation, think about whether it is morally permissible to favour his wife over a stranger. This is what Williams says:

> . . . this construction provides the agent with one thought too many: it might have been hoped by some (for instance, by his wife) that his motivating thought, fully spelled out,

would be the thought that it was his wife, not that it was his wife and that in situations of this kind it is permissible to save one's wife.

(Williams, 1981, p.18)

The upshot of this point, if we accept it, is that there are some situations in which it is better not to think about the moral status of one's actions. Sometimes at least, having moral scruples makes you a worse person than you would have been without them.

This is a result which has been taken up with some enthusiasm by moral philosophers. For example:

> . . . we often do not want ethics to intrude into practical living, not because we feel guilty about what we are doing, but because it introduces 'one thought too many'. In a personal relationship, for example with one's partner or children, the last thing one wants is that people are acting with an eye to behaving well, or out of a sense of duty. Parents are to cherish children out of spontaneous love of them, not because they feel they ought to do so... A partner who realises that the other is meeting them not because they want to, but out of a sense of duty, thereby recognises that the relationship is lost. We do not want anything specifically ethical to intrude: a lover or parent who acts out of love, but at the same time is always checking what ethics requires of them or is mainly pleased that he or she is acting dutifully, is inadequate. [. . .] There are places, it seems, where only spontaneous emotion will do, and where ethical thinking should not intrude.
>
> (Blackburn, 1999, pp. 21–22)

Blackburn's claim about duty intruding into relationships signalling their loss seems to me deeply implausible, and certainly not warranted by Williams' original claim. I am not sure whether Blackburn has been extraordinarily lucky in his relationships, or whether he just sets himself very high standards, but my intuitions fail to match his in this case. It seems to me that most relationships are likely from time to time to require thoughts of duty to bolster temporarily flagging inclination. For instance, suppose I am away from home overnight after a meeting, and that I promised my wife before I left that I would call her. By the end of the meeting, which was long and argumentative, running well over time and sapping my energy, I wish that I had not made that promise, for all I want to do is go to bed. Nevertheless, that I promised to call my wife tonight provides me with a reason to call her even though I feel no inclination to do so. I don't feel (and I hope my wife doesn't either) that occasional occurrences of this sort, when thoughts of what I ought to do are necessary to motivate me, herald the imminent collapse of our marriage. This illustrates, I think, the need to be sure not to place more weight on the one thought too many point than it can bear.

Smith too exaggerates the scope of the one thought too many point, treating it as though it established that having any motive derived from thoughts of duty is sufficient to render the agent non-virtuous. He claims that good people are people who care *non-derivatively* about other people's welfare, justice etc. (Smith, 1994, p. 75).

In response, consider the following sort of case, similar to one discussed by Kant. Suppose that one of these good people finds one day that thoughts about others' welfare no longer motivate him as they used to. He has become soured or inured, so that considerations of other people's welfare do not matter to him as they once did. But suppose also that this person is conscientious. That is to say, he does not wish to fail to do his moral duty. Because of this, he is still motivated to help others, but now in a derivative fashion, because of his motive of duty, and his conviction that it is right to help others who are in need. Isn't he still a good person nonetheless? Note also that there is nothing contradictory in supposing that someone can possess the general motive to do their duty and also possess non-derivative motives to do various things such as help others, etc. Presumably, when he was in his earlier condition of caring directly about others' welfare, the moral motive was nonetheless present. But it was unapparent, since its motivational assistance was not required.

This discussion of 'one thought too many' defends the view that acting out of duty may be good. This appears to be in tension with the thought that depression involves a lack of virtue. But this appearance is misleading. Williams' point in its original form only claimed to show that there are some situations in which having 'one thought too many' is indicative of alienation and ethical shortcoming. The mistake Smith and Blackburn make is to extend the point beyond this limited scope. It is not very hard to come up with situations in which the thoughts one has about one's duty are clearly not 'too many' at all. To take a trivial example, suppose I am deciding who should win a scholarship, and one of the candidates is my son. Wondering whether it is morally permissible to favour my son in such a case is appropriate. Or imagine that you decide that the education your child would receive in a private school would be better than that she would receive in a state school. Having moral scruples does not make you a bad parent in this case, even if we think that in situations such as this, it is permissible to send one's child to a private school (just as in Williams' original example it is permissible to give preference to one's wife over a stranger). Most importantly, having the moral scruples does not mean that you love your child any less. Nor, indeed, would acting on your scruples in the case of the scholarship candidate. Although love might motivate you to give your own child the prize, not giving it to him is not evidence of a failure of love. Blackburn and Smith, and perhaps Williams, seem to think that any explicit moral thinking is a sign that things have gone wrong in some way. I do not think that this is always the case.

All this said, consideration of Williams' point about having one thought too many does illustrate that there are some things one should be motivated to do, at least most of the time without recourse to thoughts of duty. While calling my wife out of duty occasionally does not establish that I am a bad person; someone who as a matter of routine has think of duty to motivate himself to play with his children or talk to his wife has fallen short of virtue.

This links with another characteristic of depression. Depressed people tend to think frequently that they have failed, or are failing to do what they ought to do. Some treatments for depression focus on eliminating 'ought-thoughts' altogether, and some writers on the subject have gone so far as to attack morality itself as a cause of depression (e.g. Gilligan, 1976). This is a viewpoint with which I cannot agree. While Gilligan asserts that morality is 'force causing . . . suicide' (Gilligan, 1976, pp. 144–145), it may equally be awareness of his moral duty that keeps the depressed person from such an act. Less extremely, we might ask which is worse, to play with your children out of a sense that you ought to, or to not play with them at all? It seems to me that the depressed person fails to distinguish between reasonable and unreasonable moral demands. They ask too much of themselves, and enter a vicious circle of self-blame and further depression. Nevertheless, continuing awareness of genuine moral demands should not be sacrificed lightly.

The conclusion that the depressed person lacks virtue is an uncomfortable one, since it appears to involve moral condemnation of the afflicted. This appearance is false. Lack of virtue does not imply wrongdoing, and need not be blameworthy, at least according to some of the modern followers of Aristotle. A major strand in the move towards virtue ethics, in addition to the focus on character, has been the rejection of deontic concepts such as obligation and blame (e.g. Anscombe, 1958, p. 1). Different philosophers reject these notions to different extents, but most agree that the aretaic evaluations of character (in terms such as *good, noble, bad*, or *base*, as opposed to *right, wrong, obligatory, forbidden*) are broader than the deontic assessments of action. Thus the fact that I lack some virtue does not imply that I have done something that I ought not to have done, or that I have failed to do something that I should have done. This means that the fact that I cannot help being depressed does not block the thought that my depression constitutes a lack of virtue.

Even Kantians can agree with this. While it may be my moral obligation to do various things, it cannot be my moral obligation to feel any particular way. What is beyond my control cannot be commanded by morality. The most that may be asked of me is that I take whatever steps are open to me to bring it about that I feel in certain ways. Marcia Baron summarizes Kantian thinking on this topic: 'There are affective responses that are incompatible with virtue; there are others whose complete absence is incompatible with virtue. It is a duty to cultivate the latter and to seek to extinguish, transform or at least weaken the former.' (Baron *et al.*, 1997, p. 47). I am thus obliged to do whatever I can to get out of my depression: it is a state which threatens the future performance of moral obligations, and as such I would be better to be rid of it. Given a cognitivist account of depression means I must try as much as I can to change the way I think about myself, etc. This is no easy task, of course, but it at least shows the way in which Kantianism can concern itself with good character, and even with feelings and desires. While such conative and affective elements of the psyche may be beyond direct control, and thus outwith the scope of a duty-based morality, if they may be indirectly affected by cognitions which are to some degree alterable by voluntary effort, such a theory has the resources to comment upon them. By arguing in this fashion, Kant too has an account of virtue, and can agree that the depressed person falls short of it.

The view that depression is or involves a lack of virtue may be bolstered in a more kindly way if we recall another major strand in ancient Greek thinking about virtue – that to be virtuous is to possess *eudaimonia*: happiness or flourishing. Certainly the depressed person is not happy in the colloquial sense. Even if we allow that this is not the sense in which Aristotle identifies virtue with happiness, it is not hard to see that depression presents a major stumbling block. Self-respect, it is often suggested, is an essential component of human well-being. Without it, even if you have many other goods (friends, family, achievement, honour, etc.) they will not benefit you fully. Your inability to acknowledge that you deserve them robs them of at least some of their value for you. This accords with what surely is everyday moral experience: if you can come out of depression you will be both better off, and a better person.

This has implications for how we should think of depression and its treatment. We should not be too quick to dismiss a depressed person's self-understanding if that is presented in ethical rather than medical terms. While it is important to avoid appearing to support any self-blame that the depressed person may be prone to, we can at the same time acknowledge that they may be correct to think that they are exhibiting ethical failings. This can be framed in a more positive light in a therapeutic context: recovering from depression will bring with it better behaviour.

I think there is a connection here with Aristotle's ideas about the acquisition of virtue. Aristotle famously says that the way to acquire virtue if you lack it is to behave as if you were virtuous (*Nicomachean Ethics,* pp. 1103a–1104b). Do the generous thing, even though you lack generosity, and you will in time through a process of habituation become generous. It is hard to see how this could work if the agent were *merely* performing the action, without any understanding of why it is the appropriate action. The agent must also practice thinking about the situation in the correct light. Iris Murdoch offers a good example. A woman disapproves of her son's choice of wife. She finds her daughter-in-law common and lacking in social graces. Despite her feelings, she is outwardly perfectly polite and welcoming. After some time, the woman decides to make an effort to look at her daughter-in-law in a different light. She re-conceives or reinterprets her daughter-in-law's behaviour so that what she once saw negatively as common and undignified she now sees positively as simple and spontaneous (Murdoch, 1970, pp. 17–23). In order to establish a settled change in one's dispositions and character traits, one should practice thinking about things in the correct way, not merely acting correctly. After all, the woman in Murdoch's example acted with perfect propriety all the way through.

What this suggests to me is that the processes by which virtue may be acquired and those by which cognitive therapists seek to cure depression are very closely related. Psychiatrists and other mental-healthcare workers should be prepared to accept, and where possible seek to take advantage of this connection.

Acknowledgements

I would like to thank Heather Widdows and the editors of this volume for their helpful comments and advice.

References

Anscombe, E. (1958). Modern moral philosophy. *Philosophy, 33,* 1–19.

Aristotle (1925). *The Nicomachean Ethics* (Tr. and ed. D. Ross,) Oxford, Oxford University Press.

Baron, M., Pettit, P., and Slote, M. (1997). *Three Methods of Ethics.* Oxford, Blackwell.

Beck, A. T., Rush, A. J., Shaw, B. F., and Emery, G. (1979). *Cognitive Therapy of Depression.* New York, Guilford Press.

Blackburn, S.(1998). *Ruling Passions.* Oxford, Clarendon Press.

Clark, D. A., Beck, A. T., and Alford, B. A. (1999). *Scientific Foundations of Cognitive Theory and Therapy of Depression.* New York, Wiley.

Gilligan, J. (1976). Beyond morality: psychoanalytic reflections on shame, guilt, and love. In *Moral Development and Behavior: Theory, Research, and Social Issues* (ed. T. Lickona), pp. 144–158. New York, Holt, Rinehart and Winston.

Haaga, D. A. F., Dyck, M. J., and Ernst, D. (1991). Empirical status of cognitive theory of depression. *Psychological Bulletin,* **110,** 215–236.

Humberstone, L. (1992). Direction of fit. *Mind,* **101,** 59–83.

Little, M. O. (1997). Virtue as knowledge: objections from the philosophy of mind. *Noûs,* **31,** 59–79.

McDowell, J. (1978). Are moral requirements hypothetical imperatives? *Proceedings of the Aristotelian Society, Supplementary Volumes,* **52,** 13–29.

McDowell, J. (1979). Virtue and reason. *The Monist,* **62,** 331–350.

McIntosh, C. N. and Fischer, D. G. (2000). Beck's cognitive triad: one versus three factors. *Canadian Journal of Behavioral Science,* **32,** 153–157.

Murdoch, I. (1970). *The Sovereignty of Good.* London, Routledge.

Sanderson, W. C. and McGinn, L. K. (2001). Cognitive-behavioral therapy of depression in M. Weissman, (ed.) *Treatment of Depression: Bridging the 21st Century,* pp. 249–280. Washington DC, American Psychiatric Association Press.

Smith, M. (1994). *The Moral Problem.* Oxford, Blackwell.

Stocker, M. (1979). Desiring the bad: an essay in moral psychology. *Journal of Philosophy,* **76,** 738–753.

Williams, B. (1973). Egoism and altruism. In *Problems of the Self* (ed. B. Williams), pp. 250–265. Cambridge, Cambridge University Press.

Williams, B. (1981). *Moral Luck.* Cambridge, Cambridge University Press.

Conclusion

The future of scientific psychiatry

Lisa Bortolotti and Matthew R. Broome

One of the central aims of this volume has been to explore the extent to which the neurosciences (including, amongst others, cognitive neuropsychology, neurochemistry, and neurobiology) can exhaust the explanatory needs of psychiatry as a branch of medicine. From the careful consideration of the arguments put forward in this volume, it is fair to conclude that the neurosciences have very significantly contributed to the understanding of psychopathologies, but that it is necessary to reconcile the neuroscientific discourse with other explanatory frameworks in order to capture all the aspects of people's behaviour that are relevant for the study of psychiatry as an academic discipline and as a branch of medicine.

Folk-psychological notions – such as belief–talk and reference to moral responsibility – that have not been fully vindicated by neuroscience can make some features of psychopathologies immediately salient. There are multiple examples of this tension between neuroscience and folk-psychology in the volume. Frankish argues that we can make sense of delusions on the basis of their similarities and dissimilarities with beliefs of a certain kind, even if we are dissatisfied with existing doxastic accounts. Kennett and Matthews, and Law claim that notions such as autonomy and motivation are central to the understanding of the way in which the behaviour of people affected by psychopathologies is perceived as divergent from the norm.

Similarly, phenomenological approaches need to be attended to, and used to inform neuroscientific research, rather than put aside and forgotten. Phenomenology focuses on that which is given, or presupposed, in neuroscience: namely, our ordinary background sense of reality and belonging. As Ratcliffe argues, it is some of this very basic fundamental experience that may be altered in those with psychiatric illness – a profound transformation of experience has been undergone. Without the tools of phenomenology, neuroscience, however sophisticated, will be blind to the subtle and far-reaching changes experienced by those with mental illness.

In this final section we shall offer two other examples (from our own work) of the way in which neurosciences, at the current stage of development, cannot do all the explanatory work in psychiatry. The first example centres on the employment of normative notions in the characterization of the manifestation of psychopathologies as deviant. The second example highlights the importance of environmental factors in the onset of psychosis. In the end, we shall explore some potential for future research in these areas.

Psychopathology as a failure of self-knowledge

The notion of authorship as the capacity to endorse a thought as one's own and justify it on the basis of reasons, has been developed by Richard Moran and discussed extensively in the philosophical and psychological literature (Moran, 2001; Carman, 2003; Ferrero, 2003; Lawlor, 2003; Moran, 2004; Tiberius, 2008; Bortolotti, forthcoming). The notion of authorship, as we see it, is not necessarily tied to the rationality of the beliefs endorsed or to the rationality of the process of formation of such beliefs. Rather, authorship lies in the capacity to endorse the content of a belief and make it one's own by justifying it with reasons. Authorship so conceived generates a form of first-person authority. By taking responsibility for the thoughts one reports, one can relate to the content of those thoughts in a way no third person can. The belief is not just self-ascribed; it is also endorsed and seen as part of a self narrative that underlies agency.

Our suggestion is that the sense that a subject with delusions has a mental disorder can sometimes be captured only by attending carefully at the quality of the subject's reason giving. So authorship of beliefs and self-knowledge more generally, are areas in which a radical failure can signal the presence of a belief that is not just badly integrated with other beliefs, and imperfectly rational, but truly pathological. Due to the mentioned features of authorship, namely its dependence upon the capacity to engage in reason giving and its contribution to self-knowledge, it is explanatorily useful to ask whether subjects with delusions are authors of their delusional beliefs. A discussion of authorship in psychopathology has the potential to clarify what makes delusions different from ordinary beliefs, if anything, and can contribute to the classification of some beliefs as delusional on the basis of the reasoning patterns of the subjects with those beliefs. But it can also have an added value. It can tell us something about self-knowledge in subjects with delusions. In what sense is authorship of a belief related to first-person authority over that belief and to self-knowledge in general? The type of self-knowledge to which authorship contributes can be defined as *agential* rather than epistemic authority, because it involves the self as an agent capable of endorsing one's mental states and taking responsibility for them. It is an active rather than passive notion. In order to enjoy epistemic authority, all the subject needs to do is to have at her disposal more information about her conscious mental life than a third person. But in order to have agential authority, the subject needs to be able to *do* something. First persons are authors if they exercise some control over their thoughts and if what they think is, to some extent, 'up to them' (Moran, 2001).

Jaspers' and subsequent accounts of the classification of delusions rely on the distinction between 'form' and 'content'. The theme of the delusion, such as persecution, control, infatuation, determines its content. The structure of the delusional belief and its relationship to reasons the subject can offer the interviewer for holding it, constitutes the form. The form of a delusion is affected by whether the reasons provided to the interviewer by the subject are 'understandable'. When these reasons are deemed 'un-understandable' the delusion is said to be primary or autochthonous. This explains why the form of a delusion has been viewed as of particular importance both in terms of diagnosis but also of prognosis: content has been seen as somewhat more 'epiphenomenal' and related to the subject's biography, concerns, and culture, whereas the form reflects the pathological processes.

The form of a belief so intended can determine: (1) whether a belief is genuine; (2) whether it is well integrated in an existing system of beliefs; and (3) to what extent the subject has self-knowledge with respect to that belief. It can help us answer questions about self-knowledge, because form concerns authorship. Only the author of a belief is in a position to make the content of a belief one's own and justify it with reasons. If subjects with delusions are unable to give reasons for their delusional states, then they cannot be regarded as their authors. Subjects might believe something quite striking, and of great consequence for themselves, and might be confident with respect to the content of their beliefs. But when asked to provide the reasons why they are committed to their belief contents, that is, to make explicit the grounds for holding the beliefs, they cannot answer. For instance, consider the case of a 21-year old man who has the sudden conviction that certain songs played on the radio used his voice in the role of lead singer, but cannot explain why (Yager and Gitlin, 2005). The significance of the belief reported make it an ideal candidate for authorship, but the subject is unable to provide any reason that might convince others that his belief is likely to be true.

A different case, even more difficult to account for on the basis of authorship, is the case of the subject who endorses a belief on the basis of some reasons, but these are reasons that others fail to regard as relevant to the content of the belief. For instance, suppose there is a man who believes that his wife is unfaithful to him because the fifth lamp-post along on the left is unlit (Sims, 2003). The subject is attempting to justify his belief, but fails to support his belief on the basis of reasons that others can share and understand. Another case is one in which the subject with delusions can come up with reasons that support the reported delusional belief, although those reasons are not objectively very good ones. Authorship here is to some extent present but there might be a failure of rationality. A good example is that of the woman who claims that her blood is being injected out of her body in her sleep because she has spots on her arms. When the interviewer says that they are freckles and that he has them too, she agrees that the spots are similar to freckles, but continue to believe that she is being injected (Sims, 2003, p. 123).

As we can see in the examples, delusions vary widely with respect to the level of commitment that subjects manifest towards the content of their delusional beliefs. Here, commitment is not supposed to track the importance of the delusion in terms of action-guidance, persistence or integration with other intentional states of the subject, but is supposed to give us clues as to whether the subject is a genuine author of her beliefs. If the subject cannot provide any reason, or any reason that maintains meaningful relations to the content of the belief, for endorsing the belief, the interviewer might either doubt that the state reported is a genuine belief (coming to challenge the intentionality of the state reported) or interpret the inability to provide reasons as a breakdown of self-knowledge.

This latter move is even better justified in situations where not only the authorship of the beliefs is compromised, but also their ownership. There are a number of disorders of the self that might affect the capacity both to recognize a thought as one's own and to endorse its content. For example, a subject might explain that there is a thought in her head that has been put there via a special device capable of transmitting thoughts. Subjects may go into greater detail as to how the machine can transmit thoughts and elaborate on the magic or technology responsible for such a device. The transmitted thoughts might be said to be created or taken from another. Whereas the delusional explanation is often well-articulated and supported with reasons by the subject, the 'inserted' thoughts are disowned and no endorsement is manifested.

The thought is known first personally by the subject and therefore the subject is aware of the content of that thought independently of behavioural evidence. But the subject also feels passive with respect to the thought and regards it as alien or out of the subject's control (Sims, 2003, p. 164). With respect to questions about ownership and authorship, lack of control and total alienation are different cases. There are cases of delusion where the subject believes that her thoughts are controlled by others: 'a university student in her second year believes that her university lecturer has implanted an electronic device in her head that can control her thoughts' (Lewis and Guthrie 2002, p. 70). And there are cases of thought insertion proper, where the thought is not only controlled but produced by others: 'One evening one thought was given to me electrically that I should murder Lissi' (Jaspers, 1959/1997, p. 579). In both cases the subjects are self-aware of the thought, but only in the former case is the thought regarded as the subject's own thought. We would describe the latter case as a case in which both ownership and authorship of the thought fail quite dramatically. We are using here a fairly rich account of ownership, according to which the subject needs to be able to ascribe the thought to herself in order to own it, and awareness of the content of the thought, or identification of the thought in her own mind, are not sufficient conditions for ownership. For different accounts, see Campbell (2002), Gerrans (2001), and Gallagher (2004).

If the capacity for self-ascription is required for ownership, then we would have to deny that the subject suffering from thought insertion owns the 'alien' thought. Authorship requires ownership, and typically subjects with thought insertion do not endorse the thoughts they find in their heads as their own and do not provide reasons to justify them. So they fail to see themselves as, and to be, the genuine authors of those thoughts. We prefer to talk about loss of both ownership and authorship in this case, rather than loss of agency, because we are not concerned with the question of actual mental causation here. In order to feel that a thought is ours we do not need to have produced that thought or formed it as a result of deliberation. Post-hoc justification is sufficient to lead us to acknowledge the thought as ours. Both ownership as self-ascription and authorship fail to apply to the subjects affected by thought insertion, because subjects cannot ascribe the thought to themselves and they cannot see themselves as endorsing the content of that thought. Subjects fail to assume responsibility for the content of the 'alien' thought, not because they have not produced it as a result of deliberation (which is the case with many 'ordinary' beliefs), but because they cannot give reasons for it and they don't recognize themselves as people who would endorse that belief.

The repercussions for judgements of self-knowledge are very significant. A thought that is disowned or that cannot be authored is not included in a coherent narrative of the self that is likely to make sense of past behaviour and guide future thought and action. If we consider the reports of subjects who are recovering from their delusion, at some intermediate stage, when they feel better but are not fully recovered, they remember the experience of thought insertion as the experience of someone having inserted a thought into their head and they start wondering whether that experience was the effect of their schizophrenia. At a later stage, if and when they are fully recovered, they regain their capacity to integrate the thoughts once regarded as alien into their restored image of themselves. This interesting correlation between the stage of their mental health and the integration of their beliefs in an accepted image of themselves reveals how important it is for the conception of delusions as mental disorders or pathological beliefs to rely on the analysis of the reason–relations between the subject's beliefs in order to predict and manage potential repercussions of changes in the subject on self-esteem and self-understanding.

What we can take from this first example is that some epistemic and normative notions, such as those of reason giving and authorship, play an important role in the concept of mental illness and in our attempts at classification. They can contribute to a characterization of delusions as pathologies of belief, and have the potential to improve our understanding of delusions and of subjects with delusions. The notion of authorship, when applied to reported delusions, can tell us something about what is puzzling about delusions, why they take us by surprise, and why we might doubt in some circumstances whether the people who report those beliefs really endorse them as beliefs. But other lessons can be learnt. First, there is no one type, 'delusion', that fits all the experiences of subjects of delusions, because the form of delusions can make a huge difference to the quality of reason giving in interviews and the extent to which we take subjects to have knowledge of their own conscious mental states. The other lesson to learn is that to describe delusions as 'pathological beliefs' does not solve the problem of demarcation. We cannot draw a sharp distinction between delusions and other beliefs that we do not regard as delusional, but are either very implausible or not well supported by evidence, because in many cases of such 'ordinary' beliefs, authorship also fails (maybe to a different extent). This failure to provide a demarcation which is qualitatively sharp is not an indication that psychological or mental notions are hopeless at contributing to classification, but that they are at the right level of conceptual sophistication to provide the tools of analysis that are needed in the analysis of mental disorders. Applying such notions does not solve all the classification problems but improves understanding and allows discriminations that other levels of analysis cannot capture.

Currently, the classification of psychopathological states and mental disorders use criteria that rely on psychological terms. These terms themselves are defined normatively. Further, mental illness itself can be thought of the kind of disorder one identifies when normal reason giving, all other things being equal, breaks down. Thus, concretely speaking, a brain scan, genetic abnormality, blood test, etc. can never *a priori* serve as the sole criteria for the diagnosis of mental illness. However, to diagnose mental illness, one talks to one's patients. To bring biological investigations into diagnostic use, we can 'eliminate' mental illness and choose to redefine psychiatric disturbances using other criteria than that which we currently employ. This approach would lead to a radical shift in both the profession (and possible existence) of psychiatry, as well as to a change in wider society's perception and understanding of mental illness. It also leads to a conceptual difficulty: it does not take an expert to recognize that someone is mentally disordered but how would one decide whether dopamine quantal size, functional MRI activations, or repeats of genetic polymorphisms were abnormal in the absence of a disordered person? And this is the crux of the issue: for biological psychiatry to have any validity, and to be anything more than applied neuroscience, the main object of study needs to be the person. The normal and the abnormal themselves are normatively defined, and are not properties of the brain.

Schizophrenia and externalism: a challenge to a cognitive neuroscientific psychopathology?

Psychiatry has recently rediscovered its roots. It seemed as if its long history of interest in the impact of society on the rates and course of serious mental illness had been forgotten, overtaken by the inexorable advance of neuroscience and genetics.

(Morgan *et al.*, 2008, p. 1)

This quote echoes the peculiar phenomenon that at the turn of the millennium, the close of the 'decade of the brain' there was a return to social psychiatry. Despite the impact neuroimaging and genetics had made on understanding mental illness, and on psychiatry's understanding of itself, the impact of society on the epidemiology and prognosis of mental illness was again a serious academic concern. As is often the case in psychiatry, it is findings around schizophrenia that dictate and determine the research in wider psychiatry and this case is no exception. It had become clear that contrary to the old WHO study, there was marked heterogeneity in the rates of schizophrenia, and that further, some of this heterogeneity could be explained by urban birth and upbringing, migration, ethnicity, and what Cantor-Graae and Selten termed 'social defeat' (Cantor-Graae and Selten, 2004; Selten and Cantor-Graae, 2005). A particularly important body of research is the MRC AESOP study that demonstrated a twentyfold rate increase in the incidence of psychosis in London, compared with Nottingham and Bristol, with the very highest rates being within the black and ethnic minority groups (Morgan *et al.*, 2005a,b, 2006a,b, 2007; Fearon *et al.*, 2006; Kirkbride *et al.*, 2006, 2007a,b). These epidemiological findings were compounded both by continuum models of psychosis (Johns and van Os, 2001), suggesting that rates of psychotic experience in a non-help-seeking population were dependent upon many of the same variables that explained cases of the disorder, and by a seeming failure in the neurodevelopmental model of schizophrenia in explaining how someone with odd ideas and developmental delay became a person with a frank psychotic disorder (Broome *et al.*, 2005). Hence, as Morgan alludes to in the quote above, for the problems the study of schizophrenia brings researchers and clinicians, the answers provided by neuroscience and genetics may not be enough. Trying to connect psychological, biological, and social models of psychosis became important, and trying to empirically test the relationships between these varieties of variables has become a focus of psychosis research.

Increasingly, accounts of psychosis relating neuropsychological function, dopamine, symptoms, stress, and social isolation have been published with ingenuous experiments testing various hypotheses.

A very influential account, and one referred to by several contributors to this volume, is the salience theory of Kapur (Kapur, 2003; Kapur *et al.*, 2005). Here, Kapur links dopamine dysregulation to the aberrant salience of both internal and external representations and to the symptomatology of psychosis. In a series of remarkable experiments, Myin-Germeys, Van Os, and other colleagues from Maaastricht (Myin-Germeys *et al.*, 2001, 2003a–c, 2005) demonstrated a relationship between psychotic experiences and stress and 'daily hassles'. This sensitivity was in part consequent upon the reactivity of the participants' dopaminergic system and their history of life events, and further, neuropsychological impairment ameliorated this sensitivity. Ellet, Freeman, and colleagues (Ellett *et al.*, 2007) demonstrated how the experience of walking through a busy urban street increased anxiety levels, negative beliefs about others, and exaggerated reasoning biases linked to the formation and maintenance of delusions. Hence, for schizophrenia and other psychotic disorders, we are left with the heterogeneity of incidence rates, the role being part of an ethnic minority group, and/ or being a migrant plays, plus data suggesting that being in the urban environment has an immediate and measurable impact upon levels of paranoia in both health controls and patients.

In contrast to much of the work of the 1990s, this rebirth of social psychiatry led to a renewed interests in external factors to the brain in the genesis of psychosis. The idea of an environment, or lived experience, that was somehow 'psychotogenic' became a consequence of some of the data outlined above that stressed how much variance in psychopathology could be attributable to context and exposure. Given these findings, and that with Morgan many commentators view them as a challenge to wholly neuroscientific or genetic accounts of mental illness, can it be suggested that psycho-pathology may be consequent upon factors external to the brain? In philosophy, exter-nalism is linked to the truth of one of two claims (Rowlands, 2003): first, the *location* claim – here the idea is that some mental phenomena are not spatially located inside boundaries of subject that has or undergoes them; and second, the *possession* claim – here, the possession of at least some mental phenomena by a subject depends on fea-tures that are external to its boundaries. Based upon how various externalist philosophers accept or reject these claims, two broad varieties of externalism are described in the literature. The first, *vehicle* externalism, is based around the location claim predominantly and suggests that the very vehicles (architecture) and processes of cognition in part exist outside the skin of mental subjects. The second, *content* externalism, is driven more by the possession claim and argues that the individuation of propositional attitudes is dependent upon properties/relations external to the skin.

Is the focus on vehicle externalism, or 'extended cognition' as Clark terms it (Clark and Chalmers, 1998; Clark, 2001, 2005), helpful for us in thinking about psychosis? Given the effect the world, and specifically urban experience, may have on both the rates and symptoms of psychosis, can external factors to the brain have a role, in terms of information processing and cognition, on the aetiology of psychosis? The idea here is that much as a list on a piece of paper may supplement the neurally encoded mem-ory we have of what we want to shop for in the supermarket, certain cognitive acts may be subserved or supplemented by physical entities or relationships in the external world. Such a theory has been linked to evolutionary concerns: if the environment can encode certain information reliably, and we can easily access and utilize such information, then it would be inefficient to develop internal mechanisms to do such work. Certainly, empirical data suggests that working memory and other neuropsychological, internal deficits may be linked to the onset of psychosis and perhaps an increasing reliance on external vehicles of cognition.

Do certain environments yield particular information if the individual is in a given 'internal' (neurochemical, affective, neuropsychological) state? As perhaps the doxastic account of delusion argues, the delusional content is in the perception of the world. It is the case that what I experience when walking down Electric Avenue bears the informational content that I am Haile Selassie, and hence God Incarnate for the Rastafarians. McDowell, an externalist, in his influential *Mind and World* argues that for the thoughts of any of us to have genuine intentionality and to be about the world requires the world itself to be conceptually structured and reality to exert a rational influence on what we can think (McDowell, 1994). The deluded are not simply mistaken and as we have discussed elsewhere (Bortolotti and Broome, 2007, 2008, in press); the world and internal events become meaningful in a non-public manner – that is why Gallagher suggests in this volume that, in some sense, those with psychosis occupy an alternate world alongside our own.

Future research

One of the goals of this volume has been to demonstrate the close interaction between philosophy and academic psychiatry, and how such an interaction can be mutually beneficial. Hence, our explicit aspiration is that both mental health researchers see the clear benefit of detailed conceptual analysis for their empirical work, and that further, philosophers find in psychiatry more than just a source of clinical vignettes. Given the complexity of psychiatric research, the available empirical data bring many challenges to current explanatory models that philosophy can help address.

Psychiatry, perhaps because of the conceptual difficulty of its subject matter, has been at the forefront of methodological developments in both genetics and cognitive neuroscience, including imaging. As can be seen from the brief outline above of recent schizophrenia research, and the papers comprising the volume, academic psychiatry and allied disciplines comprise a sophisticated body of work. For philosophers it is a daunting prospect indeed to engage with these developments. As Cooper suggests, psychiatry is not a unitary science, but rather promiscuously, takes what it can get from a variety of methodologies to try and explain the data at hand. As individuals, researchers may specialize in epidemiology or pharmacogenetics, but as a discipline, psychiatry remains pluralistic. Although cognitive neuroscientific conceptions of psychopathology are dominant, they are by no means hegemonic: the chapters here point to the scope and limits of psychiatry as (wholly) cognitive neuroscience.

Future research in philosophy and psychiatry, we hope, will build upon some of the work begun here. A crucial area remains the status of our 'folk-psychopathological' concepts and the scope for studying them scientifically: the chapters by Samuels, Frankish, and Aimola Davies and Davies on delusions all address this theme. Other contributions address the pluralistic, multi-paradigm nature of psychiatry described earlier: Campbell and Thornton try to reconcile personal understanding with the causal mechanisms of science. Building on this, and something Campbell too addresses, is how philosophy can help clinicians and researchers think around or undercut prejudices such as the marked distinction between the social and the biological. Schizophrenia research has demonstrated the futility of thinking along 'either/or' lines; yet for many, the biological level of explanation remains more 'real'. Philosophy, in the therapeutic conception of the subject, can help allay these fears and insecurities and encourage researchers to maintain an open mind and a critical attitude towards the dominant methodological and explanatory frameworks. Further, philosophy has a crucial role in bringing disparate discourses and variables into relation with one another into a whole which aims at coherence.

References

Bortolotti, L. (forthcoming). The epistemic benefits of reason giving. *Theory and Psychology*.

Bortolotti, L. and Broome, M. (2008). Delusional beliefs and reason giving. *Philosophical Psychology*, **21**, 821–841.

Bortolotti, L. and Broome, M. (in press). A role for ownership and authorship in the analysis of thought insertion. *Phenomenology and Cognitive Sciences*.

Bortolotti, L. and Broome, M. R. (2007). If you did not care, you would not notice: recognition and estrangement in psychopathology. *Philosophy, Psychiatry, and Psychology*, **14**, 39–42.

Broome, M. R., Woolley, J. B., Tabraham, P., *et al.* (2005). What causes the onset of psychosis? *Schizophrenia Research*, **79**, 23–34.

Cantor-Graae, E. and Selten, J. (2004). Schizophrenia and migration: a meta-analysis. *Schizophrenia Research*, **67**, 63.

Carman, T. (2003). First persons: on Richard Moran's authority and estrangement. *Inquiry*, **46**, 395–408.

Clark, A. (2001). Reasons, robots and the extended mind. *Mind and Language*, **16**, 121–145.

Clark, A. (2005). Intrinsic content, active memory and the extended mind. *Analysis*, **65**, 1–11.

Clark, A. and Chalmers, D. (1998). The extended mind. *Analysis*, **58**, 7–19.

Ellett, L., Freeman, D., and Gartey, P. A. (2007). The psychological effect of an urban environment on individuals with persecutory delusions: the Camberwell walk study. *Schizophrenia Research*, **99**(1), 77–84.

Fearon, P., Kirkbride, J. B., Morgan, C., *et al.* (2006a). Incidence of schizophrenia and other psychoses in ethnic minority groups: results from the MRC AESOP Study.[see comment]. *Psychological Medicine*, **36**, 1541–1550.

Fearon, P., Morgan, C., Fearon, P., and Morgan, C. *et al.* (2006b). Environmental factors in schizophrenia: the role of migrant studies. *Schizophrenia Bulletin*, **32**, 405–408.

Ferrero, L. (2003). An elusive challenge to the authorship account. *Philosophical Psychology*, **16**, 565–567.

Jaspers, K. (1959/1997). *General Psychopathology*. Baltimore, MD, Johns Hopkins University Press.

Johns, L. C. and van Os, J. (2001). The continuity of psychotic experiences in the general population. *Clinical Psychology Review*, **21**, 1125–1141.

Kapur, S. (2003). Psychosis as a state of aberrant salience: a framework linking biology, phenomenology, and pharmacology in schizophrenia. *American Journal Psychiatry*, **160**, 13–23.

Kapur, S., Mizrahi, R., and Li, M. (2005). From dopamine to salience to psychosis-linking biology, pharmacology, and phenomenology of psychosis. *Schizophrenia Research,* **79,** 59–68.

Kirkbride, J. B., Fearon, P., Morgan, C., *et al.* (2006). Heterogeneity in incidence rates of schizophrenia and other psychotic syndromes: findings from the 3-center AeSOP study. [see comment]. *Archives of General Psychiatry,* **63,** 250–258.

Kirkbride, J. B., Fearon, P., Morgan, C., *et al.* (2007a). Neighbourhood variation in the incidence of psychotic disorders in Southeast London. *Social Psychiatry and Psychiatric Epidemiology,* **42,** 438–445.

Kirkbride, J. B., Morgan, C., Fearon, P., *et al.* (2007b). Neighbourhood-level effects on psychoses: re-examining the role of context. *Psychological Medicine,* **37,** 1413–1425.

Lawlor, K. (2003). Elusive reasons: a problem for first-person authority. *Philosophical Psychology,* **16,** 549–564.

McDowell, J. (1994). *Mind and World.* Cambridge, MA, Harvard University Press.

Moran, R. (2001). *Authority and Estrangement: An Essay on Self-knowledge.* Princeton, NJ, Princeton University Press.

Moran, R. (2004). Precis of authority and estrangement. *Philosophy and Phenomenological Research,* **69,** 423–426.

Morgan, C., Mallett, R., Hutchinson, G., *et al.* (2005a). Pathways to care and ethnicity. 1: Sample characteristics and compulsory admission. Report from the AESOP study. *British Journal of Psychiatry,* **186,** 281–289.

Morgan, C., Mallett, R., Hutchinson G., *et al.* (2005b). Pathways to care and ethnicity. 2: Source of referral and help-seeking. Report from the AESOP study. *British Journal of Psychiatry,* **186,** 290–296.

Morgan, C., Abdul-al, R., Lappin, J. M., *et al.* (2006a). Clinical and social determinants of duration of untreated psychosis in the AESOP first-episode psychosis study. *British Journal of Psychiatry,* **189,** 446–452.

Morgan, C., Fearon, P., Hutchinson, G., *et al.* (2006b). Duration of untreated psychosis and ethnicity in the AESOP first-onset psychosis study. *Psychological Medicine,* **36,** 239–247.

Morgan, C., Kirkbride, J., Leff, J., *et al.* (2007). Parental separation, loss and psychosis in different ethnic groups: a case-control study. *Psychological Medicine,* **37,** 495–503.

Morgan, C., McKenzie, K., and Fearon, P. (eds.) (2008). Introduction. *Society and Psychosis.* Cambridge, Cambridge University Press.

Myin-Germeys, I., van Os, J., Schwartz, J. E., Stone, A. A., and Delespaul, P. A. (2001). Emotional reactivity to daily life stress in psychosis. *Archives of General Psychiatry,* **58,** 1137–1144.

Myin-Germeys, I., Krabbendam, L., Delespaul, P., and van Os, J. (2003a). Can cognitive deficits explain differential sensitivity to life events in psychosis? *Social Psychiatry and Psychiatric Epidemiology,* **38,** 262–268.

Myin-Germeys, I., Krabbendam, L., Delespaul, P., and van Os, J. (2003b). Do life events have their effect on psychosis by influencing the emotional reactivity to daily life stress? *Psychological Medicine,* **33,** 327–333.

Myin-Germeys, I., Peeters, F., Havermans, R., *et al.* (2003c). Emotional reactivity to daily life stress in psychosis and affective disorder: an experience sampling study. *Acta Psychiatrica Scandinavica,* **107,** 124–131.

Myin-Germeys, I., Delespaul, P., and van Os, J. (2005). Behavioural sensitization to daily life stress in psychosis. *Psychological Medicine,* **35,** 733–741.

Rowlands, M. (2003). *Externalism: Putting Mind and World back Together Again.* Chesham, Acumen.

Selten, J.-P. and Cantor-Graae, E. (2005). Social defeat: risk factor for schizophrenia? [see comment]. *British Journal of Psychiatry,* **187**, 101–102.

Sims, A. (2003). *Symptoms in the Mind.* London, Saunders.

Tiberius, V. (2008). *The Reflective Life: Living Wisely with Our Limits.* Oxford, Oxford University Press.

Yager, J. and Gitlin, M. J. (2005). Clinical manifestations of psychiatric disorders. In *Kaplan and Sadock's Comprehensive Textbook of Psychiatry Eighth Edition* (eds. B. J. Sadock, and V. A. Sadock). Philadelphia, PA, Lippincott Williams and Wilkins.

Index

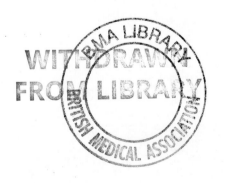

Lightning Source UK Ltd.
Milton Keynes UK
20 January 2010

148840UK00003B/1/P